Dosage Form Design

Dosage Form Design

Gayathri V. Patil

Harpal Singh

SHREE PUBLISHERS & DISTRIBUTORS
NEW DELHI-110 002

Edition : 2009

Published by :
SHREE PUBLISHERS & DISTRIBUTORS
4735/22, Prakash Deep Building
Ansari Road, Darya Ganj,
New Delhi–110 002

ISBN : 978-81–8329–311–2

Printed by :
Tarun Offset
Delhi–110 053

Preface

Pharmacy is a service within the health-care system that is related to drugs, their preparation, and their proper use to treat illness by cure, control and prevention. Intimately related to this field is the industry of pharmaceuticals, which comprises of hundreds of companies that discover, develop, produce and sell drug products. Together, the tow fields have initiated a revolution in human history wherein medical care in no longer bound by the connections of local apothecary, but is dispensed, in the form of drugs, to millions worldwide. Up until about 100 years ago, scientific principles where completely missing from the preparation of medicines. Today, as technology has progressed and science has growth in leaps and bounds, pharmaceutics has become one of the most critical contributions of science to humanity.

This book in the series on pharmaceutics brings to the reader a panoramic view of the whole field, aerating to the readers the history behind drug preparation, and the practices, processes and principles which define their preparation. Embarking on a comprehensive journey of understanding the barriers that separate designing of drugs from their dosage, the book is meant to serve as a useful referral for students, making them comprehend the potential, regulations, and implications that lie underneath the surface of pharmaceutics. In addition, it brings within its purview the current trends and developments which have taken over the pharmaceutics field, and what they hold for the future.

The comprehensive and insightful content of the book, it is hoped, serves well for both students and teachers.

Gayathri V. Patil

Harpal Singh

ACKNOWLEDGEMENT

Book writing-whether original or compilation is a complicated job requiring academic labour.

The present work is purely a research compilation of literature from authoritative publications/readings/ excerpts/notes/reviews/researches/literature, authored by eminent scholars/distinguished writers.

During research and compilation, the author has also taken assistance/references/literature from various Websites through Internet.

The author, therefore humbly, acknowledges the contributions of all those eminent writers/scholars alongwith their respective publishers and Websites from whose learned writings/displays references/ literature have been taken while preparing this book.

Contents

Chapter 1

Physical Properties of Drugs

The pharmaceutical industry's mission for the material is to rapidly advance development programmes with good confidence that form and formulation problems are unlikely to arise and to maximise a compounds' potential as a therapeutic. This commentary seeks to raise the profile of crystal form studies and the emerging topic of crystal engineering in pharmaceutical science by discussing the "state-of the-art" relating to pharmaceutical crystals and by expanding on possibilities that exist for future developments.

Crystal Polymorphism

The phenomenon of crystal polymorphism, where the same chemical compound exists in more then one unique crystalline form, has been appreciated for over a century. Polymorphs of pharmaceuticals and drug candidates can occur in all types of phases, though there is no way to predict the practical extent of polymorphism of any given compound. Based on recent reviews and commentaries, many strides have been taken towards better understanding of crystal polymorphism of pharmaceuticals.

According to lore and some published examples, the puzzling and unpredictable phenomenon of crystal polymorphism has affected many projects in pharmaceutical research and development over the last few decades. Although most accounts of polymorphic transformation during product development remain anecdotal, there exist published examples of the problem from both early stage compounds and marketed drugs.

The impact of crystal polymorphism and solvation state on pharmaceutical product value has been illustrated by costly product failures and protracted patent litigation examples. The former was most notably exemplified by the Norvir capsule product failure in 1998, which was recounted and rationalised by solving the crystal structures of the Ritonavir polymorphs. In theory, all pharmaceuticals are vulnerable to such an unexpected and unlucky event which in the case of Ritonavir resulted in enormous cost and inconvenience for the innovator and impacted the patients' use of this important HIV drug for roughly one year when no capsule formulation was available.

Recently a new, meta-stable form of 5-fluorouracil was reported highlighting the potential for even very old drugs to unexpectedly reveal new polymorphs. On the litigation side, early entry of generic versions of some notable drugs has been enabled based on the use of a patently distinct but pharmaceutically equivalent polymorphs. Ranitidine HCl and Paroxetine HCl hemihydrate are but two prominent examples where patent strategy and gaming created significant uncertainty about the value of a drug franchise. In response to these challenges, the pharmaceutical industry has developed processes and techniques for the identification and characterisation of polymorphs and solvates of compounds of interest.

Academics are contributing with both experimental and theoretical insights into crystal form study, prediction and engineering. Regulatory agencies also joined the effort in the 1990's, as exemplified by the decision-tree approach to evaluating the impact of polymorphism on product performance. It seems fair to conclude that developments in the late 1980's and many more during the 1990's have brought the industry's level of awareness, detection capability and decision making regarding polymorphs and solvates to new heights.

Amorphous State

Another phase type of interest in pharmaceutical systems is the amorphous state of a compound. Amorphous drug preparations of small molecule drugs exist in the marketplace, and they usually represent deliberate efforts to avoid crystalline forms in order to meet a delivery objective. This is done when a crystalline form is unsuitable for oral absorption due to insufficient aqueous solubility and inadequate dissolution rate, particularly when particle size reduction does not ameliorate the impact of the latter to a satisfactory degree.

Infrequently, however, no suitable crystalline forms of a compound can be found making the amorphous material the only viable option. Examples include itraconazole, quinapril HCl, zafirlukast, cilastatin and nelfinavir mesylate. In such cases, it would seem important to gain insights into the structural factors that lead to the outcome, in an effort to assess risk of eventual crystallisation events. The characterisation and application of amorphous pharmaceutical compounds and dispersions have been topics of review elsewhere, and will not be further discussed, given that the focus of the present contribution is on crystalline compounds.

Particle size reduction of poorly absorbed compounds is a proven approach to enhance biopharmaceutical performance. Milling to progressively smaller sizes can be considered a progressive approach towards amorphous, highenergy states. A special case of such crystal size modification is the advent of the nano-dispersion approach in pharmaceutical products. A key technology development in this regard is NanoCrystals, which has been successfully applied in three oral products to date: Rapamune, Tricor and Emend. The latter two compounds are excellent examples of the impact of media milling and physically stabilising a crystalline dispersion of nanometer dimensions (100's of nm) particles with the ultimate goal of significant bioavailability improvement.

The physical challenge is one of re-growth of particles, which is addressed by the use of specific surface stabilisers in formulation development. The active ingredient in Tricor, fenofibrate, is a low-melting, oil soluble substance. The bioavailability of this compound is increased by decreasing particle size, with the nano-dispersion being close to optimal. In addition, the NanoCrystal formulation of Tricor shows a decreased dependence of oral bioavailability on food compared to the previous formulation of Tricor In the case of Emend, the solubility of the drug substance, aprepitant, is on the order of 0.3 μg/mL and the doses are in 100's of mg/day. Oral bioavailability of this drug is a strong function of the particle size, with the smallest achievable crystals being optimal. The example illustrates that size modification is a viable strategy to be considered alongside form modification.

Salt Selection

Pharmaceutical developers have focused efforts on finding and formulating a thermodynamically stable crystalline form with acceptable physical properties for a given compound. This is reasonable, given the need to avoid cascading from a meta-stable form to a more stable one in unpredictable fashion. Occasionally certain physical properties, such as low aqueous solubility, are limiting to performance of the compound, leading to poor oral bioavailability or insufficient solubility for an injection formulation. One of the main strategies used to affect physical performance of a compound and one that is often employed by pharmaceutical scientists is the practice of salt selection.

At least half of compounds in marketed products are in the form of a salt for one reason or another. This fact alone speaks to the versatility of the salt selection approach. Salt forms of a pharmaceutical can have many benefits, such as improved stability characteristics, optimal bioavailability and aqueous solubility for an injectable formulation. Salts, like all other crystalline forms, are subject to polymorphism and solvate formation, thus requiring the same form identification studies as are needed for a neutral compound.

A remarkable example of co-optimisation of properties is indinavir (HIV protease inhibitor), which is marketed as the sulfate salt ethanol solvate. The crystalline free base has variable oral bioavailability in dogs and humans. While acidic solutions of the base compound showed good oral pharmacokinetics, the stability of the drug in acidic solution is not consistent with a product. Therefore, the discovery of the salt form ensured both shelf stability and robust bioavailability performance.

The salt selection strategy is limited in two ways. First, salt formation relies on the presence of one or more ionisable functional groups in the molecule; many drugs and development compounds lack this feature. Second, the ability to predict a priori whether a given compound will form a crystalline salt (or salts) is non-existent. The ability to actively identify crystalline salt forms has been confined to manual empirical evaluation using multiple salt formers for a given acid or base.

Recently advances have been made in the area of high-throughput salt selection and crystal engineering strategies associated with salt formation. In one case, we have advocated the simultaneous assessment of polymorphism as a way to help rank the developability of different crystalline salts. While salt forms will continue to have a prominent place in pharmaceutical science, the need for enhanced productivity dictates that every advantage must be sought to aid the design of an appropriate crystalline form of an active molecule. Specifically, the ability to design scaffolds into crystalline forms will enhance this capacity to convert interesting molecules into effective drugs. Crystal engineering offers some additional tools in this regard.

Crystal Engineering

Crystal engineering is generally considered to be the design and growth of crystalline molecular solids with the aim of impacting material properties. A principal tool is the hydrogen bond, which is responsible for the majority of directed intermolecular interactions in molecular solids. Cocrystals are multi-component crystals based on hydrogen bonding interactions without the transfer of hydrogen ions to form salts – this is an important feature, since Brønsted acid-base chemistry is not a requirement for the formation of a co-crystal.

Cocrystallisation is a manifestation of directed selfassembly of different components. Co-crystals have been described of various organic substances over the years and given various names, such as addition compounds molecular complexes and heteromolecular co-crystals. Regardless of naming convention, the essential meaning is that of a multi-component crystal where no covalent chemical modification of the constituents occurs as a result of the crystal formation. Pharmaceuticals co-crystals have only recently been discussed as useful materials for drug products.

Co-crystals

Pharmaceutical co-crystals can be defined as crystalline materials comprised of an active pharmaceutical ingredient (API) and one or more unique co-crystal formers, which are solids at room temperature. Co-crystals can be constructed through several types of interaction, including hydrogen bonding, ð-stacking, and van der Waals forces. Solvates and hydrates of the API are not considered to be co-crystals by this definition. However, cocrystals may include one or more solvent/water molecules in the crystal lattice.

An example of putative design, a construction and preparation ratio is the 5-fluororuracil:urea 1:1 cocrystal. This real example neatly illustrates the opportunity and challenge that exists currently with designing pharmaceutical co-crystals. Firstly, the 'design' is challenging because we have no ability to predict the exact crystal structure that may result from a crystallisation attempt. By analogy to the challenge of deriving protein structure from first principles, the primary sequence is known and elements of secondary structure are somewhat discernible from primary information.

Prediction of the actual 3-D folded conformation (tertiary structure or obtained by self-assembly) is not possible. In other words, while we currently have the ability to project which things associate in what approximate manner on the secondary level, crystal structure prediction is essentially an intractable proposition. By extension, and just as the exact function of a protein and quantitative parameters of activity are not predictable from primary and secondary structure, the prediction of crystal properties is not possible in the absence of structural information and measurements.

There is early evidence that practitioners were aware that apparent co-crystallisation of drugs could lead to useful preparations. In fact, a 'chemical compound' composed of sulfathiazole and proflavin dubbed flavazole was used to treat bacterial infection during the Second World War. The case of flavazole reveals insight into how two different molecules might interact in a putative co-crystal:"… flavazole is definitely a chemical compound containing equimolar proportions of sulphathiazole and proflavin base.

It is believed that combination occurs through the acidic sulphonamide group (SO_2NH) of the sulphathiazole and the basic centres of the proflavin. Perhaps the most realistic expression of the formula would be to place proflavin and sulphathiazole side by side with a comma between them." In the second half of the 20th century, interest in co-crystals evolved into the directed study of intermolecular interactions in crystalline solids. The technical development of routine single-crystal structure determination led to a watershed of data, now largely accessible through the Cambridge Structural Database (CSD).

The structural data have become useful for understanding the intermolecular interactions in co-crystals in atomic level detail. Using insight gained from analysis of the CSD and directed experimentation, scientists attempt design of co-crystals with specific properties, such as colour or non-linear optical response, by selecting starting components with appropriate molecular properties likely to exhibit specific intermolecular interactions in a crystal. However, even when chemically compatible functional groups are present it is not possible to accurately predict if a co-crystal, a eutectic mixture or simply a physical mixture will result from any given experiment. As a result of these complexities, attention has been directed at the identification and characterisation of intermolecular packing motifs with the goal of developing principles for co-crystal materials.

Crystal Engineerging and Pharmaceutical Co-Crystals

At the beginning of the 21st century, the field of crystal engineering has experienced significant development. Importantly, crystal engineering principles are now being actively considered for application to pharmaceuticals to modulate the properties of these valuable materials. Because the physical properties that influence the performance of pharmaceutical solids are reasonably well appreciated, there is a unique opportunity to apply crystal engineering techniques and the appropriate follow-up studies to solve real world problems, such as poor physical and chemical stability or inadequate dissolution for appropriate biopharmaceutical performance of an oral drug.

As structures and series of pharmaceutical co-crystals have begun to appear, we again find that properties cannot be predicted from the structures. Nevertheless, occasional trends have been suggested. For example, insoluble drug compounds co-crystallised with highly water soluble complements tend to achieve kinetic solubilities in aqueous media several times greater than the pure form. There are also more possible phases for each given active compound to consider, thus there will arguably be a greater opportunities for property enhancement.

In terms of stability enhancement and solubilisation, the example of the series of itraconazole co-crystals with pharmaceutically acceptable 1,4-diacids suggests a strategy alternative to amorphous drug formulation. The co-crystal options presented retain the stability inherent in a crystalline state, while allowing for solubilisation that significantly exceeds that of crystalline itraconazole base and rivals the performance of the engineered amorphous bead formulation.

From recent literature it appears that knowledge gained over the past century and increasingly sophisticated screening techniques developed within the last decade are paving the way towards design of co-crystals with potentially improved pharmaceutical properties. In terms of the application to pharmaceutical systems, the field of crystal engineering is developing the retro-synthetic understanding of crystal structure using reasoning that is analogous to that applied by organic chemists.

For example, the retro-synthetic approach in covalent synthesis operates on the level of a single molecule, while the analogous effort in crystal engineering focuses on the "supermolecule": The assemblies that define the crystalline arrangement of the molecules as they self-organise into the solid-state. The parallels between the development of crystal engineering and synthetic organic chemistry run still deeper. Methodologies for carrying out these crystallisations are being developed alongside the development of new robust motifs.

The importance of the solubility and dissolution relationships of the components of a putative cocrystal is becoming a matter of significant investigation. The same can be said for the roles of additives in templating novel forms. Mechanical milling of materials has also been documented as a means to make co-crystals, and a recent example of polymorphic forms of caffeine:glutaric acid illustrates the opportunities of this type of processing to influence crystal form. With an increase in the understanding of the modes of self-assembly, one can start to address the design aspect towards making pharmaceutical cocrystals. There remain several limitations to the application of what is currently known to the design of useful materials. As mentioned earlier, it remains intractable to reliably predict crystal structure.

Multi-component crystals are well out of reach for prediction due in part to complex energetic landscapes, lack of appropriate charge density models and a large number of degrees of freedom, making computation unfeasible. Moreover, there is only a qualitative understanding of the interplay between intermolecular interactions and materials performance, especially for properties relevant to pharmaceuticals such as solubility, dissolution profile, hygroscopicity and melting point. But the saving grace of the co-crystal approach comes in two guises: Complementarity and diversity.

On the topic of complementarity, it is possible, by way of CSD database mining for instance, to identify trends of hetero-synthon occurrence in model systems. As for the diversity aspect, the space of possible co-crystal formers is large, limited only by pharmaceutical acceptability. Coupled with parameters such as stoichiometry variation and increase in the number of components, the opportunities appear vast.

Future of Crystal Engineering

In the 21st century, practitioners of pharmaceutical chemistry need to enumerate and exploit the opportunities of crystal form design that nature affords us, and thus gain increasing ability to design the materials we need from the molecules that we seek to convert into pharmaceuticals.

Learning will be facilitated by advances in crystallisation automation, microscopy-spectroscopy techniques and new techniques such as terahertz spectroscopy and AFM, along with increasingly sophisticated X-ray diffraction lab instrumentation. In addition, further enhancements in the data mining tools associated with the CSD operating on an ever increasing number of highquality crystal structures will undoubtedly lead to new knowledge and principles of interaction.

The challenge placed before pharmaceutical scientists, now and in the future, is the following:

(i) to understand the requirement of a particular compound in terms of materials structure and properties, and

(ii) to creatively integrate crystal engineering within the limits of pharmaceutical acceptability of components to obtain new forms of active ingredients with desirable properties for formulation and delivery.

It should become the collective mantra of medicinal chemists, process engineers and pharmaceutical scientists to "design and make the material we need." This mantra can form the common aspiration for an industry that is in significant need of innovation and productivity enhancement.

PREDICTING DRUG METABOLISM

To decrease the costly and time-consuming development of active compounds ultimately doomed by hidden pharmacokinetic or toxicological defects, medicinal chemists now integrate metabolic considerations into drug design and lead optimisation strategies. As a result, many aspects of drug metabolism are of interest to medicinal chemists, including:

— the chemistry and biochemistry of metabolic reactions;

— the consequences of such reactions on activation and inactivation, toxification and detoxification;

— predictions of drug metabolism based on quantitative structure–metabolism relationships, expert systems, and molecular modeling of enzymatic sites;

— prodrug and soft drug design; and

— changes in physicochemical properties (acidity, basicity, lipophilicity, etc.) resulting from biotransformation.

Major reasons for the ever-increasing significance of biotransformation in drug discovery and development are its frequent pharmacodynamic and pharmacokinetic consequences, as resulting from the formation of:

— active metabolites from active drugs;These reasons have created a strong incentive for medicinal chemists to be able to anticipate the biotransformation of any given compound, including the generation of reactive metabolites. Whereas human expertise is irreplaceable, there is now a clear need for expert systems aimed at providing reliable and versatile metabolic predictions.

In their recent study on the needs and goals of metabolic predictions in early drug research, B. Testa *et al.*, Institute of Medicinal Chemistry, University of Lausanne, Switzerland, described more deeply about the various substrate and product selectivities characteristic of drug metabolism and they also classify and summarise the major in silico methods used to predict drug metabolism. In the following section we will discuss their findings on predicting drug metabolism in detail.

Goals of Metabolic Prediction

"Metabolic prediction" in itself is a fuzzy and broad concept which calls for definition and clarification. A number of stepwise goals toward predicting the metabolism of a given compound are listed here:

Goal 1. A list of all reasonable phase I and phase II metabolites

Goal 2. Same as above, organised in a metabolic tree

Goal 3. Same as above, plus a warning for reactive/adduct-forming metabolites

Goal 4. Same as above, plus (a) a probability of formation based on molecular factors, and (b) a filter against improbable metabolites

Goal 5. Same as above, plus a probability of formation under different biological conditions

Predicting all reasonable metabolites (Goal 1) represents the simplest goal. For want of a better definition, Testa *et al.* take "a reasonable metabolite" to be one that can be postulated on the grounds that the substructural motif (functional group) undergoing the biotransformation has a precedent in the metabolic chemistry literature, i.e., one not postulated solely on a mechanistic hypothesis. Classifying the predicted metabolites into a metabolic tree (Goal 2) calls for additional rules, as does the identification of potentially reactive and/or adduct-forming metabolites or metabolic intermediates (Goal 3).

The difficulty reaches new heights when semi-quantitative predictions are sought, based on molecular properties of the substrate (Goal 4). The necessary rules must also originate in existing knowledge, but they should be derived from structure–metabolism relationships using such statistical tools as multivariate analyses and neural networks. The same is true for the highest level of difficulty, when biological factors are taken into account to modulate the predictions according to animal species, genetic factors, age, etc. (Goal 5). In other words, the goal of the ultimate expert system would be to generate condition-dependent, semi-quantitative metabolic trees, a goal that will only be met very progressively.

Challenges to reliable drug product selectivities

There are a number of challenges to reliable drug metabolism prediction, foremost among which are the many biological factors:

— interindividual factors (i.e., which remain invariable for a given organism): animal species, genetic factors, gender;

— intraindividual factors (i.e., which vary for a given organism): age, biological rhythms, disease, stress, pregnancy, nutrition, influence of inducers and inhibitors.

Another major challenge in reliable prediction of metabolism, and one which deserves more interest than it receives, arises from the various selectivities characteristic of metabolic processes. Whereas there is only one type of selectivity at the receptor level, namely, the quantitatively or qualita-tively different responses elicited by various pharmacodynamic agents, two different types of selectivity exist in xenobiotic metabolism, namely, substrate selectivity and product selectivity (Table 1).

Table 1 Types of selectivity seen in xenobiotic metabolism.

Substrate selectivity (broad sense)	*Product selectivity*
Distinct substrates are metabolised: —at different rates —under identical conditions	Distinct metabolites are produced: — from a single substrate — at different rates — under identical conditions
Substrate selectivity (narrow sense) (nonisomeric substrates)	Chemoselectivity (chemically distinct reactions)
Substrate regioselectivity (regioisomeric substrates)	Product regioselectivity (regioisomeric products)
Substrate stereoselectivity (stereoisomeric substrates)	Product stereoselectivity (stereoisomeric products)
Substrate-product selectivities	

Substrate selectivity is defined as the differential metabolism of distinct substrates under identical conditions; its analogy with pharmacodynamic processes is clear. In contrast, product selectivity (defined as the differential formation of distinct metabolites from a single substrate under identical conditions)has no known correspondence in receptor-mediated events.

Both types of selectivity can be subdivided into subtypes depending whether substrates (or products) are nonisomeric (e.g., homologs, analogs, or congeners), regioisomeric (i.e., positional isomers), or stereoisomeric (diastereomers or enantiomers). These subtypes are listed and defined in Table 1. Product selectivity may also vary among substrates, i.e., it may be substrate-selective (substrate-product selectivity). Both substrate and product selectivity are of utmost significance when attempting to predict biotransformation.

Indeed, substrate selectivity offers the conceptual framework to rank substrates according to their relative rate of biotransformation by a given enzyme, in a given reaction, in a given organ, in a given organism, etc. Product selectivity is even more important when a single substrate is considered, since it allows them to make sense of the relative rates of formation of metabolites generated by different routes, different enzymes, or even resulting from attack by the same enzyme at different positions in the molecule.

Thus, chemoselectivity will be observed when different types of atoms are attacked (e.g., of O- vs. N-glucuronidation, N- vs. S-oxygenation, Csp^3 vs. Csp^2 hydroxylation), whereas regioselectivity implies that the same type of atom exists in the two or more positions being attacked (e.g., ortho- vs. para-hydroxylation). There is even some overlap between chemoselectivity and regioselectivity, e.g., phenol vs. alcohol glucuronidation, the chemical difference between the ether glucuronides so formed being small.

In Silico Systems to Predict Metabolism

In a schematic manner (Table 2), one can distinguish between two types of algorithms to predict drug and xenobiotic metabolism, namely, "local" systems and "global" systems.

"Local" systems

"Local" systems apply to single enzymes or to single metabolic reactions, and they are usually restricted to rather narrow chemical series. Such systems include quantitative structure–metabolism relationships (QSMRs) based on structural and physicochemical properties. Quantum mechanical calculations may also shed light on SMRs, revealing correlations between rates of metabolic oxidation and energy barrier in cleavage of the target C-H bond.

Table 2. A classification of in silico methods to predict biotransformation.

(A) "Local" methods

Applicable to simple biological systems (single enzyme, single reaction, ...) and/or to series of compounds with "narrow" chemical diversity.

— QSAR (linear, multilinear, multivariate, …)
⇒ affinities, relative rates, …
(depending on the physicochemical properties considered)

— 3D-QSAR (CoMFA, Catalyst, GRID/GOLPE, …)
⇒ substrate behavior, relative rates, inhibitor behavior, …

— Molecular modeling and docking
⇒ ligand yes/no (substrate? inhibitor?), regioselectivity, …

— Quantum mechanical (MO) methods (ab initio, semi-empirical)
⇒ regioselectivity, mechanisms, relative rates, …

(B) "Global" methods

Applicable to versatile biological systems (many enzymes, many reactions, ...) and/or to series of compounds with "broad" chemical diversity.

— Databases (MDL Metabolite Database, Biotransformations, ...)
⇒ nature of metabolites, reactive/adduct-forming metabolites, …

— Expert systems and their databases (META, MetabolExpert, METEOR,...)
⇒ nature of major and minor metabolites, metabolic trees, reactive/adduct-forming metabolites, relative importance of these metabolites depending on biological factors, …

Three-dimensional QSMRs (3D-QSMRs) methods yield a partial view of the binding/catalytic site of a given enzyme as derived from the 3D molecular fields of a series of substrates or inhibitors (the training set). In other words, they yield a "photographic negative" of such sites, and will allow a quantitative prediction for novel compounds structurally related to the training set. Two popular methods in 3D-QSARs are CoMFA (comparative molecular field analysis) and Catalyst.

The molecular modeling of xenobiotic-metabolising enzymes affords another approach to rationalise and predict drug–enzyme interactions. Its application to drug metabolism was made possible by the crystallisation and X-ray structural determination of cytochromes P450. Given the assumptions made in homology modeling and the lack of accurate scoring functions, such pharmacophoric models cannot give quantitative affinity predictions. However, they can afford fairly reliable yes/no answers as to the affinity of test set compounds, and even the regioselectivity of metabolic attack.

The pharmacophoric models of a large number of mammalian and mostly human CYPs are now available, as well as other xenobiotic-metabolising enzymes such as DT-diaphorase and glutathione S-transferases. The crystallisation and X-ray structural elucidation of mammalian cytochromes P450 is a breakthrough that removes the set of assumptions inherent in homology modeling and will thus improve the predictive power of molecular modeling.

Quantum mechanical methods are also classified as local in Table 2. Here, a word of caution is necessary, since such methods are in principle applicable to any chemical system. However, they cannot handle more than one metabolic reaction or catalytic mechanism at a time, and as such can only predict metabolism in simple biological systems, in contrast to the global methods presented in the next subsection.

"Global" Systems

As reviewed by Hawkins, one approach to predict metabolism is to use databases in the form of either knowledge-based systems or predictive expert systems. Existing knowledge-based systems include the MDL Metabolite Database, and the book series Biotransformations, which has been produced as a software product called Metabolism.

These databases can be searched to retrieve information on the known metabolism of compounds with similar structures or containing specific moieties. Predictive databases attempt to portray the metabolites of a compound based on knowledge rules, defining the most likely products. Existing systems of this type are MetabolExpert, META, and METEOR.

Meteor

A brief presentation

METEOR is a computer system which uses a knowledge base of structure–metabolism rules (biotransformations)to predict the metabolic fate of a query chemical structure. METEOR's biotransformation rules are generic reaction descriptors rather than simple entries in a reaction database. The system uses a rich internal structure representation language. The expression of specific functional group transformations can, therefore, be made context-sensitive.

Unconstrained analyses of query structures can give rise to a combinatorial explosion of results data. To overcome this problem, METEOR has an integrated reasoning engine, based on a system of non-numerical argumentation, which uses a repository of higher-level reasoning rules. The reasoning model built into METEOR allows the system to evaluate the likelihood of a biotransformation taking place. METEOR is provided with a link to an external log P calculation program.

The likelihood of biotransformation can modified by the reasoning engine according to the general, global relationship between lipophilicity and drug metabolism. The system can also make comparisons between potentially competing biotransformations. The user of the system can choose to analyse queries at a number of available search levels. At high levels, only the more likely biotransformations are requested for display. At lower levels, the more putative metabolites are also selected for display.

Input into the system is by graphical means or by molfile import. Output from the system is also flexible. Results can be viewed from within the program where individual metabolites can be selected and processed to deeper levels or sent to DEREK for Windows for a toxicological assessment. The metabolic tree can be searched by molecular mass, molecular formula, or structure. Reports can be generated in rich text format, and metabolites can be exported in SDfile format. The system is also supplied with a knowledge base editor so that users can build their own biotransformations and rules. The predictive capability of the system is constantly being evaluated, and the knowledge base and rule base are continuously being developed and improved.

Evaluation

The study team have recently completed an evaluation study of the now outdated version 6.0 of METEOR, comparing its predictions ("retrodictions" or "retrospective results" would be more appropriate here) with the published fate of nine drugs and one industrial chemical. Criteria for the selection of these 10 substrates were impeccable biological data available from the literature, the chemical diversity of the substrates, and extensive metabolism with multiple pathways. The 10 substrates were acenocoumarol, diclofenac, esonarimod, etoperidone, galantamine, gemifloxacine, n-hexane, indinavir, omapatrilat, and tramadol.

The results for acenocoumarol are summarised in Figs. 1A and 1B. There was a full qualitative agreement between experiment and algorithm for seven reactions (Fig. 1A), five of which are clearly mediated by cytochromes P450. Three reactions were predicted, but not seen (false positives). Reactions mA8 and mA9 are reasonable ones which may have escaped experimental detection due to low levels.

In contrast, hydrolytic ring opening of functionalised coumarins (mA10) is poorly documented if at all, suggesting that additional structural constraints need to be implemented in the software. Cytochrome P450-mediated reactions of dehydrogenation are rare, but greatly facilitated for highly delocalised metabolites, as is the case here (eA11). This false negative offers a valuable example of how an evaluation can help update the biotransformation dictionary of global systems. For the 10 substrates, 130 first-generation metabolites were predicted and/or seen experimentally.

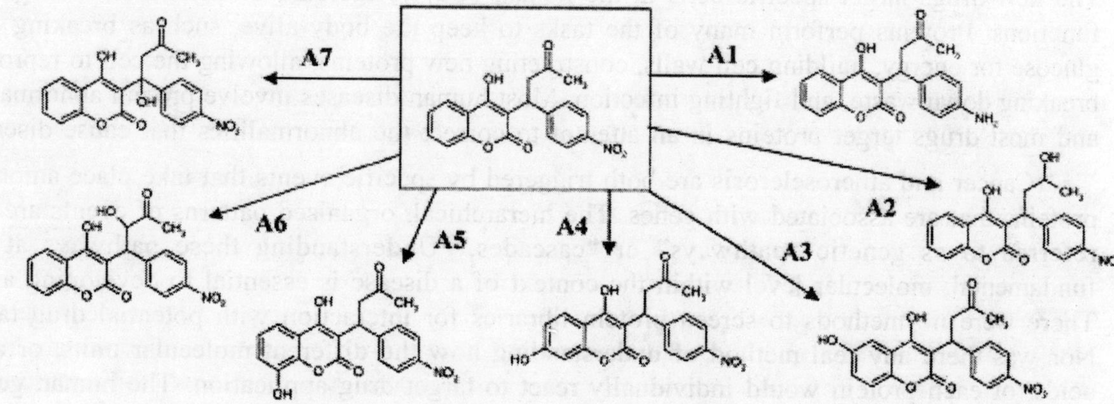

Figure 1A Metabolic scheme of acenocoumarol, comparing the experimental results with the predictions of METEOR version 6.0.

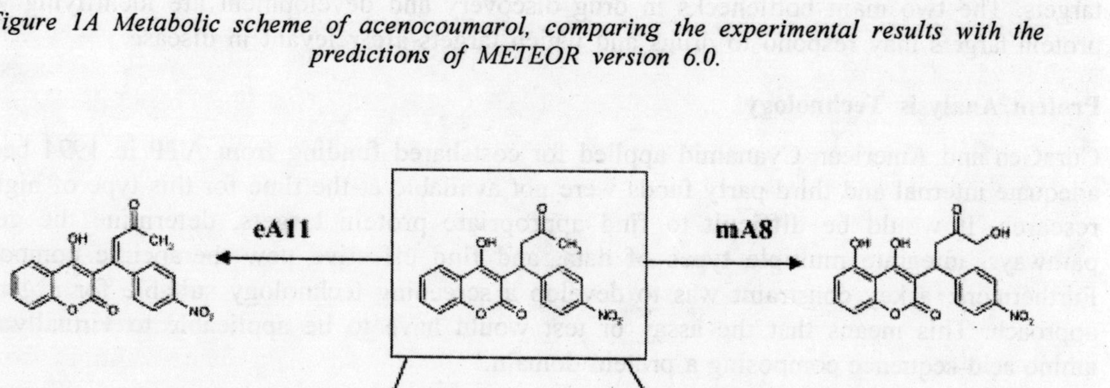

Figure 1B Metabolic scheme of acenocoumarol, comparing the experimental results with the predictions of METEOR version 6.0

Correct predictions represented 30 % of these reactions, apparently false positives 62 %, and false negatives 8 %. These 70 % discrepant results could be subdivided into 20 % apparently false positives due to molecular constraints not being taken into account, 3 % false negatives due to missing reactions in the biotransformation dictionary, and 47 % most probably due to the complexity of biological factors. As stated, such results are of considerable interest in improving and updating the algorithm.

DESIGN PROTEIN-SPECIFIC DRUGS

The new drugs target specific cells in the human body to increase or decrease certain protein functions. Proteins perform many of the tasks to keep the body alive, such as breaking down glucose for energy, building cell walls, constructing new proteins, allowing the cell to reproduce, breaking down waste, and fighting infection. Most human diseases involve protein abnormalities, and most drugs target proteins in an attempt to correct the abnormalities that cause disease.

Cancer and atherosclerosis are both triggered by specific events that take place among the proteins that are associated with genes. The hierarchical, organised patterns of events are often referred to as genetic "pathways" or "cascades." Understanding these pathways at their fundamental, molecular level within the context of a disease is essential to developing a cure. There were no methods to screen protein libraries for interaction with potential drug targets. Nor was there any real method of understanding how the different molecular units, or amino acids, of each protein would individually react to target drug application. The human genome contains about 60,000 genes. However, only certain subsets of these genes are suitable drug targets. The two main bottlenecks in drug discovery and development are identifying which protein targets may respond to drugs and which targets are relevant in disease.

Protein Analysis Technology

CuraGen and American Cyanamid applied for costshared funding from ATP in 1994 because adequate internal and third-party funds were not available at the time for this type of high-risk research. It would be difficult to find appropriate protein targets, determine the genetic pathways, integrate multiple types of data, and find effective new therapeutic compounds. Furthermore, a key constraint was to develop a screening technology suitable for a genomic approach. This means that the assay or test would have to be applicable to virtually every amino acid sequence composing a protein domain.

CuraGen, founded in 1991, was an emerging biotechnology firm located in Branford, Connecticut. The company's mission was to systematically catalogue disease-related proteins and to develop the tools needed to rapidly produce chemical compounds specific to these targets. American Cyanamid was acquired by American Home Products Corp. (AHP) in 1995. AHP (later renamed Wyeth Pharmaceuticals) was a publicly held, Fortune 100, chemical and life sciences company that discovered and developed medical and agricultural products and manufactured and marketed these products throughout the world. Of AHP's five major medical research efforts, its most important work related to oncology and cardiovascular disease.

Traditional functional genomic methods screened a single protein target for interaction against a library of proteins. CuraGen intended to develop tools to screen multiple proteins simultaneously. CuraGen's approach had two tiers. The first was to identify short protein segments (protein building blocks known as amino acids), called peptides, connected with the problematic protein–protein interactions related to disease. They would create enormous combinatorial libraries of peptides by mixing and matching the 20 kinds of amino acids, and they would then identify those peptides in the libraries that bind to the disease-related proteins.

The second tier was to develop unique computational and structural analysis techniques to determine the salient chemical and physical features of the selected peptides that enable them to block the disease-related proteins. The principles learned from that exercise would serve as technical guidelines for designing future therapeutic drugs carrying the same biomedical functions.

The approach directly applied to understanding and diagnosing multiple disease processes including genetic disorders, cancer, and viral infections. To pursue the development of their "molecular recognition technology," CuraGen assembled a staff with expertise in molecular biology, spectroscopy, statistical mechanics, nanofabrication, and computational methods. AHP provided medicinal chemists and structural biologists to develop three-dimensional search techniques for small molecules, called organic mapping.

The structural biology and organic-mapping tools that CuraGen hoped to create with ATP's help were enabling technologies. These tools could stimulate substantial industrial investigation in these high-risk areas, and success would have a significant impact on the process by which therapeutics are discovered.

CuraGen intended to develop new drugs to treat major diseases by identifying molecules that block abnormal protein–protein interactions. As a direct consequence of the speed and high-resolution three-dimensional structural information provided by the molecular recognition technology, the costs of developing such drugs were expected to be lower, and the time to clinical trials would be reduced. Moreover, the use of molecular recognition technology, together with other state-of-the-art technologies, had the potential to result in the discovery of breakthrough drugs for treating uncured diseases. The impact of these uncured diseases on the economy vastly exceeded the aggregate annual revenues of the pharmaceutical/biotechnology industry.

Molecular recognition technology was expected to accomplish the following:

— Reduce the time and cost of identifying novel, small organic molecules (new drugs) that bind to diseaserelated target proteins as well as the interactions between drugs and proteins

— Reduce preclinical experimental failures resulting from the application of unrefined drug design tools by focusing on protein–protein interactions

— Reduce failure rates through an understanding of molecular recognition, and, as a result, (1) enable better choices of target protein modules for which therapeutics can be designed and (2) ensure greater target module specificity (reduced sideeffects)

AHP estimated that CuraGen's process would reduce lead development from two years to six months. The process had the potential to reduce costs by 88 percent. CuraGen hoped to develop a process that would reduce drug development time by approximately 60 percent and reduce the cost of development by approximately 70 percent. If successful, this would result in a savings of $1.5 million in preclinical costs for every successful drug. Cost and time savings could benefit millions of cancer and heart disease patients awaiting new drug therapies.

The ATP-funded project addressed four primary focus areas:

— *Molecular biology*. The CuraGen team needed to construct a library of proteins, understand how to recognise biochemical targets, select biochemical controls, and analyse target interactions.

— *Experimental structure*. CuraGen intended to synthesise peptides and measure distances between atoms within a molecule.

— *Computational modelling*. The team would develop experimental constraints and predict relevant molecule conformations (arrangements of molecules in space). They would confirm protein–protein interactions by genetic testing.

— *Organic mapping*. AHP would develop threedimensional search programmes to select molecules from a database with similar arrangements of atoms.

CuraGen would confirm results by analysing the structural basis for biological functions of proteins coded by a specific gene, genetically testing protein–protein interactions, and by conducting in vitro and in vivo tests. Yale University performed experiments using radioisotopes to measure the efficiency of in vitro translations.

CuraGen studied interactions between pairs of proteins that have been linked to cancer in humans (RAS and RAF, vEGF and KDR). Researchers introduced the genes encoding those proteins into bacteria and yeast cells as a means for reproducing the proteins. They tested the proteins produced by the modified cells against their diversity library, looking for substances that interrupt interactions between the pairs of proteins.

CuraGen collaborated with Pennsylvania State University to measure distances between nuclei. They developed a method to simultaneously measure multiple distances in a single experiment. The purpose was to pick out the active form of a peptide, search for similar molecules in the database, and design new molecules. The final focus areas were called Multiplexed Interaction Method (MIM), protein inhibitor screening, molecular structure, and organic mapping. MIM, which derived from the molecular biology focus area, screened protein–protein interactions and observed metabolic pathways in order to determine disease-specific targets for drug screens.

AHP generated two new genetic databases for data mining, as well as algorithms to search for pharmacophore similarities (three-dimensional substructure of a molecule that carries the essential features responsible for a drug's biological activity). CuraGen also developed a tool, the CombiGen system, to efficiently identify small-molecule drugs that can potentially bind to protein targets or block diseaserelated protein–protein interactions. The key advance of this system is that it can screen thousands of targets simultaneously.

The project's structure analysis led to developing a bioinformatics software, called PathCalling, that extracts consensus information from MIM data. PathCalling identifies biological pathways that play a role in disease. The process starts with a set of genes that are associated with a disease. High-throughput biological methods search for other genes that are part of the same pathway. These genes are then reintroduced into the PathCalling system to extend the pathway. The key technical advance of PathCalling is the capability of the high-throughput operation to identify genes whose protein products interact with each other.

The second structural advance was another software tool, HitCalling, that screens the proteins associated with a particular gene identified by PathCalling against small-molecule diversity libraries. HitCalling identifies both binding and inhibition in protein–protein interactions with a potential drug.

Small molecules identified in the screens are drug candidates that can be optimised using traditional technologies, then advanced into preclinical and clinical trials. HitCalling provides a uniform assay or sample format, without the need for individual assay development, for every drug-screening target. This allows all the proteins in a pathway to be screened and permits multiple targets to be screened simultaneously. As a result, researchers can screen more molecules faster compared with existing drug screening technologies.

Building on techniques developed under the ATPfunded project, CuraGen collaborated with Yale University and received another award in 1996 from Connecticut Innovations, Inc. to pursue nuclear magnetic resonance (NMR) applications. (NMR spectroscopy provides information on the position of specific atoms within a molecule by using the magnetic properties of the cell nuclei.) The new work complemented the ongoing development of highthroughput methods for structural analysis of the ATPfunded project. They extended NMR methods from peptides to general organics, which offered greater diversity for drug screening.

Identification of Possible Protein Targets

CuraGen successfully developed tools to screen multiple proteins simultaneously. The key performance criterion for the project was to reduce the rate of false positives, which is the incorrect identification of possible protein targets. Reducing the false-positive rate provides several benefits:

— The system sampled 10 to 100 proteins at a time, rather than 1 at a time (searching through a library of millions of other proteins for interactors).

— Entire libraries could be screened against each other to discover a large set of protein–protein interactions, each a potential drug-screening target.

— The cost of generating information would be greatly reduced. Much of the cost arises from sequencing the DNA of all the genes that express the protein to analyse the interacting proteins. Reducing the falsepositive rate reduces the sequencing cost by a factor of 10.

The cumulative effect of these advances enables the molecular recognition technology to systematically identify new targets for drug screening. These are novel, pharmaceutically relevant genes and expressed proteins that are associated with specific diseases.

By the end of the ATP-funded project, the PathCalling database contained several thousand proprietary protein interactions, approximately five times more interactions than the closest industry competitor had compiled. Results from PathCalling indicated that it would be possible to use consensus information to identify the protein domain that participated in protein–protein interactions, which would aid in structure-based drug design against these targets.

The company's technology development has had the following additional benefits:

— The infrastructure for PathCalling provides a system for identifying proteins that are in the same pathway as known disease-related proteins.

— Many of the protein domains discovered through PathCalling are novel coding sequences.

CuraGen met or exceeded all of its technical goals for the ATP-funded project. The goals were to reduce the time and cost of identifying novel small organic molecules that bind to disease-related target proteins (new drugs), reduce experimental failures by focusing on protein–protein interactions, and increase understanding of molecular recognition in order to (1) better select target protein modules for which therapeutics can be designed and (2) ensure greater specificity (reduced side-effects). By project completion in 1998, CuraGen's propriety MIM, PathCalling, and HitCalling technologies met or exceeded the technology project goals:

— Construct one genomic library per month (met goal)

— Construct 4,000 samples for testing against the libraries per month (exceeded goal of 48 per month)

— Prepare 20,000 templates per month (exceeded goal of 2,000 per month)

— Sequence 20,000 samples per month (exceeded goal of 2,000 per month)

— Confirm 1,000 protein–protein interactions per month (exceeded goal of 100 per month)

— Discover 200 new interactions per month (exceeded goal of 50 per month)

CuraGen is using MIM, PathCalling, and HitCalling in several modes:

— Screening genome versus genome for simple organisms, such as microbial pathogens. These types of screens were previously impractical because true interactions would be overwhelmed by a background of false positives.

— Screening tens to hundreds of protein domains versus protein libraries in order to identify protein–protein interactions relevant to human disease. The improved technology for preparing the protein domains and libraries has allowed the implementation of a systematic workflow to generate and capture information.

— Completely screening interactions between proteins in the yeast genome (initiated in collaboration with Dr. Stanley Fields, inventor of the yeast two-hybrid system). Interactions discovered in yeast often mirror interactions between homologous proteins in humans. A database of the complete set of yeast interactions could therefore be a valuable asset for drug discovery.

— Patenting protein–protein interactions for use as targets in drug screening.

The CuraGen relied on a combination of hypothesisdriven disease models, drug-response models, gene-and pathway-mining approaches, and human genetics. The company is developing a broad pipeline of protein, antibody, and small-molecule drugs in the areas of oncology, inflammatory diseases, obesity, and diabetes.

With HitCalling, CuraGen developed a high-throughput protein analysis tool that can accept targets directly from upstream genomics processes such as PathCalling. This removes the bottleneck in creating a new assay or sample for each target. Furthermore, the number of targets entered into screens can keep pace with the number of targets discovered through genomics. In addition to screening targets identified through PathCalling, the HitCalling assay system can also be used to screen other targets.

After the ATP-funded project, CuraGen initiated a collaboration with the Massachusetts Institute of Technology to continue developing HitCalling technology. CuraGen has also sought collaborations with academic groups engaging in combinatorial synthesis as a source of drug-screening libraries.

Molecular Recognition Technologies

CuraGen sold subscriptions to the PathCalling database to Genentech and Biogen. CuraGen obtained numerous patents for protein–protein interactions discovered by PathCalling. The patents cover more than 90 protein-protein interactions as targets in identifying potential drugs. Moreover, the company obtained additional drug-screening libraries from ArQule, a leader in combinatorial chemistry, to further utilise CuraGen's protein-screening technologies.

CuraGen has shared these technologies through research collaborations, database subscriptions, and internal programmes. In one research collaboration, CuraGen analyses disease-related genes and applies its MIM research services in conjunction with PathCalling to reveal additional proteins in the same pathway. CuraGen then uses HitCalling to identify drug candidates.

Database subscriptions permit subscribers to search through the company's database of biological pathways to identify proteins that could be licensed for use in drug discovery assays. CuraGen has established research collaborations and, for a time, provided database subscriptions that provided access to PathCalling. As of 2005, CuraGen was using PathCalling and HitCalling in internal programmes to identify targets and drug candidates for its own drug discovery and development programmes.

Other dissemination efforts include delivering information over the Internet to collaborators. GeneScape is CuraGen's web-based bioinformatics system that incorporates real-time process management, data analysis, and data visualisation. GeneScape provides access to CuraGen's complete technology platform, including GeneCalling (developed under a separate ATP award) to discover disease-related genes and CuraTools for web-distributed bioinformatics. CuraGen is currently collaborating with leading life science companies Genentech, Biogen, and Pioneer Hi-Bred International.

CuraGen announced its initial public offering in 1998 for $34.5 million. Without ATP funding, CuraGen would not have had the resources to pursue PathCalling in parallel with other programmes. According to company representatives, the development of PathCalling and

HitCalling would have been delayed by at least two years. CuraGen worked with ATP on this project, as well as on two others (94-05-0027, Integrated Microfabricated DNA Analysis Device for Diagnosis of Complex Genetic Disorders; 96-01-0141, Programmable Nanoscale Engines for Molecular Separation), so ATP has played an integral role in the development of CuraGen's potential commercial drug offerings.

Since its inception, CuraGen's stated strategy has been to discover new ways to treat disease by understanding how the expressed proteins from genes function within the human genome. With the help of ATP, the company has identified disease-related genes and their therapeutic targets that has led to the development of unique pharmaceutical products.

CuraGen was restructured beginning in late 2002, because the business strategy of supplying tools and services to the pharmaceutical industry was no longer viable. Profit margins were too thin, and financing was shifting to companies pursuing proprietary pharmaceuticals.1,2 According to Johnathan M. Rothberg, CEO, "CuraGen competed successfully in the race to discover drug targets from the human genome and…has emerged with a wealth of knowledge about the molecular basis of disease…We must now focus our resources with greater intensity on drug-development projects that are designed to turn these targets, and this knowledge of disease, into cures for unmet medical needs."

As a result of CuraGen's accomplishments, the company has collaborated with numerous companies, including Abgenix, Biogen, Genentech, Seattle Genetics, and Bayer, and now has an extensive pipeline of protein, antibody, and small therapeutics to treat cancer, inflammatory disease, and diabetes. The company's most advanced projects are in clinical development.

In December 2004, CuraGen received its first "fast track" designation from the U.S. Food and Drug Administration for a novel protein therapeutic being developed for the treatment of oral mucositis (a complication of chemotherapy, which leads to painful ulceration of the mouth and throat).

CuraGen is collaborating with a biopharmaceutical company, TopoTarget A/S, to develop a second small-molecule drug, a histone deacetylase (HDAC) inhibitor. HDAC inhibitors appear to restore a normal balance in the expression of genes in cancer cells, making them susceptible to radio and chemotherapy to directly treat solid and hematological cancers. This drug is currently in a Phase II clinical trial for the treatment of multiple myeloma.

Two additional clinical development programmes are ongoing in 2006: a third antibody has completed Phase I testing for kidney inflammation; and a fourth antibody drug candidate is beginning clinical trials for metastatic melanoma. CuraGen is also using the ATP-funded technology to select promising candidates from TopoTarget's extensive library of HDAC inhibitors for clinical development.

Colonic Drug Delivery

The colonic region of the gastrointestinal tract is one area that would benefit from the development and use of such modified release technologies. Although considered by many to be an innocuous organ that has simple functions in the form of water and electrolyte absorption and the formation, storage and expulsion of faecal material, the colon is vulnerable to a number of disorders including ulcerative colitis, Crohn's disease, irritable bowel syndrome and carcinomas. Targeted drug delivery to the colon would therefore ensure direct treatment at the disease site, lower dosing and fewer systemic side effects.

In addition to local therapy, the colon can also be utilised as a portal for the entry of drugs into the systemic circulation. For example, molecules that are degraded/poorly absorbed in the upper gut, such as peptides and proteins, may be better absorbed from the more benign environment of the colon. In addition, systemic absorption from the colon can also be used as a means of achieving chronotherapy for diseases that are sensitive to circadian rhythms such as asthma, angina and arthritis.

Successful colonic drug delivery requires careful consideration of a number of factors, including the properties of the drug, the type of delivery system and its interaction with the healthy or diseased gut. For instance, regardless of whether a local or systemic effect is required, the administered drug must first dissolve in the lumenal fluids of the colon. Overall, there is less free fluid in the colon than in the small intestine and, hence, dissolution could be problematic for poorly water-soluble drugs.

In such instances, the drug may need to be delivered in a presolubilised form, or delivery should be directed to the proximal colon, as a fluid gradient exists in the colon with more free water present in the proximal colon than in the distal colon. Aside from drug solubility, the stability of the drug in the colonic environment is a further factor that warrants attention.

The drug could bind in a nonspecific manner to dietary residues, intestinal secretions, mucus or general faecal matter, thereby reducing the concentration of free drug. Moreover, the resident microflora could also affect colonic performance via degradation of the drug. In terms of systemic therapy via the colon, the small lumenal surface area and relative 'tightness' of the tight junctions in the colon could restrict drug transport across the mucosa and into the systemic circulation. To a certain extent, the longer residence time in the colon (up to five days) may compensate for these limitations.

There is also evidence to suggest that the activity of the cytochrome P450 3A class of drug metabolising enzymes is lower in the mucosa of the colon than the small intestine. Therefore, colonic delivery may lead to elevated plasma levels and improved oral bioavailability for drugs that are substrates for this enzyme class. In relation to delivery, modified release formulations are usually based on either a single unit (tablets and capsules) or multi-unit (pellets and granules) platform design.

The biopharmaceutical performance of the two designs are very different: multi-unit systems tend to exhibit more uniform gastrointestinal transit and absorption characteristics due to their small size and divided nature. Also, the slower rate of passage of multi-units through the colon would be advantageous for colonic delivery. From the perspective of cost, however, single unit systems are usually more costefficient to manufacture.

Targeting drugs to the colon

By definition, an oral colonic delivery system should retard drug release in the stomach and small intestine but allow complete release in the colon. The fact that such a system will be exposed to a diverse range of gastrointestinal conditions on passage through the gut makes colonic delivery via the oral route a challenging proposition. Nevertheless, a variety of approaches have been used and systems have been developed for the purpose of achieving colonic targeting. These approaches are either drug-specific (prodrugs) or formulation-specific (coated or matrix preparations). The most commonly used targeting mechanisms are:

— pH-dependent delivery;
— time-dependent delivery;
— pressure-dependent delivery; and
— bacteria-dependent delivery.

pH-sensitive enteric coatings have been used routinely to deliver drugs to the small intestine. These polymer coatings are insensitive to the acidic conditions of the stomach yet dissolve at the higher pH environment of the small intestine. This pH differential principle has also been attempted for colonic delivery purposes, although the polymers used for colonic targeting tend to have a threshold pH for dissolution that is higher than for those used in conventional enteric coating applications.

Most commonly, copolymers of methacrylic acid and methyl methacrylate that dissolve at pH6 (Eudragit L) and pH7 (Eudragit S) have been investigated. This approach is based on the assumption that gastrointestinal pH increases progressively from the small intestine to colon. In fact, the pH in the distal small intestine is usually around 7.5, while the pH in the proximal colon is closer to 6. These delivery systems therefore have a tendency to release their drug load prior to reaching the colon.

To overcome the problem of premature drug release, a copolymer of methacrylic acid, methyl methacrylate and ethyl acrylate (Eudragit FS), which dissolves at a slower rate and at a higher threshold pH (7–7.5), has been developed recently. A series of in vitro dissolution studies with this polymer have highlighted clear benefits over the Eudragit S polymer for colonic targeting.

A gamma scintigraphic study comparing the in vivo performance of these various polymers revealed that Eudragit FS (coated onto tablets) was superior to the older polymers in terms of retarding drug release in the small intestine, although, in some subjects, the coated tablets did not break up at all. Intrasubject variability in polymer performance was also apparent as marked differences in the times and sites of tablet disintegration were observed on separate occasions.

The inter and intrasubject variability in gastro-intestinal pH and possibly certain other intrinsic variables such as electrolyte concentration and transit time will therefore impact on the in vivo behaviour of pH-responsive systems, ranging from early drug release in the small intestine to no release at all, with the formulation passing through the gut intact. The latter situation will also arise when the pH of the colon, and possibly the small intestine, is considerably lower than normal, as is the case in patients with ulcerative colitis. In spite of their limitations, pH-sensitive delivery systems are commercially available for mesalazine (5-aminosalicylic acid) (Asacol and Salofalk) and budesonide (Budenofalk and Entocort) for the treatment of ulcerative colitis and Crohn's disease, respectively.

Time-dependent delivery has also been proposed as a means of targeting the colon. Time-dependent systems release their drug load after a preprogrammed time delay. To attain colonic release, the lag time should equate to the time taken for the system to reach the colon. This time is difficult to predict in advance, although a lag time of five hours is usually considered sufficient, given that small intestinal transit time is reported to be relatively constant at three to four hours.

One of the earliest systems to utilise this principle was the Pulsincap™ device. Somewhat complex in design, the system consists of an impermeable capsule filled with drug and stoppered at one end with a hydrogel plug. On contact with gastrointestinal fluids, the plug hydrates and swells and, after a set lag time, ejects from the capsule body, thereby allowing drug release to occur.

The lag time is controlled by the size and composition of the plug. Hebden, et al. investigated the behaviour of the Pulsincap™ system, preprogrammed with a five-hour time delay, in fasted human subjects using gamma scintigraphy. While drug was released in all subjects approximately five hours post-administration, the position of the device at the time of release varied considerably, with some still present in the stomach.

To reduce the influence of gastric emptying on the performance of the Pulsincap™, the system was modified by application of an outer enteric coat. This double barrier concept forms the basis of most current time release systems. The outer enteric coat dissolves on entering the small intestine to reveal an inner polymeric barrier that delays drug release by either swelling, eroding or dissolving over a period of time equivalent to small intestinal transit.

Although the use of an outer enteric coat overcomes, to a certain extent, the variability in gastric emptying, the intrinsic problem with such systems is the overall inter and intrasubject variability in transit. Moreover, gastrointestinal transit is prone to diurnal rhythms, with transit being appreciably slower in the evening as compared with the morning. The basic fact that such systems are unable to sense and adapt to an individual's transit time and merely release their drug load after a preset lag time, irrespective of whether the formulation is in the colon or not, clearly limits their utility.

Gastrointestinal pressure has also been utilised to trigger drug release in the distal gut. This pressure, which is generated via muscular contractions of the gut wall for grinding and propulsion of intestinal contents, varies in intensity and duration throughout the gastrointestinal tract, with the colon considered to have a higher lumenal pressure due to the processes that occur during stool formation. Systems have therefore been developed to resist the pressures of the upper gastrointestinal tract but rupture in response to the raised pressure of the colon. Capsule shells fabricated from the water-insoluble polymer ethylcellulose have been used for this purpose.

The system can be modified to withstand and rupture at different pressures by changing the size of the capsule and thickness of the capsule shell wall. Proof of concept studies have been conducted in dogs and, to a limited extent, in humans. Although the results appear promising, it has not been proven definitively that rupture occurs in the colon. One must also question the influence of co-administered food on performance, as fed state contractions may be sufficiently powerful to disintegrate the capsule in the stomach.

The resident gastrointestinal bacteria provide a further means of effecting drug release in the colon. These bacteria predominantly colonise the distal regions of the gastrointestinal tract where the bacterial count in the colon is 10^{11} per gramme, as compared with 10^4 per gramme in the upper small intestine. Moreover, 400 different species are present. Colonic bacteria are predominantly anaerobic in nature and produce enzymes that are capable of metabolising endogenous and exogenous substrates, such as carbohydrates and proteins that escape digestion in the upper gastrointestinal tract. Therefore, materials that are recalcitrant to the conditions of the stomach and small intestine, yet susceptible to degradation by bacterial enzymes within the colon, can be utilised as carriers for drug delivery to the colon.

This principle has been exploited commercially to deliver 5-aminosalicylic acid to the colon by way of a prodrug carrier. The prodrug sulphasalazine consists of two separate moieties, sulphapyridine and 5-aminosalicylic acid, linked by an azo-bond. The prodrug passes through the upper gut intact, but, once in the colon, the azo-bond is cleaved by the host bacteria, liberating the carrier molecule sulphapyridine and the pharmacologically active agent 5-aminosalicylic acid. This concept has led to the development of novel azo-bond-based polymers (azo-polymers) for the purpose of obtaining universal carrier systems. However, issues with regard to the safety and toxicity of these synthetic polymers have yet to be addressed.

To overcome such concerns, natural materials, essentially those that are polysaccharide-based, offer a viable alternative to the problem. Such potential materials include amylose, chitosan, chondroitin sulphate, dextran, guar gum, inulin and pectin. These materials are not, however, without their limitations. They are hydrophilic in nature, which renders them either soluble or prone to swelling in an aqueous environment and hence unsuitable as drug carriers. To fully realise the potential of these polysaccharides for colonic delivery, some form of structure modification and/or formulation strategy is required. In the case of pectin, for example, a highly methoxylated and poorly water-soluble derivative has been utilised in the form of a relatively thick compression coating on tablets.

On testing in human volunteers, the coated tablets remained intact in the stomach and small intestine, but disintegrated on reaching the colon. Pectin, in the form of calcium pectinate, has also been used in the form of a matrix for colonic delivery, although the relatively open structure of such systems renders them liable to drug release prior to colonic arrival. Colon specificity has also been achieved using a delivery system based on the polysaccharide amylose (COLAL™).

Amylose is one of the two major components of starch, the other being amylopectin. In comparison with other polysaccharides, amylose and amylopectin are degraded by a broader range of colonic bacteria. While amylopectin is metabolised by pancreatic enzymes in the small intestine, amylose, in its glassy amorphous state, is resistant, but, at the same time, susceptible to digestion by amylaseproducing bacteria residing within the colon.

This material, in combination with the water-insoluble polymer ethylcellulose, which is necessary to control the swelling of amylose, has been exploited as a film coating. After application to solid dosage forms, these film coatings have been shown to withstand simulated gastric and small intestinal conditions and allow drug release specifically within a colonic environment.

A number of gamma scintigraphic studies have provided confirmatory evidence for the targeting performance of the COLAL™ delivery system in humans. Moreover, the system has come through a Phase II study successfully in which the antiinflammatory agent prednisolone metasulphobenzoate was delivered to the colon of patients with active ulcerative colitis, thereby providing proof of concept data in diseased subjects.

Challenges and Opportunities of Discovery Pharmaceutics

The main reasons for attrition in drug discovery and development are safety or tolerability concerns, poor absorption, disposition, metabolism, and excretion (ADME) properties, and lack of efficacy. In an effort to reduce these attrition rates, most pharmaceutical companies are now evaluating their lead molecules for druglike properties much earlier in the discovery process. The data generated at this early stage allow upfront assessment and identification of development challenges and provide the possibility of optimising druglike properties at the lead optimisation stage, thus enabling the selection of the best candidate for lead nomination.

Even though pharmaceutics alone is not a major attrition factor, many drugs in development are affected by their poor biopharmaceutical properties. When a compound with suboptimal biopharmaceutical properties is selected for development, considerably more time needs to be spent on formulation and process development, ultimately leading to higher costs and delays.

Selection of lead compounds that have the appropriate physicochemical properties and adequate chemical and physical stability, and that can readily be formulated to give appropriate bioavailability from a relevant dosage form, can ultimately lead to faster development timelines, reduced cost, and diminished complexity of the development process.

Physicochemical Properties

The aqueous solubility of a drug substance is a fundamental property that should be evaluated early in discovery. Lack of solubility can affect the results of early high-throughput screening assays and the ability to achieve efficacious and toxicologically relevant exposures in animals. This characteristic will also affect the future developability of and formulation efforts for the compound.

Solubility depends on the solvation energy of the solute in the solvent overcoming both the crystal lattice energy of the solid and the energy to create space in the solvent for the solute. Thus, the solubility of a compound depends not only on properties of the drug molecule itself, such as polarity, lipophilicity, ionisation potential, and size, but also on properties of the solvent and the solid, such as the crystal packing and presence of solvates.

Solubility measurements throughout discovery range from methods that dilute dimethylsulfoxide (DMSO) stock solutions in aqueous buffers and mimic the methods in which high-throughput assays are run, to those measuring pseudoequilibrium solubility using crystalline solids and aqueous buffers. Detection methods include turbidimetric methods, UV plate readers, liquid chromatography (LC)/UV, and LC/mass spectrometry (MS). The solubility method chosen depends on the desired turnaround time, the quantity of compound, and the quality of the results required.

In the early stages of discovery, when many compounds are synthesized in small quantities for high-throughput screening, high-throughput solubility methods can provide an early rank-ordering that can help weed out the lowest solubility compounds, which would be expected to give rise to the highest development hurdles. These methods typically are those that involve dilutions starting with the compounds dissolved in DMSO.

As compounds move to later stages of discovery, a more reliable assessment of solubility is required. These solubility measurements should ideally start with the solid compound, preferably crystalline, and the experiments should run for a long enough time that they approach equilibrium.

A crystalline form is desired as compounds get closer to lead selection, because although the crystalline form available in discovery may not be the final form chosen for development, the likelihood that the solubility of 2 crystalline forms differs by more than ~2 fold is slight, whereas the difference in apparent solubility between an amorphous and a crystalline form of a compound can be many orders of magnitude. The crystallinity of a sample can be assessed by polarised light microscopy, or, if enough compound is available, a more detailed characterisation can be obtained by powder x-ray diffraction and thermal analysis.

Ionisation constant (pKa)

For a compound containing basic or acidic functional groups, solubility at a given pH is influenced by the compound's ionisation characteristics. The solubility of a compound in aqueous media is greater in the ionised state than in the neutral state. Thus, solubility of ionisable compounds is dependent on the pH of the solution. Many drugs are weak acids or bases and thus are ionisable within the pH range of the gut. Solubility and dissolution, and therefore absorption, of a weak base can be altered by changes to gastric pH (eg, when coadministered with antacids).

While a weakly basic compound might fully dissolve in the acidic environment of the stomach and result in high exposure levels under such conditions, coadministration of drugs that raise the stomach pH can lead to greatly decreased solubility, leading to significantly lower exposure. Other considerations for an ionisable compound include the impact of ionisation on stability and permeability and for compounds containing both acidic and basic functional groups the formation of zwitterions, for which the solubility at the isoelectric point is typically the lowest over the entire pH range.

If a compound is ionisable, a salt can be formed, which may have better dissolution or an improvement in other physical properties such as hygroscopicity, solid-state stability, or the potential for polymorphism. The solubility product, K, needs to be taken into consideration in predicting the solubility of a salt in a particular environment that contains other salts with a common counterion.

Lipophilicity

Lipophilicity affects solubility and permeability as well as other ADME properties such as protein binding and tissue distribution. The partitioning of a compound is dependent on its ionisation state and thus is dependent on pH.

The most commonly used method to measure lipophilicity is the shake-flask method to determine the octanol/water partition coefficient. After an adequate equilibration time, the concentration of compound in an octanol layer (or another lipophilic phase) and the concentration in an aqueous layer are measured. More recently, this method was adapted to a 96-well plate format by Analiza (Cleveland, OH). Additionally, high-performance liquid chromatography (HPLC) methods have been developed.

Many drugs are surface active, that is, they have both a hydrophilic part and a hydrophobic part and are therefore capable of micelle formation. Surface activity can increase solubility in aqueous media because of micelle formation or other aggregation, where the hydrophobic groups of the molecule are not exposed to the aqueous environment. Surface-active compounds can also disrupt membranes and can thus lead to toxicity.

If the solute is a hydrophobic drug molecule, addition of surfactants to aqueous solvent can increase solubilisation by incorporating the solute into micelles. This solubilisation effect can be seen with simulated gastrointestinal fluids, which typically contain bile salts or other surfactants. The surface tension of solutions of surface-active compounds, as well as their critical micelle concentration, can be measured using several different techniques. These methods include detachment methods such as DuNuoy ring and Wilhelmy plate, maximum bubble pressure, and pendant drop. More details on these methods can be found in physical chemistry textbooks such as Adamson and Gast.

Stability Screening

The stability screening of drug candidates plays an important role in drug discovery. The goal of a stability study at this stage is to obtain an overview of the stability of the compound in a variety of pharmaceutical situations and therefore to identify potential liabilities that may affect drug development. The information obtained from these studies can be used to

— provide feedback to the research team for modification of the labile groups to improve stability;
— help the development scientists to determine the developability of the compound;
— provide guidelines on compound handling and storage; and
— provide information to guide stabilisation strategies.

The revised parent drug stability test guideline Q1A (R2) issued by the International Conference on Harmonisation (ICH) requires that the drug substance be tested under different stress conditions that are indicative of environmental challenges to which the drug will be exposed. It is suggested that stress testing include the effect of pH, temperature, humidity, light, and oxidising agents.

To generate high-quality data, a robust, stability-indicating assay needs to be developed. Frequently, a reverse-phase HPLC assay that allows direct injection of stability samples suffices. While not always practical at the discovery stage, an ideal assay should allow detection of degradation peaks equivalent to 0.1% of the parent peak, which is consistent with the ICH impurity guidelines. This level of detection allows the quantitation of the appearance of degradation products instead of the disappearance of the parent compound, which provides a more precise measurement of degradation.

In recent years, automated systems capable of performing and analysing multiple degradation experiments on drug substances under various stress conditions have been reported. These automated workstations can provide structural and kinetic information on the degradants during the experiment. They also are much faster than manual approaches and are amenable to high-throughput measurements in a 96-well format.

pH-Dependent stability in solution

Information on the stability of a compound in solution is needed to understand its characteristics under physiological conditions and to develop solution dosage forms. The pHdependent stability of a drug substance can be tested at 37°C at pH 1, pH 4, pH 7, and pH 9 for 1 day up to 1 month by HPLC analysis. The studies should be initiated at a reasonable concentration to detect even minor decomposition products in the range of detection. For compounds with low solubility, organic solvents such as acetonitrile and methanol can be added.

The hydrolytic degradation of a compound in acidic and alkaline conditions can be studied by refluxing the drug in 0.1N HCl and 0.1N NaOH for 8 to 12 hours. If the drug is found to degrade completely, both the time and the temperature of the study can be decreased.

Solid-state stability of drug

The solid-state stability of drug substances as a function of temperature and humidity should be studied at the candidate selection stage. Solid-state reactions that occur in drug substances include solid-state phase transformation, dehydration/ desolvation, and chemical reactions. Solid-state degradation of pharmaceuticals is often related to molecular mobility, and common degradation pathways include oxidation, cyclisation, and hydrolysis.

The chemical stability of a drug substance in the solid state can be evaluated under various temperature and humidity conditions. Preweighed samples are stored in stability cabinets at 40°C, 60°C, 25°C/85% relative humidity (RH, open vials), and 40°C/75% RH (open vials) for 2, 4, and 8 weeks. At predetermined time intervals, samples are removed, dissolved in appropriate solvent, and analysed by HPLC.

It is usually difficult to assess the solid-state phase transformation during discovery because of the limited amount of drug material. Solids from the above-mentioned studies should be evaluated at the end of the experiment by differential scanning calorimetry (DSC), thermogravimetric analysis, and powder x-ray diffraction to determine whether there are any changes in polymorphic forms across the conditions tested. Preliminary results obtained from this study can help the development scientists to design full-scale solid-state stability tests.

Oxidation is one of the most common degradation pathways for organic compounds. Oxidation can occur through chain processes that involve initiation, propagation, and termination steps and are catalysed by heat, light, metals, or free radicals. It can also occur via electron-transfer reactions to form reactive radicals of anions or cations. In the solid state, oxidation occurs where molecular oxygen diffuses through the crystal lattice to the labile sites.

Certain functional groups show particular sensitivity toward oxidation. For chain processes, oxidative degradation is linked to the lability of hydrogen atoms within the molecular framework. For example, substituted aromatics such as toluenes, phenols, and anisoles are susceptible to hydrogen abstraction because the aromatic group can stabilise the resulting radical through resonance. For electron transfer reactions, nitrogen (amines), sulfur heteroatoms (sulfides, disulfides, and sulfoxides), and oxygen-based anions (phenol anions) are common sites for electron-transfer-induced oxidation, producing final products such as N-oxides, sulfoxides, sulfones, and ketones.

At the drug candidate selection stage, oxidative stability can be tested in solution in the presence of 100-200 ppm hydrogen peroxide or other free radical initiators such as 2,2 '-azobis (2-amidinopropane) dihydrochloride. While it may not be necessary and is rather difficult to test solid-state oxidative stability in discovery, a recent report by Simon et al demonstrated a rapid method that may be useful for rankordering the oxidative stability of solids. In this method, parameters describing the lengths of oxidation induction periods were obtained from nonisothermal DSC measurements based on the dependence of onset temperature of the oxidation peak on heating rate.

Exposure of a drug to irradiation can influence its stability, and a test of a compound's photostability should be performed at the discovery stage. The information about the compound's photoreactivity is needed to provide information for handling, packaging, labeling, and use of the drug substance or product.

At the candidate selection stage, photostability should be evaluated both in the solid state and in solution. For solidstate photostability, the preweighed drug substance is stored at high-intensity light (HIL)/UV conditions at 25°C in a photostability chamber according to the ICH guidelines (1.2 million lux hour exposure to visible light and 200 W hour/m 2 to UV). At the end of the experiment, the solid is dissolved in appropriate solvent and analysed by HPLC. For solution photostability, solutions at appropriate concentration are stored at ICH HIL/UV conditions and analysed by LC. For both solid and solution photostability, samples protected from light are stored under the same condition and used as controls.

While it is not always feasible in drug discovery to identify all degradation products and elucidate degradation mechanisms, preliminary studies on these aspects will guide de velopment scientists in solving the stability problems and designing a strategy for stabilisation. Traditional methodologies, which use spectral and elemental analysis, are often slow and resource-consuming. The modern approach is to integrate systems in which LC/MS or LC/MS/MS is employed to obtain molecular weight and fragmentation information or to use LC/nuclear magnetic resonance to obtain further detailed structural information. The integrated approach provides rapid and unambiguous identifi- cation of several degradation products at one time.

PREFORMULATION

Vehicle selection for preclinical in vivo studies can be a major challenge for discovery scientists. In preparing, scientists must determine the objective of the in vivo studies since the type of constraints placed on the vehicle can be very different for different objectives. For example, if the goal of the study is to get an initial idea of the oral efficacy of the compound, it is essential that the excipients selected for the vehicle not interfere with the measured end points.

The easiest way to get this initial evaluation of efficacy may be to use solution formulations rather than suspensions and in that way reduce the complexity of the studies. If, on the other hand, the main goal of the in vivo study is to get an idea of whether the compound is developable, a more complex crossover design using both solution and suspension dosing may be needed.

In selecting a solution vehicle the solubility of the compound in aqueous and nonaqueous systems is determined first to identify the various vehicle possibilities. At the same time, the chemical stability in these solvents should be evaluated. Several strategies can be used to increase the solubility of compounds with low aqueous solubility. If the compound is ionisable, it may be possible to achieve the target concentration through pH adjustment. If pH adjustment does not give the desired results, a cosolvent can be used. Polyethylene glycol 400 (PEG 400) is a good example of a commonly used inert cosolvent that has wide application across several therapeutic areas for both oral and parenteral administration.

If the in vivo model for preclinical pharmacology testing precludes the use of vehicles such as PEG 400 and propylene glycol, then other, more exotic vehicles such as N-methyl-2-pyrrolidone, Labrafil, and vitamin E TPGS (d-alpha tocopheryl polyethylene glycol 1000 succinate) may be considered. In other instances a complexing agent such as cyclodextrin can be used to increase the compound's solubility. Care should be taken to ensure that compounds are soluble in cyclodextrin solutions at the target concentration, especially when the discovery programme has vast diversity in their chemical structures. Otherwise, instead of screening compounds for biological efficacy it is possible that the efficacy study is inadvertently screening for the ability of the compound to form cyclodextrin complexes.

It is often desirable to give a drug parenterally in solutions at a concentration that exceeds its aqueous solubility. For intravenous administration, there are numerous approaches that may be adopted for solubilising the compound. Use of cosolvent is most often the preferred route to increase the solubility of these compounds. When this approach is used, care has to be taken not to exceed toxicity levels for the cosolvent. Furthermore, the formulation may cause hemolysis or the drug may precipitate out of the formulation immediately after injection. Yalkowsky and his group have developed an in vitro precipitation model to predict the potential of compounds to precipitate upon intravenous administration. This simple model can be used to predict whether precipitation of a compound might occur on dilution or injection.

Suspension dosing

An important part of candidate selection is the design of pharmacokinetic (PK) studies that explore potential problems and define the probability of success of formulation approaches to enable future clinical studies. An early evaluation of potential formulation options aids in the assessment of factors that could lead to increased development time and costs and can be critical for decision making and prioritisation of development resources.

Most drugs are developed for oral administration of a solid dosage form. The impact of solubility and dissolution rate of the solid drug substance on the rate and extent of oral drug absorption should, therefore, be evaluated and compared with the absorption achieved after solution administration. Because of limited compound availability and time constraints that are usually experienced in discovery settings, a simple suspension formulation is most often chosen for this purpose. Crystalline material should be used for this suspension dosing, since amorphous drug is likely to have significantly higher solubility and a significantly higher dissolution rate in the gastrointestinal (GI) tract, potentially leading to unrealistic absorption levels that cannot be reproduced once a crystalline form of the drug has been identified at a later stage of the development process.

In a case where dissolution of the solid drug is much faster than absorption of the dissolved drug into the body, permeability, not dissolution, is the rate-limiting step for absorption. Suspension and solution dosing should result in the same systemic exposure levels in such a case. However, more commonly the dissolution of the solid drug proceeds slowly, and once the drug is dissolved it readily permeates through the gut wall. Here, drug absorption is therefore dissolutionrate-limited, and dosing a suspension will result in signifi- cantly reduced exposure compared with solution dosing.

Any changes in dissolution rate that can be achieved through formulation approaches, such as reduction of particle size of the solid drug or administration of a salt in the case of an ionisable compound, can lead to a profound effect on the rate and degree of drug absorption. If, however, the solubility of the drug in the GI fluid is extremely low and saturation of the intestinal fluid with the drug is achieved at low concentrations, reduction of particle size will not have the desired effect of increased exposure. Absorption in this case is not dissolution-rate-limited but solubility-limited. Which of these 2 phenomena is responsible for low drug absorption after administration of a suspension often depends on the dose administered.

At low doses, saturation of the GI fluid with drug might not be reached, and a decrease in particle size might result in increased systemic exposure, indicating dissolution-rate-limited absorption. An increasc in dose at a given particle size will result in dose-related increases of systemic exposure up to a certain level. Above this level, drug concentrations in the GI fluid reach saturation, and a further increase in dose or reduction of particle size will not lead to increased exposure. In this scenario, drug absorption changes from being dissolution-rate-limited to solubilitylimited and exposure levels reach a plateau, indicating the need for more complex formulation technologies such as the generation of high-energy, amorphous drug substance or the design of a solubilised, precipitation-resistant formulation to overcome solubility-limited absorption.

In vivo crossover studies during drug discovery for comparison of the performance of suspension and solution formulations are especially important during the evaluation of potential candidates with low aqueous solubility. An early idea of the highest exposure that can be reached from a simple suspension dosing of a given drug candidate and how this exposure compares to projected efficacious levels in humans is essential for the early identification of potential development hurdles. Once these data have been obtained, suitable approaches and adequate resources can be planned when the compound is moved into development to minimise surprises during clinical development.

Chapter 2

Chemical Properties of Drugs

The phrase "chemical property" is context-dependent, but generally refers to a material's quality which becomes evident during a chemical reaction; this is, which can only be established by changing a substance's chemical identity. Simply speaking, chemical properties typically cannot be determined by just viewing or touching the substance; the substance internal structure must be affected to investigate its chemical property.

Chemical properties can be contrasted with physical properties. However, for many properties within the subject and methods of physical chemistry (and many other disciplines at the border of chemistry and physics), the distinction may be a matter of researcher's perspective. The properties can often be viewed as supervenient, i.e., secondary to the underlying reality (several layers of superveniency are possible).

Physicochemical characterisation deals with the skills and techniques needed to provide research and development staff with the basic chemical information that is germane to successful design and development of a suitable formulation to deliver a drug to its site of action. This information includes measured solubility in different solvents, acid-base equilibria, oil-water partition coefficients, critical micelle concentration ranges and concentration-time profiles from which degradation rate constants may be extracted. Drugs which are to be formulated as solids require extensive information on the solid state, such as melting point, enthalpy and entropy of fusion, crystal morphology, surface properties and particle analysis. Acquisition of such data is also critically important in characterising the excipients that may be needed in formulations. In addition to characterisation data on the individual drugs or excipients, methods for characterising the interactions between drugs, or between drugs and excipients, is also important in formulation design, and in accounting for the biopharmaceutical properties of drugs. Another aspect of the characterisation of drugs and excipients includes their spectroscopic characteristics, especially UV-VIS, fluorescence, infra-red, nuclear magnetic resonance and mass.

Macromolecular drugs and excipients present special difficulties in characterization, mainly due to their potential for highly organized and relatively weakly stabilised structures. The same may be said for complex delivery systems, such as micelles, microemulsions, liposomes and vesicles. While full elucidation of such complex organised structures requires specialities outside Pharmaceutics (e.g., molecular modelling, nuclear magnetic resonance and X-ray diffraction methods), available skills and facilities for characterisation of these more complex compounds and systems include scanning microcalorimetry, hot-stage microscopy and temperature-controlled circular dichroism spectrometry.

Chemical Properties of Racemic Drugs

In the IUPAC rules the word "racemic" is applied to an optically inactive product in any state of matter and "racemic mixture" would appear to be the correct terminology for a 1:1 mixture of enantiomers in any physical state. However, in the solid state, the rules specifically refer to a racemic mixture as "a mixture of equimolar amounts of enantiomeric molecules present as separate solid phases". Perhaps in recognition of the historical significance of Pasteur's observations, sodium ammonium tartrate was the material chosen in the IUPAC rules to distinguish between a racemic mixture as defined above and a racemic compound. The IUPAC rules define a racemic compound as "any homogeneous solid composed of equimolar amounts of enantiomeric molecules". Sodium ammonium tartrate when crystallised below 27.8°C from an aqueous solution gives equal amounts of dextrorotatory and laevorotatory mirror-image crystal forms, i.e. a racemic mixture. The crystals separating out above 27.8°C constitute a homogeneous solid phase in which each symmetrical crystal contains an equal amount of the two salts, i.e. a racemic compound. If the temperature of Pasteur's solution had been above 27.8°C, he would have been unable to recrystallise the racemic mixture and conduct the classic first resolution by hand separation into two distinct phases.

The choice of sodium ammonium tartrate in the rules to distinguish between a racemic mixture and a racemic compound was probably unfortunate since it may give the impression, firstly, that any given material can be recrystallised either as a racemic mixture or as a compound simply by changing the experimental conditions and secondly, that in a racemic mixture the two mirror-image crystallographic phases can be identified by visual inspection and possibly separated by hand. This combination of properties is very rare and is probably unique to sodium ammonium tartrate. For most racemic materials the solid recrystallises either as a racemic mixture or as a racemic compound of which the latter is by far the most common. For those materials which do recrystallise as a racemic mixture, the individual crystal phases usually occur in conglomerates and not as distinct separate crystals. Jacques et al., prefer the term racemic conglomerate to racemic mixture since this avoids ambiguities in the definition of racemic mixture and more accurately describes the physical appearance of the solid. Although the term racemic compound is free from ambiguity the term "racemate" is commonly used to describe racemic compounds.

This is in agreement with the IUPAC 1970 definition: "Any homogeneous solid containing equimolar amounts of enantiomeric molecules is termed a racemate". In the 1979 revision, however, the phrase "any homogeneous solid" was changed to "any homogeneous phase". This had the effect of expanding the definition of racemate to include an equimolar mixture of enantiomers in any physical state. Thus in the gaseous and in the liquid (melt or solution) states the terms "racemic mixture" and "racemate" can be used interchangeably. In the gaseous and liquid states, both types of racemic modification will behave as ideal or nearly ideal mixtures with physical properties which are indistinguishable from those of the pure enantiomers.

However both the 1970 and 1979 rules agree that in the solid state, the term "racemic mixture" refers to a heterogeneous mixture of two separate solid phases while the term "racemate" refers to a homogeneous single phase. A survey of recent literature reveals a tendency to use "racemic mixture" interchangeably with "racemate". For solids this is incorrect.

Until advances in technology made possible the largescale synthesis and analysis of single enantiomers, the question of using an enantiomeric drug rather than its racemic modification was largely academic. Synthesis of a chiral drug from achiral precursors always leads to a racemic modification. Now that the preparation of pure enantiomers is a commercial reality the decision whether to market a pure enantiomer or the racemic drug depends on many factors of which clinical efficacy and safety are of overriding importance. Pure enantiomers often show different pharmacodynamic and pharmacokinetic behaviour.

Very often one isomer possesses the desired pharmacological properties whilst the other isomer may be inert, completely different in its pharmacological activity or even toxic. Another problem which is becoming acute with the increasing number of chiral drugs is that the approved drug names and accompanying monographs very often fail to give any indication of enantiomeric composition. As pointed out by Lee and Williams, Martindale's Extra Pharmacopoeia lists 39 beta-adrenergic blockers, only 14 of which are identified as being either the racemic drug or the pure enantiomer. Of the drugs not identified, at least two have two chiral centers (i.e. four isomers) and one has three chiral centers (i.e. eight isomers). Gal suggested there is an urgent need for the adoption of an explicit system for naming stereoisomeric drugs such as that proposed by Simonyl. Where clinical efficacy and safety are not compromised, a racemic drug may still be preferred to an enantiomer on the basis of considerations such as lower cost and more desirable physical properties.

The solid state properties of racemic mixtures and racemic compounds are likely to be very different from their corresponding enantiomers. Such differences in physical properties must be considered both for new chemical entities as well as for established drugs where the racemic modification is in current use, but where stereoselective synthesis provides an opportunity to use a pure enantiomer. One other racemic modification is encountered in the solid state, namely the pseudoracemate. These three racemic modifications originate from differences in the packing forces in the crystal lattice. In a racemic mixture, each enantiomer has a greater affinity for molecules of its own kind than for those of the other enantiomer and the two enantiomers crystallise in separate phases.

In a racemic compound, each enantiomer has a greater affinity for molecules of the opposite type than for its own kind. The unit cell of the crystal thus contains an equal number of molecules of each enantiomer and the product is a true addition compound. In cases where there is little difference in the affinity between enantiomers of like or opposite configuration, the two enantiomers exist in an unordered manner in the crystal., i.e. the racemic modification shows nearly ideal mixing and forms a racemic solid solution.

Racemic mixtures, racemic compounds and pseudoracemates can be differentiated from one another on the basis of their melting point behaviour. Provided either both enantiomers or the racemic drug and at least one pure enantiomer are available, a two component phase diagram is readily constructed using differential scanning calorimetry (DSC).

Racemic modifications are frequently hydrated and transformations from one racemic modification to another with increases in temperature can be associated with a reduction in the degree of hydration. For example, below 27.8°C, sodium ammonium tartrate ('Pasteur's salt') recrystallises as a racemic mixture with four waters of crystallisation, but the racemic compound which recrystallises above 27.8°C, contains only one molecule of water of crystallisation. Conversely, histidine hydrochloride recrystallises as a dihydrate racemic compound below about 45°C but, at temperatures of 45°C and above, recrystallises as an anhydrous racemic mixture. It is apparent from these examples of polymorphism and solvation that, depending on the temperature of crystallisation, it is possible for a racemic drug to crystallise in more than one racemic modification and vary in its extent of hydration.

Other elements of chirality in the molecule have been excluded. Furthermore, only molecules with one asymmetric carbon atom have been considered. However, drugs may have two or more chiral centers. Thus, labetalol has two asymmetric centers and therefore has four stereoisomers, i.e. two racemic pairs RR and SS; SR and RS. The RR and SS isomers are enantiomers of each other as are the SR and RS isomers. other combinations of pairs of isomers are not mirror images.

A melting point phase diagram has not been reported but, on the basis that racemic compound formation is the most common racemic modification, it may be speculated that labetalol is a racemic mixture of two racemic compounds i.e. a simple eutectic mixture containing two solid phases namely the racemic pair, RR and SS, and the racemic pair SR and RS. However, the possibility of other racemic modifications cannot be excluded. Labetalol is now clinically available as the RR isomer and it is apparent that the solid state properties of the RR isomer will be different from those of the racemic drug. Since the number of stereoisomers increases geometrically with the number of chiral centers, the complexities possible in the solid state become readily apparent particularly when the possibilities of polymorphism and hydrate formation are included.

CHIRALITY OF DRUGS

Chiral defined as, "Not superposable … with its mirror image, as applied to molecules, conformations, as well as macroscopic objects, such as crystals". Mislow gave a shorter but essentially equivalent definition: "An object is chiral if and only if it is not superposable on its mirror image; otherwise it is achiral". Thus, it is clear that chiral refers to a spatial property of objects, including molecules.

Therefore, the term describes that nature of a molecule which makes it non-superposable on its mirror image, and does not refer to the stereochemical composition of bulk material, i. e., drugs, compounds, substances, etc. Thus, "chiral drug" does not tell us whether the drug is racemic, single-enantiomeric, or some other mixture of the stereoisomers. In the present article, therefore, chiral will be used strictly according to the definitions cited above, i. e., to refer to the chirality of individual molecules or other chiral objects. Thus, "chiral drug", "chiral substance", etc., will be used to indicate that the drug in question is composed of chiral molecules, but the enantiomer composition is not specified by this terminology.

There is however a great and obvious need for a convenient term to refer to chiral substances that are composed of only one of the two enantiomers. Numerous terms for this purpose have been introduced over many years, but the issue remains complex and largely unresolved. The present author recently discussed this issue in detail and introduced a new term for the purpose: unichiral. In the present chapter unichiral will be used to specify the stereochemical composition of a chiral drug, substance, compound, sample, etc, as stereochemically homogeneous, i. e., consisting of a single-enantiomer (in the context where the term is used and within the limits of measurement).

For thousands of years, remedies from nature obtained from vegetable, animal, or mineral sources were relied upon for relief from human diseases. Such folk medicine was, by its very nature, inaccurate and unscientific and often had no rational basis. Moreover, the toxicity of many of the products was a serious problem; indeed, some of the pharmacologically active preparations were used as poisons. The advent of the printing press in the 15th century resulted in the wide dissemination of knowledge about natural medications and this in turn produced a considerable increase in the use, and misuse, of such remedies. More rational therapy with purified natural products did not begin until the 1800s.

Despite the problems, however, some of the natural preparations were effective in relieving the symptoms and at times even eliminating the disease. In fact, we know today that the number of pharmacologically active substances produced by nature is large and the spectrum of biological activities of natural products is extraordinarily broad; for example, antimicrobial, antineoplastic, CNS-active, anti-inflammatory, cardiovascular, etc., are only a few of the therapeutic classes of drugs from nature.

Chirality is a hallmark of many molecules from nature. Indeed, the number of chiral natural molecules is very large and the structural variety they represent is vast. Among such substances - be they small molecules or macromolecules - an overwhelming majority occur in unichiral form. For example, chiral α-amino acids and the peptides and proteins containing them, sugars and their polysaccharides, steroids, antibiotics, and many other compounds from nature are unichiral. Another important aspect of many chiral molecules from nature is their homochirality. This means that related chiral molecules in the same chemical class usually have the same sense of chirality. For example, with rare exceptions α-amino acids occurring in nature consistently have the L configuration; similarly, monosaccharides are of the D configuration. Thus, both unichirality and homochirality are typical for compounds from nature: most of them occur in enantiomerically homogeneous form, and closely related molecules usually have the same sense of chirality.

In the light of the above, then, it is not surprising that many of the compounds used as therapeutic agents in natural remedies over the centuries andmillennia have been chiral and that the vast majority of such substances occur in unichiral form. For thousands of years and until the beginning of the 19th century most such natural remedies were used as crude plant extracts rather than purified active principles. Obviously, in that "pre-scientific" era, the remedies were used without any clue as to the nature or identity of the active ingredient(s) within, let alone any understanding of the chirality of themolecules involved. Recognition of the existence of chiral drugs had to await a better understanding of chemical structure, i. e., the advent of modern organic chemistry and the discovery ofmolecular chirality.

The number of pharmacologically active agents now known to be present in various old remedies is large and many of these compounds are based on chiral molecules. Information about some of the earliest herbal remedies that contain chiral active ingredients goes back nearly 5000 years. A few examples of old therapies with chiral active ingredients are presented below.

In a book about herbs, the Chinese scholar-emperor Shen Nung described in 2735 BC the beneficial effects of Ch'ang Shan in the treatment of "fevers". This preparation is the powdered root of a plant, Dichroa febrifuga Lour. Modern medicinal chemistry has identified several alkaloids with antimalarial properties in the plant, and it is therefore clear that the ancient use of Ch'ang Shan in fevers was not entirely without basis. One of the antimalarial compounds from Ch'ang Shan is februgine (β-dichroine), a relatively simple unichiral compound 1. Modern attempts to develop these agents as antimalarial drugs failed, due to significant toxicity.

1

Shen Nung also observed the stimulant properties of another Chinese plant, Ma Huang, now known as Ephedra sinica. The chief active ingredient, ephedrine, is a sympathomimetic amine, and therefore it is clear in this case also that the use of Ma Huang as a stimulant had a rational basis. The ephedrine molecule is simple and contains two chiral centers; the compound from ephedra is unichiral and has the 1R,2S configuration 2. Ephedrine was first isolated from Ma Huang in 1887, i. e., more than 4600 years after the effects of the compound were recorded. Ephedrine was introduced into medical practice during the 1920s and for decades was widely used - as a CNS stimulant in narcolepsy, as a bronchodilator, in the treatment of Adams-Stokes syndrome with complete heart block, as a stimulant in some forms of depression, and in some other disorders - but more recently it has been largely replaced in most of these indications by other treatment modalities.

Ephedrine has also been widely available in "dietary supplements" for weight loss, increased energy, body building, etc. However, in the early 1990s concern arose over potentially serious adverse effects from such use of ephedrine, including cardiovascular, nervous-system, and other toxic effects, and in April 2004 the U.S. Food and Drug Administration (FDA) banned the sale in the United States of dietary supplements containing ephedrine or closely related compounds.

Another millennia-old unichiral drug is the opioid agent morphine. Opioid refers broadly to all compounds related to opium (a more recent definition states that the term opioid includes any compound that interacts with the brain's opioid receptors). Opium powder is the dried juice from the unripe seed capsule of the poppy Papaver somniferum and its name is derived from the diminutive of the Greek word opos, i. e. juice. Opium has analgesic, euphoric, and other effects and contains many alkaloids, including morphine 3 and codeine 4. Poppy juice is mentioned in the writings of the Greek philosopher and naturalist Theophrastus, but evidence has been found suggesting that opium may have been known much earlier, to ancient civilisations in Egypt and Mesopotamia.

Within the Arab-Islamic civilisation, whose rise began in the 7th century, opium came to be used mainly as a constipant to control dysentery. The arrival of the Islamic armies and their influence in Europe in the 16th century brought opium to Europe. Laudanum, a somewhat purified opium concentrate, was compounded by Paracelsus, a Swiss alchemist and physician, and the smoking of opium became openly popular during the 1700s; however, opium may have been extensively but less openly used in Europe in earlier times.

Morphine, the most important alkaloid in opium, was obtained as a purified powder from opium in 1805 by Friedrich Wilhelm Sertürner (1783-1841), a German pharmacist's assistant. He named it morphium after Morpheus, the Latin god of dreams, so named by Ovid using a Greek word. Later, the great French chemist and physicist Joseph-Louis Gay-Lussac (1778-1850), who was a strong supporter of Sertürner in his priority claim for the isolation of the substance over French pretenders, renamed the drug morphine, against the wishes of Sertürner. The morphine molecule is a pentacyclic tertiary amine with five chiral centers 3 and the natural product is the levorotatory enantiomer.

The invention of the hypodermic needle and syringe in the middle of the 19th century resulted in the widespread use of morphine, and addiction became a common problem. An early - and false - hope to circumvent the addiction liability of morphine was provided by a most unlikely candidate: heroin.

This compound, the diacetyl derivative of morphine 5, is a potent opiate narcotic first synthesised in 1874 via acetylation of morphine, and was introduced into medical practice in 1898 as a cough suppressant. Heroin is a semisynthetic drug, i. e., a chemically modified derivative of a natural product, and retains the stereochemistry of morphine. Heroin may have been the first synthetic unichiral drug introduced in clinical medicine.

H_3C N H H_3C O O CH_3 O O O

5

Heroin was actively marketed to physicians by its manufacturer, as an advertisement from ca. 1900 shows. The drug was touted as a "non-addicting" morphine analog that could safely replace morphine and thereby eliminate the latter's addiction problem. This claim turned out to be tragically mistaken and today heroin is the most important abused opioid, with grave social, economic, and medical consequences. Another chiral drug, methadone, a totally synthetic opiate agonist, has been recruited to fight heroin addiction. Methadone was first synthesized, in the racemic form, in the 1940s and was later shown to have stereoselective opioid agonist properties, concentrated nearly exclusively in the (R)-(-) enantiomer 6.

O CH_3 CH_3 N H_3C CH_3

6

Methadone is used in the racemic form in the U.S. as an analgesic and in the treatment of opiate addiction, but in some other countries the pharmaceutical product is the unichiral levo form. Perhaps the most fascinating old chiral drug, from a historical point of view, is quinine. Its earliest history is obscure, but it is known that by the early 1600s it was being used by South

American natives in Peru, Ecuador, and neighboring regions as a crude preparation from the bark of the cinchona tree for the treatment of malaria. In 1633 Antonio de la Calancha, an Augustinian monk in Lima, wrote a pamphlet describing the native use and fever-curing powers of cinchona and by the middle of 1600s the extract of "Jesuit's bark" was being used in Europe indiscriminately for a variety of fevers.

Cinchona was, however, effective only against malaria, an infectious disease widespread in many regions of Africa and Asia, and even in Europe for centuries. Cinchona was the first effective treatment for malaria, and in 1820 the French pharmacists Pierre Joseph Pelletier and Joseph Bienaimé Caventou isolated quinine, the main antimalarial ingredient, from cinchona bark. The quinine molecule contains four chiral carbon centers and the natural product is the levorotatory unichiral compound 7.

CH2
H
HO
N
H3C-O
N
7

The name cinchona was coined by the Swedish botanist Linnaeus in honor of Doña Francisca Henriquez de Ribera, the fourth Condesa of Chinchón and wife of the viceroy of Peru, a Spanish colony at the time. According to legend, in 1638 she was cured of malaria by the bark and, impressed with the cure, she took samples of cinchona to Spain, thereby launching the European career of the miracle remedy. However, as has been frequently pointed out, there are problems with Linnaeus' nomenclature. First, he misspelled cinchona, leaving out the first h in the countess' name; second, she died in South America before she could return to Spain. Be that as it may, cinchona has stuck in the official names of several species. As for quinine, this name is derived from quina quina, the Spanish spelling of a native Quechua name that was sometimes used for the cinchona tree in Peru, and was given by Pelletier and Caventou to their new substance.

After its isolation in 1820, purified quinine quickly replaced the crude cinchona preparations in the treatment of malaria. Supplies of quinine were limited and the need was great, as the drug was in demand for the treatment of malaria not only in Europe but also in various parts of Africa and Asia, where European powers were engaged in establishing or strengthening their colonial control. Chemists in Europe were responding to the need with attempts to synthesize quinine in the laboratory. In England in 1856 an 18-year old chemistry student named William Henry Perkin (1838-1907), working with August Wilhelm von Hofmann (1818-1892), a German professor of chemistry appointed director of the newly established Royal College in London, attempted to synthesize quinine by oxidising N-allyltoluidine with potassium dichromate. The reaction, predictably in hindsight, did not produce quinine, but Perkin's further studies of the reaction led to the discovery of mauveine, a purple dye which in turn launched the artificial, "aniline" or "coal-tar", dye industry. The invention of mauveine not only revolutionised the dye and textile industries but also produced an intense stimulatory effect on chemical research in general, on the pharmaceutical industry, and on medicine (Perkin's mauveine is a mixture of two compounds neither of which is chiral).

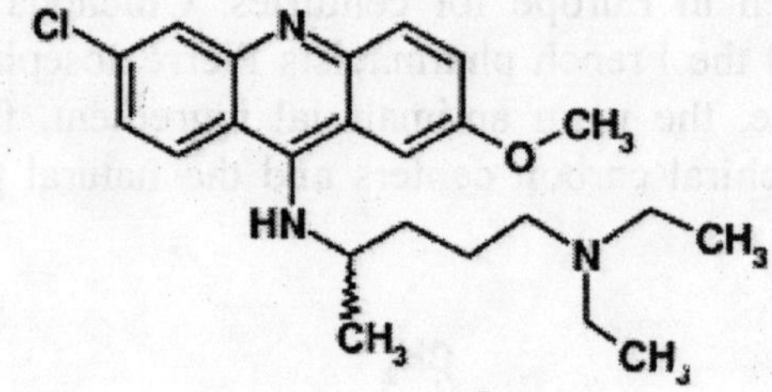

The need for effective antimalarial drugs has persisted over the nearly two centuries since quinine was first isolated. Modifications of the quinine molecule have produced many useful antimalarial agents, including the chiral drugs quinacrine 8, primaquine 9, and chloroquine 10. These compounds were introduced during the 20th century, in racemic form. Chloroquine was particularly useful inasmuch as it was cheap and effective, but more recently resistance by the malaria parasites to this drug has made it ineffective in many parts of the world where the disease is endemic. Quinine remains a useful antimalarial agent in the treatment of chloroquine- and multidrug-resistant falciparum malaria today, but increasing resistance by the parasites may result in a re-duction in the drug's importance in the future. Malaria remains one of the great killers, with about 1-1.5 million victims dying of the disease every year, the majority of them African children.

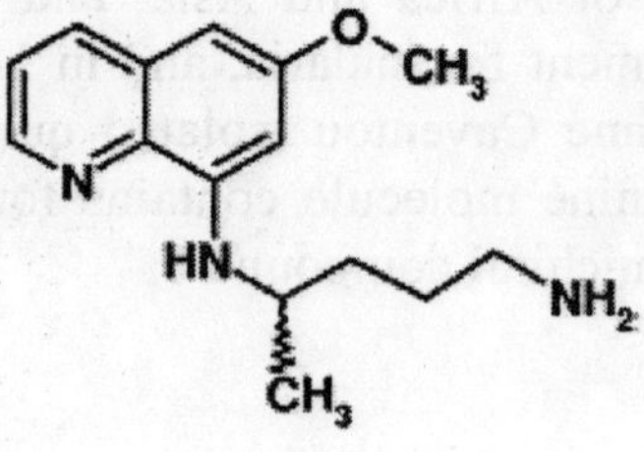

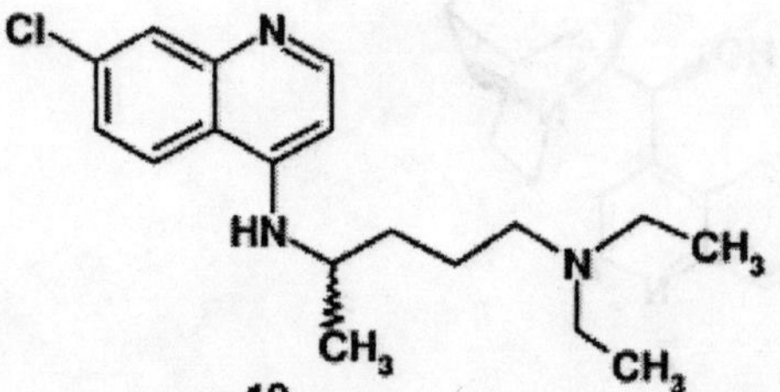

The devastating disease scurvy is caused by insufficient amounts of l-ascorbic acid 11 (vitamin C) in the diet. After the 15th century, exploration, expanding trade, and colonisation by European powers required long sea voyages, usually undertaken without foods rich in vitamin C on board. The result was the decimation of ships' crews by scurvy. In a remarkable study in 1747 that can be described as the first serious clinical therapeutic trial, British physician James Lind (1716-1794), a surgeon in the Royal Navy and the "father of naval hygiene", demonstrated that fruits such as oranges and lemons can reverse and prevent the disease. However, it was nearly 50 years later, in 1795, that the British Admiralty finally took notice of these findings and instituted an appropriate diet on board Royal Navy ships to prevent scurvy.

Ascorbic acid was isolated by the Hungarian biochemist Albert Szent-Györgyi from fruit juices in 1928 and, in part for this work, he was awarded the Nobel Prize in Physiology or Medicine in 1937. In that same year one half of the Nobel Prize in Chemistry went to the English chemist Walter Norman Haworth for the proof of the structure and synthesis of ascorbic acid.

The above examples of old chiral drugs from natural sources are but a handful from a long list of many examples. Others include (some plant origins given in parentheses) tetrahydrocannabinol 12 (marihuana, hashish), digoxin (foxglove, digitalis lanata Ehrh.), cocaine 13 (erythroxylon), cathinone (khat, Catha edulis Forsk.), nicotine 14 (tobacco, Nicotiana tabacum), atropine (deadly nightshade, atropa belladonna L.), reserpine (Rauwolfia), colchicine 15 (autumn crocus, meadow saffron), and emetine (ipecac), to name only a few. Each of these chiral compounds has an interesting history but these accounts are beyond our scope here.

The chemical structures encompassed by just these relatively few chiral molecules are highly varied. Stereochemically, atropine is an interesting case: this racemic substance is believed not to occur naturally, but its levorotatory form, (S)-(-)-hyoscyamine 16, occurs in several Solanaceae plant species and is racemised to atropine during isolation. This facile racemisation reaction is the result of the stereochemical lability of the chiral center due to the presence of the adjacent carbonyl group and the β-hydroxy group, in combination with its benzylic position.

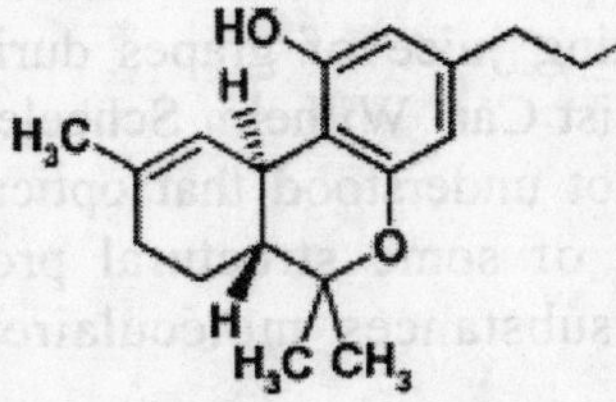

12

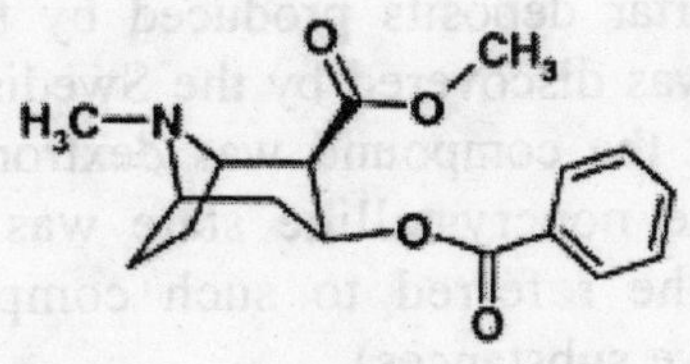

13

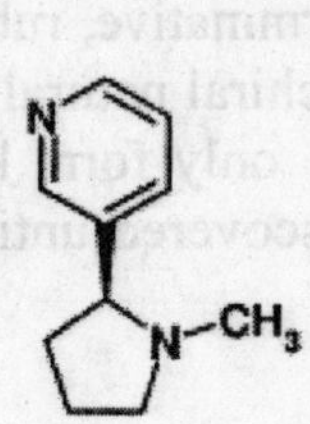

14

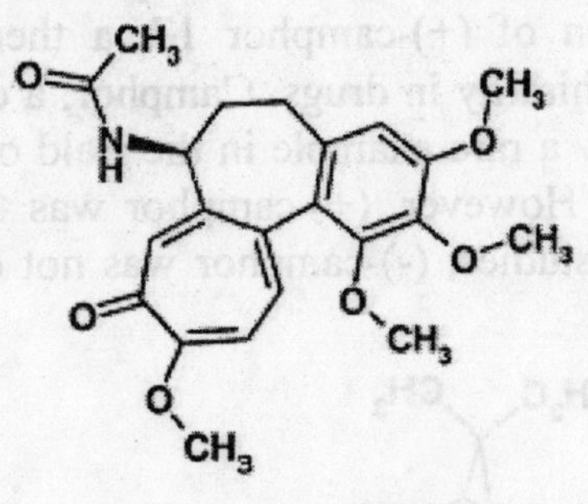

15

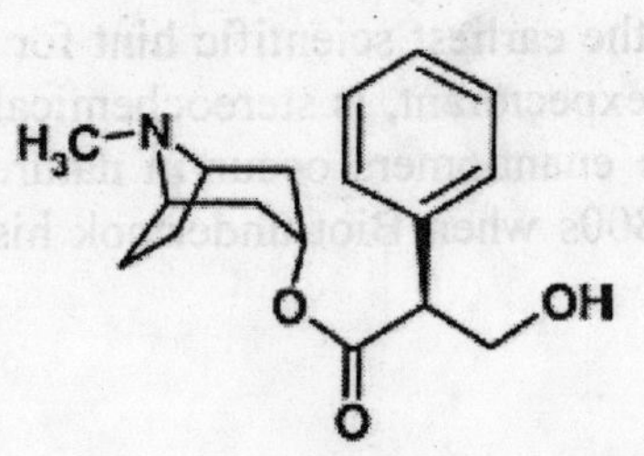

16

The vast majority of chiral drugs present in the old remedies were unichiral: Mother Nature is not even-handed. All in all, chiral drugs have been of great importance in the development of pharmacotherapy, from the earliest plant remedies of millennia ago to the modern age. Many of these ancient chiral drugs are still in use today, and many new and important drugs have been developed by modifying the molecules of natural products identified in old remedies. The "pre-science" era of pharmacotherapy based on crude natural remedies came to an end as the 19th century was drawing to a close. The dawn of the modern era of therapeutics did not mean, however, the end of the therapeutic use of natural compounds, chiral or achiral; only the science and technology became different. Beginning with the first decades of the 20th century, natural products were routinely purified from their sources and their chemical structures were elucidated. Chirality, when present, was now recognised.

Recognition of Chirality in Drugs

The earliest recognition of chirality in drugs was intimately linked to the discovery of molecular chirality. The relevant background work that led to the discovery was accomplished mainly in France during the first half of the 19th century. Hemihedrism in crystals - those of quartz - was first reported by René-Just Haüy, a French priest and crystallographer, in 1801. Circularly polarised light (often referred to as plane-polarised light) was discovered in 1809 by Étienne Louis Malus, and the physicist François Arago made the first observation of optical rotation by a substance when he studied the effects of quartz crystals on polarised light.

French physicist Jean-Baptiste Biot discovered beginning in 1815 that certain organic compounds rotate polarised light in the noncrystalline state, e. g., in the liquid or solution state. Among these compounds were sucrose, turpentine, camphor, and tartaric acid. Tartaric acid obtained from tartar deposits produced by the fermenting juice of grapes during the wine-making process was discovered by the Swedish pharmacist Carl Wilhelm Scheele in 1769, and Biot showed that the compound was dextrorotatory. Biot understood that optical rotation by substances in the noncrystalline state was the result of some structural property of the molecules, and he referred to such compounds as substances moléculairement actives (molecularly active substances).

This realisation by Biot of a molecular-structural cause of optical rotation, coupled with his discovery in 1815 of the optical rotation of (+)-camphor 17, a therapeutic agent, may be considered the earliest scientific hint for chirality in drugs. Camphor, a carminative, rubefacient, and a mild expectorant, is stereochemically a rare example in the field of chiral natural products in that both enantiomers occur in nature. However, (+)-camphor was the only form known in the early 1800s when Biot undertook his studies; (-)-camphor was not discovered until 1853.

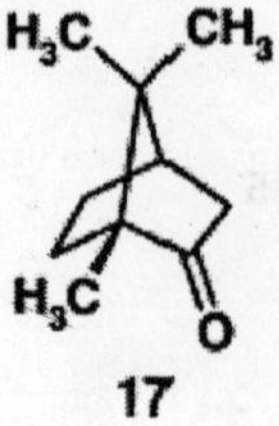

H_3C CH_3

H_3C O

17

A fuller appreciation of the existence of chiral drugs was achieved a few decades later by the celebrated French chemist (and later microbiologist) Louis Pasteur. Pasteur was familiar with the above-outlined work of Biot on optical rotation by organic compounds. In 1848 he found that the crystals of sodium ammonium tartrate (from dextro-tartaric acid) were hemihedral, i. e., there were small facets at alternate corners of the crystals. He recognised that these facets rendered the crystals chiral.

Pasteur then examined the sodium ammonium salt of another, related, acid. That acid had been obtained in 1820 - unexpectedly and on a single occasion - as a side-product during the manufacture of (+)-tartaric acid from tartar at a chemical plant in Thann, Alsace, France. The mysterious new acid intrigued chemists. In 1826 Gay-Lussac obtained a sample for study and named it racemic acid, from racemus, Latin for cluster of grapes. Racemic acid was found to be identical with (+)-tartaric acid, with the exception that - inexplicably at the time - it did not rotate polarised light, a fact first shown by Biot.

Pasteur obtained a sample of the new acid and found - to his initial dismay - that the crystals of sodium ammonium racemate, like those of the corresponding (dextrorotatory) tartrate, were hemihedral. To his surprise, however, he observed that there were two different crystals present in the salt of racemic acid. That is, in some of the crystals the hemihedral facets were inclined to the right and some to the left (as in quartz), and Pasteur recognised that the two crystals were related to each other as the two hands, i. e., they were enantiomorphous. Pasteur then manually separated the two kinds of crystals and found that they rotated polarised light in solution, the rotations by the two being equal in absolute value but opposite in direction.

The dextrorotatory salt thus obtained was identical in all respects to the corresponding salt of the known (+)-tartaric acid and could be converted to a free acid that was identical in all respects with (+)-tartaric acid, while the levorotatory salt gave an acid that was identical with the natural acid except that it rotated polarised light in the opposite direction. These results led Pasteur to the realisation that its crystals were enantiomorphous and the molecules of the two substances in racemic acid must be chiral, due to some 3-dimensional feature of their molecular structure, and that they are mirror-image (i. e., enantiomeric) molecules. This was the discovery of molecular chirality - the year was 1848 and Pasteur had not yet turned 26 years old. The discovery also opened the road toward an appreciation and development of drug chirality.

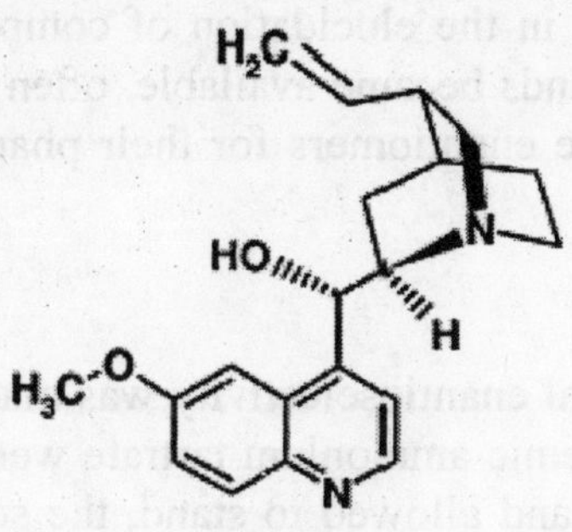

18

The first steps on that road were taken by Pasteur himself. In the early 1850s he went on to study many chiral compounds, among them quinine, quinidine 18, etc. He recognised that these molecules were chiral and that the substances isolated from their natural sources were unichiral, and he measured their optical rotation and described their crystal habit. Quinine was already wellknown as an antimalarial agent at the time and we may therefore consider Pasteur's description of this drug as chiral to have been the first clear recognition of molecular chirality in a therapeutic agent. Later, in a lecture in 1860 on the dissymmetry of natural products, Pasteur stated the essence of the matter: ... morphine, codéine, quinine, strychnine, brucine, ...Tous ces principes immédiats sont moléculairement dissymétriques. Clearly, Pasteur was the first to appreciate that certain drug molecules are chiral.

From the chirality standpoint the next fundamental development occurred in 1874, when the tetrahedral carbon atom was proposed as a basis for molecular chirality by the Dutch and French chemists Jacobus Henricus van't Hoff (1852-1911) and Joseph Achille LeBel (1847-1930), respectively, independently and almost simultaneously. The discovery of the "asymmetric carbon atom" finally provided the explanation for the existence of "optical isomers" and for the chiral nature of the molecules of optically active substances, including many drugs. In his original 1874 pamphlet proposing the tetrahedron van't Hoff listed camphor as a chiral molecule, but the structure he gave was incorrect.

C_3H_7

O

CH_3

19

Advances in organic chemistry during the second half of the 19th century began the era of the elucidation of the structures of organic molecules, including many chiral molecules. By the early 1880s the 2-dimensional structures of many relatively simple organic compounds were elucidated, but the structures of more complex molecules were not known. By the end of the 19th century, despite limitations in the elucidation of complex organic structures, many chiral pharmacologically active compounds became available, often in both enantiomeric forms. This in turn led to studies comparing the enantiomers for their pharmacological actions and biological fate.

Enantioselectivity

The first observation of biological enantioselectivity was made by Pasteur himself. He found, in 1858, that when solutions of racemic ammonium tartrate were fortified with "organic matter" (i. e., a source of microorganisms) and allowed to stand, the solution "fermented" and (+)-tartaric acid was consumed rapidly while (-)-tartaric acid was left behind unreacted. Eventually the (-)-

enantiomer was also metabolised, but considerably more slowly than (+)-tartrate. In later experiments Pasteur showed that the common mold Penicillium glaucum metabolised (+)-tartaric acid with high enantioselectivity. He correctly theorised that the enantioselective destruction of tartaric acid by microorganisms involves selective interaction of the tartrate enantiomers with a key chiral molecule within the microorganism.

21

Towards the end of the 19th century the role of chirality in biological activity began to receive serious attention. Two lines of investigation were pursued: one focused on the metabolic fate of chiral compounds while the other examined their pharmacological activity. The first report of enantioselectivity in what may be considered a pharmacological effect appeared in 1886, when (+)-asparagine was found to have a sweet taste while (-)-asparagine was without taste. Pasteur, aware of the finding, interpreted the results as an indication of the presence of a unichiral compound in the nervous system of taste, suggesting that the interactions of the asparagine enantiomers with the chiral biological mediator were different.

During the period from the mid-1880s to the mid-1920s many studies comparing the enantiomers of pharmacologically active compounds were carried out, and many examples of enantioselective pharmacological effects were ob-served. As an example, (-)-hyoscyamine 16 was found to be ca. 12-20 times more potent than the dextro enantiomer in a variety of pharmacological effects, e. g., mydriasis in the cat, salivary secretion in the dog, and at cardiac myoneural junctions. Interestingly, (+)-hyoscyamine was the more potent enantiomer in CNSexcitatory effects.

By the 1890s stereoselective action by enzymes on substrates was known, in large measure as a result of the monumental work of the great German chemist Emil Fischer (1852-1919) on sugars which spanned the period 1884-1907. Fischer first demonstrated that microbial fermentation of sugars displayed considerable enantioselectivity. Later Fischer extended these studies to the action of enzymes isolated from the microorganisms, and, here too, profound enantioselectivity was found in the reaction of sugars. From his structural and stereochemical studies of sugars as enzyme substrates Fischer concluded that overall shape and stereochemical configuration strongly influence the suitability of a molecule to serve as substrate for an enzyme. He condensed these spatial requirements in the statement that for an enzyme to act on a substrate the two must fit like a lock and its key.

It was against this background that a variety of in vitro investigations of enantioselectivity in the metabolism of a variety of chiral compounds were undertaken in the late 1800s and early 1900s. Enantioselective enzymatic reactions were shown in vitro for many physiological compounds, e. g., amino acids, peptides, lactic acid, etc., but some foreign compounds were also studied. For example, it was found that racemic β-(α-naphthyl)alanine 20 was enantioselectively metabolised by bacteria, the levo enantiomer being consumed while the dextro enantioform was untouched. A complex picture of enzymatic stereoselectivity emerged from these studies: depending on the substrates and enzymes, in some cases no enantioselectivity was found while in others one of the enantiomers was selectively acted upon; moreover, in some cases the direction of enantioselectivity changed for the same substrate, depending on the enzyme.

Many in vivo studies of enantioselective metabolism were also carried out in the same period. For example, when (±)-camphor was fed to dogs or rabbits more of the levo enantiomer was converted to a glucuronyl conjugate than of the dextro enantiomer. When (±)-malic acid was injected subcutaneously into the rabbit larger amounts of (+)-malate appeared in the urine, indicating that (-)-malate (the naturally occurring form) was more extensively metabolised.

In 1926 Arthur Robertson Cushny, a Scottish pharmacologist, reviewed the studies of enantioselective pharmacology and metabolism pub-lished during the previous ca. 40 years. The review, which was the first extensive, detailed, and critical discussion of enantioselectivity in pharmacology, reveals a great deal of insight into the nature of chirality and its biological implications. Cushny also made important experimental contributions to the field and was a true pioneer of chirality in pharmacology. All in all, it is clear that early in the 20th century it was known that drug action and metabolism can be enantioselective. However, this knowledge remained largely in the academic halls of pharmacology, medicinal chemistry, and biochemistry and its broader implications for the creation of safer and more effective drugs were largely ignored until the last 20 years of the century.

By the beginning of the 20th century examination of the role of chirality in drug action and disposition had begun and enantioselectivity was found in many cases. Such studies continued at an accelerated rate during the rest of the century. In 1933 Easson and Stedman proposed a fundamental model as the basis for enantioselective drug-receptor interactions. This model was deduced from studies of the pressor effects of the enantiomers of epinephrine which showed a 300 : 1 enantioselectivity, the natural ®-(-) form being the more potent enantiomer 21. It was concluded that three groups in the molecule - the amino group, the aliphatic hydroxyl group and the electron-rich aromatic ring -interact with three complementary sites on the (chiral) receptor, and it was argued from the 3-dimensional geometry of contact between two chiral entities (the drug and the receptor) that if all three groups of one enantiomer of the drug fit three complementary sites on the receptor, the other enantiomer will not be able to interact fully or in the same manner with the same three bonding sites on the recep-tor. Thus, the binding of the two drug enantiomers to the receptor can be significantly different, which in turn may produce different biological effects by the enantiomers.

The 3-point-interaction model, originally proposed for a specific effect of epinephrine, was later broadened to explain biological enantioselectivity of chiral drugs in general, be it in drug-receptor interactions, enzyme-substrate interactions, protein binding, etc. Moreover, the 3-point-interaction model of enantioselectivity has also been used in chromatography to explain enantioselective retention arising from interactions of the chiral analyte molecules with the molecules of the chiral stationary phase or other chiral selectors.With the advances in organic chemistry in the early decades of the century the more complex drugs began to yield their chemical structures. For example, the structure of morphine was proposed in 1923; the drug was synthesized in 1952, and its absolute configuration was determined in 1955. (+)-Morphine was synthesized in 1960 and was shown to differ significantly from the natural (-)-morphine in that it lacks analgesic activity. (+)-Morphine does possess antitussive activity, albeit to a lesser extent than (-)-morphine.

The correct connectivity of the atoms of the quinine molecule was determined early in the 20th century by Rabe but without establishing the stereochemistry of the molecule. Attempts were made by several groups over subsequent decades to synthesize quinine stereoselectively, but success was not obtained until 2001, 181 years after the compound was first isolated. It should be pointed out here that the firm establishment of the absolute configuration of chiral drugs, as of other chiral molecules, by an experimental method had to await the famous experiment of 1951 in which Bijvoet et al. determined the absolute configuration of sodium rubidium tartrate using the technique of anomalous X-ray scattering. This milestone in stereochemistry opened the door to the elucidation of the absolute configuration of thousands of compounds, including many drugs.

Chirality continued to occupy pharmacologists and chemists during the remainder of the century. Enantioselectivity in the effects or disposition of chiral drugs was found in a large number of cases, for a large variety of pharmacological effects and chemical structures. To mention a few examples, in 1940 significant biological differences between the enantiomers of sex hormones, e. g., those of the steroid equilenin 22, were reported; the β-adrenergic-antagonist activity of propranolol, the first commercially successful beta blocker, was determined to be lopsidedly in the (S)-(-) enantiomer 23, and similar selectivity was found in several other, related, β-adrenergic antagonists. Examples of enantioselective toxicity were also found, e. g., levodopa (L-3,4-dihydroxyphenylalanine 24).

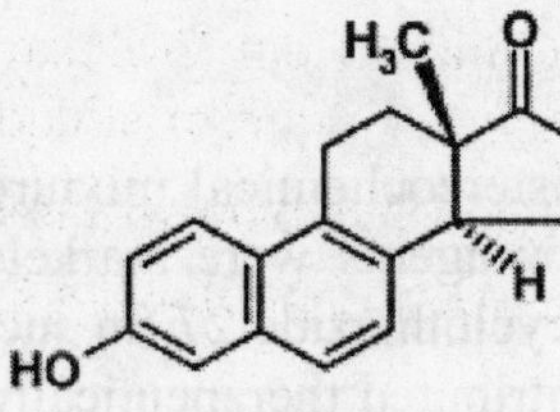

H_3C, O, H, HO — **22**; OH, NH, H_3C, CH_3 — **23**; HO, O, OH, NH_2, HO — **24**

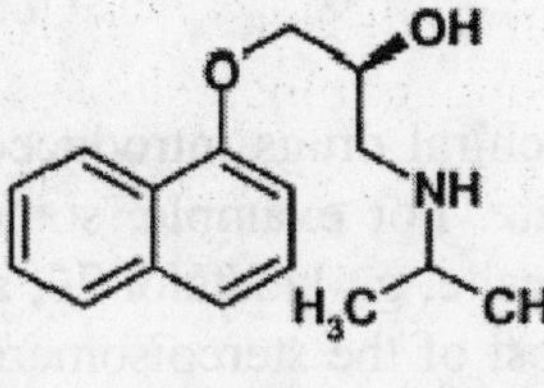

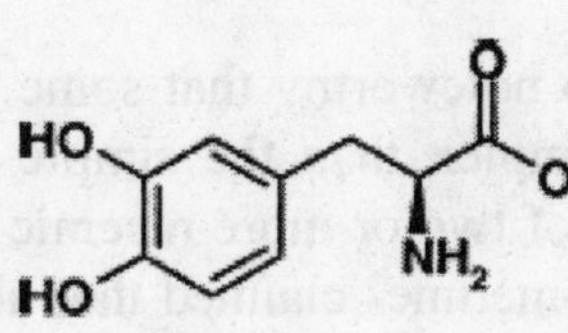

Initial clinical trials in the 1960s of this breakthrough treatment for Parkinson's disease used the racemic mixture but it quickly became clear that unacceptable toxicity was present in the D-enantiomer, and the drug was therefore developed in the unichiral, L, form. By the 1970s a large body of information had accumulated on the role of chirality in drug action and metabolism, and many reviews and monographs on the subject appeared during the last ca. 30 years of the century, for example.

In 1973 a seminal review of stereoselectivity in drug biotransformations and metabolism was published by Jenner and Testa.Modern pharmacotherapy came of age during the 20th century. Many new pharmacologically active natural products were isolated and identified, thousands of new compounds (many of them chiral) were synthesized and examined for pharmacological effects and therapeutic potential, and a large number of new drugs were introduced into the armamentarium of the physician. As mentioned above, by 1987 ca. 55% of all clinically used drugs were based on chiral molecules.

Many of the new chiral drugs introduced were natural products or semisynthetic derivatives thereof and, as Ariens and Wuis pointed out, a vast majority, ca. 98%, of such drugs were introduced in unichiral form. Atropine was one of the few exceptions. As the racemised derivative of the naturally occurring (-)-hyoscyamine, atropine may be considered a semisynthetic agent and may have been the first synthetic racemic drug introduced into medical practice. The drug was first isolated in 1833, its pharmacological properties studied in the 1880s, and the compound was synthesized in 1901.

With time, entirely synthetic chiral drugs began to form a major segment of the new therapeutic agents. This trend began slowly early in the century, but by the 1950s the number of such drugs was increasing rapidly. The vast majority of synthetic chiral drugs introduced by 1987, ca. 88%, were racemic, and by the late 1980s roughly a quarter of the drugs on the market were chiral and racemic. Among the earliest entirely synthetic racemic drugs were several anticonvulsant or sedative barbituric-acid derivatives, e. g., pentobarbital 25, for which a preparation patent was issued in 1916.

O CH$_3$ HN n-C$_3$H$_7$ O N O CH$_3$ H

25

It is also noteworthy that some of the chiral drugs introduced as stereochemical mixtures were more complex than the simple racemate. For example, some new agents were marketed as a mixture of two or more racemic mixtures, e. g., labetalol 26, and cyclothiazide 27. In such cases it was sometimes claimed that all or most of the stereoisomers contributed therapeutically useful activity, but it is difficult to avoid the conclusion that synthetic considerations and their cost implications weighed heavily in the decision to market the complex mixture. A few other chiral drugs were mixtures of epimers, resulting either from the stereochemical instability of a chiral center within the molecule, e. g., carbenicillin 28 or from nonstereoselective synthesis, e. g., the prodrug cefpodoxime proxetil.

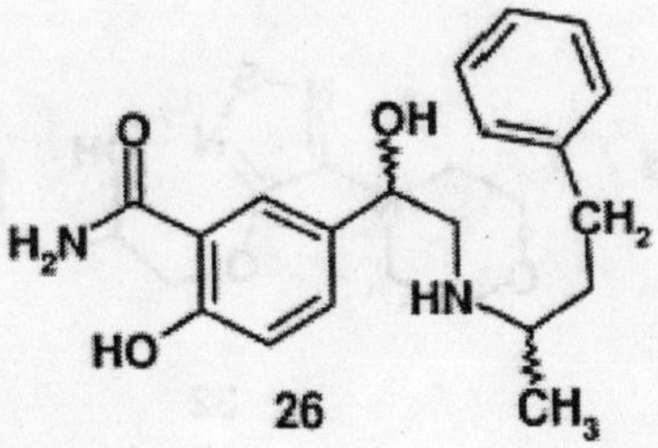

Overall, then, a vast majority of synthetic chiral drugs were introduced during the 20th century in racemic (or, in a few cases, in other stereoisomeric mixture) form, as discussed above. It is relevant in this regard that the clinical use of some racemic drugs was stopped or severely curtailed due to toxicity that became evident only after introduction of the drug on the market, e. g., the antiarrhythmic agent tocainide 29 and the analgesic and anti-inflamniatory drug benoxaprofen 30. One may wonder whether in such cases the adverse effects in question may be enantioselective, i. e., whether a unichiral version (that excludes the more toxic enantiomer) would have been a safer drug.

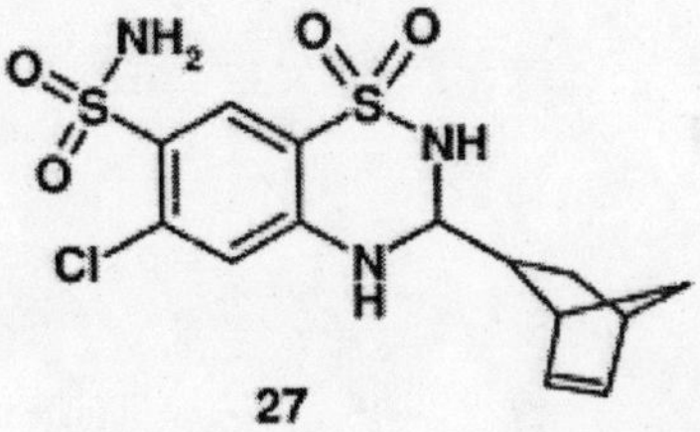

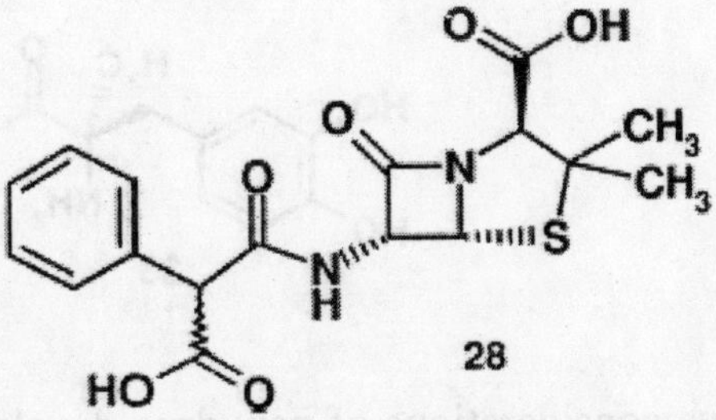

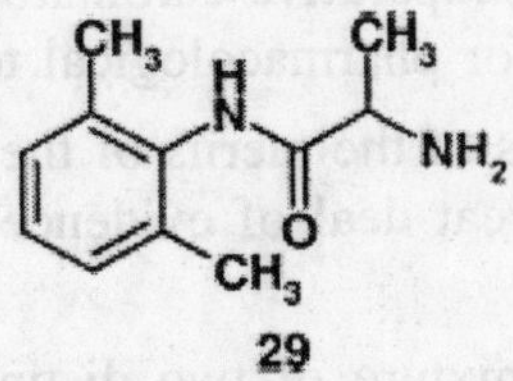

It should be noted, however, that despite the general preference for the marketing of synthetic chiral therapeutic agents in racemic form, a few synthetic chiral drugs were introduced in a unichiral form. Such exceptions included the abovementioned levodopa and also d-penicillamine 31, (-)-timolol 32, methyldopa 33, etc, and it is clear that in most such cases the choice of developing a unichiral form was dictated by overt serious toxicity present predominantly in the other enantiomer.

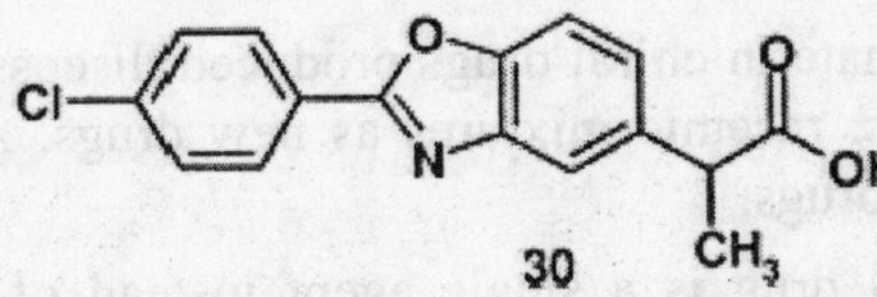

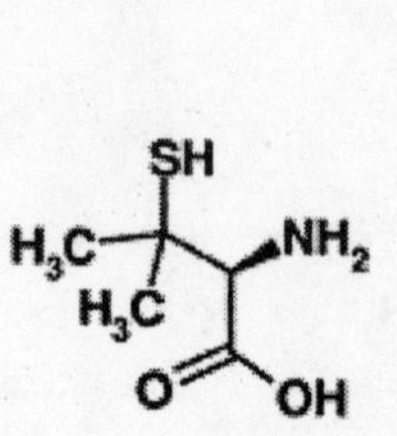

31 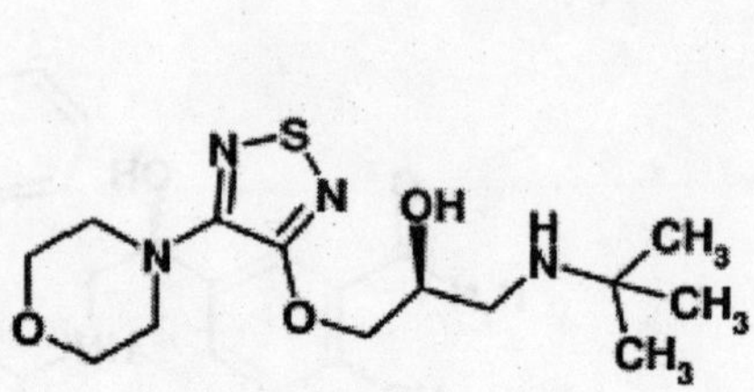 32

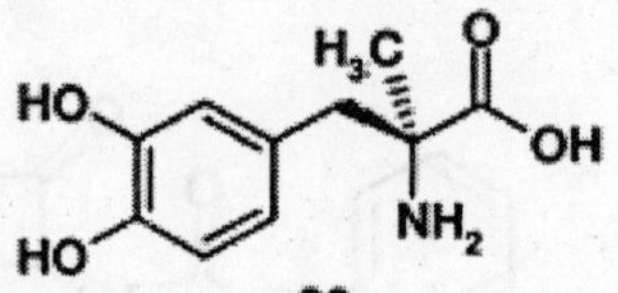

33

From the above considerations of new-drug development in the 20th century a clear conclusion can be drawn: during most of the century pharmaceutical firms did not make an effort to study the role of chirality in new-drug candidates and did not have a great deal of interest in developing unichiral drugs if nature did not provide them. This lack of interest in chirality from the industry may have been the result of a lack of interest in chirality from governmental drug-regulatory agencies. For example, until 1987 the FDA did not explicitly require the inclusion of information on the enantiomer composition of chiral substances in new-drug applications.

A broad and serious examination of the role of chirality in new-drug development only began during the 1980s. The driving force behind this change in attitudes must be ascribed to the advent of enantioselective analytical methods capable of selectively detecting and measuring the individual enantiomers in the presence of each other; to the development of powerful new methods for the synthesis of unichiral compounds, and to preparative chromatographic methods for the separation of drug enantiomers on a useful scale for pharmacological testing.

The new climate in chiral drugs produced discussions of the merits of the development of unichiral agents vs. racemic mixtures as new drugs. A great deal of evidence accumulated in favor of unichiral drugs.

The unichiral drug is a single agent instead of a mixture of two distinct drugs, which simplifies the interpretation of the basic pharmacology, therapeutic and toxic effects, pharmacokinetic properties, and the relationship of plasma concentrations to effects. Other advantages may include reduced dosage, reduced drug interactions, and reduced toxicity.

This, however, is a complex matter and each drug must be judged on its own merits; indeed, the preference for unichiral drugs is not absolute, and in several cases a unichiral form proved to be less safe than the racemic (or some other) mixture of stereoisomers, e. g., fluoxetine 34, labetalol 26, and sotalol 35.

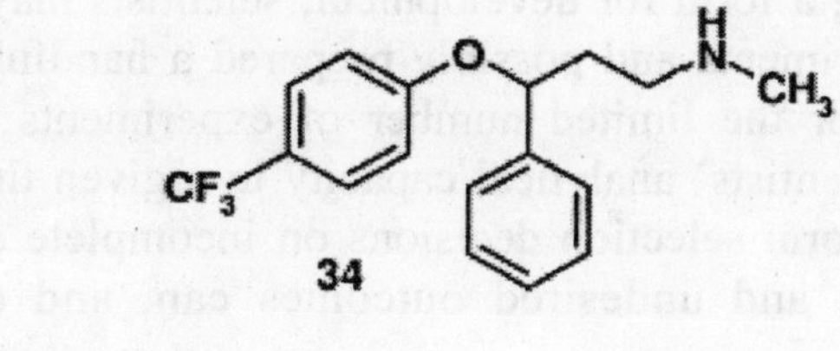

The explanation for this phenomenon may be a direct pharmacodynamic or pharmacokinetic competition/interaction between the stereoisomers which results in the prevention by one stereoisomer of toxicity by another (as is likely to be the case for labetalol), or a specific protective effect provided by one of the enantiomers in the racemic mixture (as in the case of sotalol). About 25 years ago a novel concept in this regard was introduced by Tobert et al. on the basis of their studies of the diuretic and uricosuric agent indacrinone 36: the non-racemic mixture of the enantiomers as an optimised drug. The optimum therapeutic effects for indacrinone were obtained with the 4 : 1 S/R mixture of the enantiomers. The broad applicability of this concept remains to be determined.

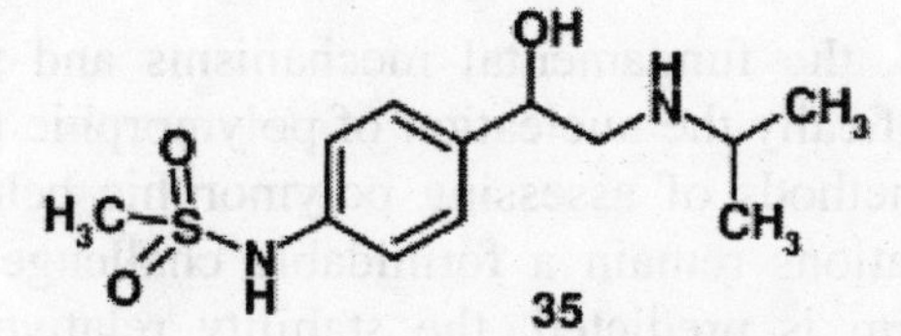

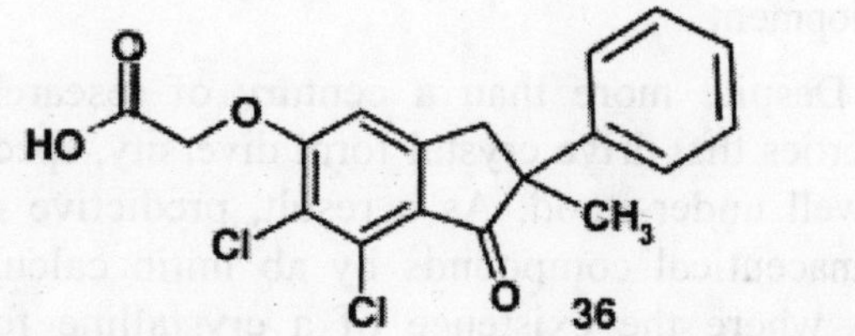

Chemical Properties of Pharmaceutical Solids

Solid form discovery and design depends on the nature of the molecule of interest and type of physical property challenges faced in its development. The preferred solid form is generally the thermodynamically most stable crystalline form of the compound. However, the stable crystal form of the parent compound may exhibit inadequate solubility or dissolution rate resulting in poor oral absorption, particularly for water-insoluble compounds. In this case, alternative solid forms may be investigated. For ionisable compounds, preparation of salt forms using pharmaceutically acceptable acids and bases is a common strategy to improve bioavailability. Like the parent compound, pharmaceutical salts may exist in several polymorphic, solvated and/ or hydrated forms. Most APIs and their salts are purified and isolated by crystallisation from an appropriate solvent during the final step in the synthetic process. A large number of factors can influence crystal nucleation and growth during this process, including the composition of the crystallisation medium and the process(es) used to generate supersaturation and promote crystallisation.

Most often a combination of solvent recrystallisation (cooling or evaporative, as well as slurry conversion) and thermal analysis (e.g., hot stage microscopy, differential scanning calorimetry) are employed for initial form screening. Such methods are inherently slow and only allow exploration of a small fraction of the composition and process space that can contribute to form diversity. Before suggesting a form for development, scientists may have carried out only a few dozen crystallisation experiments and possibly prepared a handful of different salts of a compound. The main reasons for the limited number of experiments are the constraints on availability of compound and scientists' analytical capacity in a given time frame, and they are therefore often forced to make form selection decisions on incomplete data. Accordingly, it is not surprising that unexpected and undesired outcomes can, and do, occur later on in development.

Despite more than a century of research, the fundamental mechanisms and molecular properties that drive crystal form diversity, specifically the nucleation of polymorphic forms, are not well under-stood. As a result, predictive methods of assessing polymorphic behaviour of pharmaceutical compounds by ab initio calculations remain a formidable challenge. Even in cases where the existence of a crystalline form is predicted, the stability relative to other crystalline packing arrangements has been difficult to estimate with accuracy. Moreover, the prediction of packing structures for multicomponent (e.g., solvates, hydrates, co-crystals) or ionic systems is not yet possible. Due to these limitations, solid form discovery remains an experimental exercise, where manual screening methods are employed to explore form diversity of a compound.

Control over solid form throughout the drug development process is of paramount importance. Reliable preparation and preservation of the desired form of the drug substance must be demonstrated, and has become increasingly scrutinised by regulatory agencies as more sensitive and quantitative solid-state analytical methods have become available. Many strategies to influence and control the crystallisation process to produce the solid form of interest have been reported. Recent studies have also begun to uncover the role of reaction by products and other impurities in determining polymorphic outcome and crystal properties, and in fact, it has been shown that in some cases such species can stabilise metastable crystal forms. In addition, new processing methods continue to be developed to improve discovery and characterisation of new forms, including precipitation by supercritical fluid, laser induced nucleation and capillary crystallisation. However, there remains a lack of fundamental understanding of the nucleation process and the specific factors that contribute to crystallisation of diverse forms of a compound. In order to fully control the crystallisation process, the link between the physical or chemical processes that influence nucleation and crystal growth needs to be better established. It is in this area that new experimental methodologies have the potential to enable development of this knowledge base.

There is reason to believe that the already complicated landscape of pharmaceutical solid forms will become even more complex in the future. It is now increasingly appreciated that hydrogen bonded cocrystal structures between active agents and molecules other than water or solvent can be prepared. For example, co-crystals of aspirin, rac-ibuprofen and rac-flurbiprofen have been prepared by disrupting the carboxylic acid dimers using 4,4V-bipyridine. These structures are formally molecular compounds (or co-crystals) but do not involve formation of covalent bonds or charge transfer from or to the active substance. Exploration of a given compound's polymorphs, hydrates, solvates, salts, co-crystals and combinations of all of these appears intractable by conventional experimental methods, and as the number of potential methods for exploring and controlling crystal form diversity continue to expand, existing strategies will become increasingly inadequate. In an effort to understand form diversity in a more comprehensive manner, high-throughput (HT) crystallisation systems have recently been developed. This methodology uses a combinatorial approach to solid form generation, where large arrays of conditions and compositions are processed in parallel. Experiments are performed at small scale to reduce the material demand and to afford the largest number of conditions possible.

The large number of crystallisation trials performed in these experiments reflects the reality that nucleation rate has an extremely non-linear dependence on the experimental conditions, and as such, the probability of a chance occurrence of a particular form is increased by a HT approach. Supersaturation (solubility) and induction time of the various possible solid forms are independently controlled by these conditions, resulting in highly non-linear time dependence of crystallisation. In addition, the combinatorial approach permits exploration of a chemical continuum, where use of many solvent mixtures may allow one to assess what underlying physical or chemical processes are required to produce a particular solid form. Once a variety of conditions that can be used to produce a given crystal form on the microscale are identified in the HT screen, scale-up studies are typically conducted to optimise the process for laboratory scale production.

HT Crystallisation Systems in Drug Design

HT crystallisation systems have been developed to more rapidly and comprehensively explore the multiparameter space that contributes to solid form diversity. In its simplest description, HT crystallisation can be broken down into three key experimental steps: design of experiment (DOE), execution of experimental protocols and analysis of data. Systems designed to carry out these experiments generally consist of both hardware and software components that drive and track experimentation, and permit data storage, retrieval and analysis. Such systems should be designed to be flexible and scalable to ensure that a variety of experimental procedures can be carried out either serially or concurrently. Thus, the system can be employed at various stages of drug development, where differences exist in the quality and quantity of compound available. While it is highly desirable to have the ability to mine and model experimental data, and to use the subsequent knowledge to guide further experiments, not all HT crystallisation systems are equipped with these features.

While the concepts of HT screening are widely applied in the pharmaceutical industry, most notably in the drug discovery arena, the application of HT approaches to drug development, in particular solid form screening, are just beginning to be realised. These latter approaches, however, are more akin to HT experimentation than HT screening. Hence, several important distinctions, which reflect on the design of HT experimental systems, need to be made. First, the goal of HT screening is to get a small number of successful outcomes, which are then passed on to the next stage of development. Little effort is typically made to learn why certain outcomes were positive and why others were negative. In contrast, HT experimentation, such as HT crystallisation, is carried out with the goal of having each point in the experiment produce multiple types of data that can be interpreted, and the interpretation used to guide the experimental process to a successful conclusion. Second, unlike traditional HT screening assays where experiments are generally conducted under constant experimental conditions, HT crystallisation experiments for solid form discovery are best conducted using a variety of process methods, each having varying experimental conditions (e.g., temperature variations as a function of time) over the course of the experiment. These additional process variables permit maximal diversity in the experimental space, increasing the likelihood that comprehensive coverage will be achieved. Finally, there is a distinction to be made in terms of relative "hit rates". In both HT screening and HT crystallisation, a "hit" can be thought of as a set of conditions that gives rise to a desired result.

In HT screening, the desired result is typically an activity, or potency, that exceeds a predefined threshold. In HT crystallisation, a hit is defined as the formation of a solid. The typical observed hit rate of HT screening is on the order of 0.1% of the total number of samples analysed. In contrast, HT crystallisation experiments can yield hit rates ranging from tens of percents to nearly 100%, depending on the type of experiment and the process mode(s) used. For example, while only a handful of compounds from a selection of thousands may exhibit the required potency, 10–50% of crystallisation trials may yield solids. In fact, the range of wells that yield solids is very wide, depending on process mode and experimental time scale. The impact of these differences is manifested in the design and operational requirements of HT experimentation systems.

A fully integrated HT crystallisation system consists of a number of components, including experimental design and execution software, robotic dispensing and handling hardware, automated highspeed micro-analytical tools, end-to-end sample tracking and integrated cheminformatics analysis software for data visualisation, modelling and mining. A schematic overview detailing the workflow of such a system is depicted in. These features are supported by a comprehensive informatics foundation that is used to handle the large quantities of data generated. Specifically, informatics tools are used to design statistically relevant and diverse experiments, drive the automation hardware to perform the specified operations, and provide an analytical function to analyse, compare and sort the results of experiments. An important feature of these systems is the ability to mine and model experimental data and use the knowledge generated to guide further experiments. These functions are supported by use of a relational database that provides a mechanism of communication between system components.

When designing a HT crystallisation experiment, or set of experiments, a large variety of parameters of composition and process are involved. Experimental designs must be aimed at covering a large multifactorial parameter space, with the goal of determining which experimental factors affect the desired outcome. In practice, it is desirable to place constraints on the experimental space, making common statistical design methods such as full or partial factorial designs inappropriate or impractical.

Doptimal design is an example of a DOE algorithm that can take a set of constraints, such as the ones described above, in combination with a target analytical model and determine the optimal set of experimental points to test. Another commonly used DOE algorithm is diversity generation, with which the experimentalist selects a set of pertinent chemical properties and uses the algorithm to evenly spread experimental points over the chosen property space. In addition, some systems utilise a solubility calculator tool to estimate the solubility of the API in the given solvent/additive mixture. The calculated information is then used to select the appropriate concentration of API in each mixture so that it is supersaturated with respect to the reference phase at the harvest temperature. Here, the driving force for crystallisation can also be varied by tailoring the composition of each sample based on the API solubility in that mixture.

Ideally, DOE algorithms should also incorporate prior knowledge or experimental results, which have been stored in a database as a set of rules or models, to limit an experimental space to have certain predicted characteristics. For example, over the course of time, a regression model may be developed between a set of known or calculated chemical properties and a parameter of experimental interest. The model could be used during the design of a new experiment in order to test only those chemicals that are predicted to give a desirable result. Since a large number of factors need to be considered during experimental design, the DOE interface available to the scientist must not only be flexible and easy to use, but must also offer tools that aid design efficiency and effectiveness and permit input of scientific knowledge generated over time.

At the end of the experimental design process, the resulting set of experimental conditions is translated into a series of commands for the HT systems, and stored in a relational database for later retrieval by the software that controls the automation. When an experiment is activated, the overall operation of the automation systems is managed by the HT informatics system, which is responsible for physical operation of the HT platforms as well as data tracking and storage.

Execution of experimental commands is carried out by automated laboratory equipment that comprises the HT crystallisation system. Specialised automated systems perform several of the functions in a sequence of events that make up the experiment. Each station is controlled through an interface to the informatics system that ensures the samples are processed at the correct stations, in the correct order, with the selected experimental parameters being followed. Parameters of operation are recorded, including the time at which an action is taken. After execution of the experimental steps, the software interface retrieves any pertinent information generated by the automated platform, such as assay results or operational parameters, stores these data in the relational database, and updates the status of the experiment to reflect the completion of operations.

In general, the hardware required for a HT crystallisation system is comprised of four major functional elements: sample preparation, solids generation, solids detection and sample analysis. Sample preparation involves adding the compound of interest (API) to the diverse set of conditions used to conduct crystallisation studies. Typically, the API is dispensed as a solution in a suitable solvent, followed by solvent removal to yield the solid API. Solvent removal can be achieved by passive evaporation or by controlled active evaporation (e.g., use of a vortex dryer). Alternatively, the API can be delivered in the solid state with suitable powder handling systems. Depending on the amount of saturation desired, the crystallisation vessel used, and the

API's solubility in solvents or solvent mixtures of interest, API masses ranging from a few hundreds of micrograms to several milligrams will be present in each vessel. Once the API has been delivered to the crystallisation vessels (tubes, vials or microwell plates), combinations of solvents and/or additives are added to each vessel. By taking advantage of the power of combinatorial approaches, large numbers of unique combinations can be dispensed from manageable sets of starting materials.

Compatibility of equipment components (syringes, dispense tips, tubing, etc.) and consumables (plates, tubes, etc.) with solvents and other compounds is a key hurdle faced in the development of combinatorial crystallisation for small molecules. Unlike protein crystallisation systems, which are commonly based on the sitting-drop method in aqueous media, small molecule crystallisation employs a range of crystallisation additives and processes.

The additives include organic solvents with varying properties, water, acids, bases and co-crystal formers, as well as other compounds. This wide range of materials needs to be handled by appropriate liquid handling techniques to enable the combinatorial assembly previously mentioned. Ideally, liquid transfers are achieved using multichannel pipettors with individually controllable channels. Depending on the crystallisation vessel design, the volumes of reagents dispensed will be as low as a few microliters to as high as several hundred microliters.

Potential for cross-contamination and tendency toward unwanted solvent evaporation from crystallisation wells are challenges that need to be addressed in a HT crystallisation system. A large number of the solvents used to crystallise small molecules have high vapor pressure under ordinary laboratory conditions. Sealing of the crystallisation vessels is key to being able to control composition during crystallisation from these solvents. Due to solvent fugacity, vessels need to be protected from ingress of the components of neighboring wells. These problems have been solved by different means, such as sealing of individual tubes with a Teflon-backed crimp seal or Orings/ gasket seals and clamped covers.

HT crystallisation must enable several process modes that are compatible with the compound. In some cases, multiple modes of operation may be combined. Less common process modes include melt crystallisation, flash or quench cooling and template-directed crystallisation. It is important to note that generation of maximal diversity in solid form requires multiple modes of operation. In thermally induced cooling crystallisation, samples created in the sample preparation process described above are subjected to temperature ramps. Prior to beginning the temperature ramp, samples are exposed to an elevated temperature for a short period of time in order to dissolve the API in the crystallisation medium. Although dissolution can be achieved most simply by diffusion and convection from the heating process, addition of external energy can speed up the process (e.g., sonication). Samples may be optically inspected and vessels that contain undissolved solids can be flagged in the database for further analysis. For instance, undissolved samples may be treated as slurry conversion experiments and monitored over time for crystal form changes. The thermal cycle is then initiated, using controlled cooling to induce supersaturation. In this mode of crystallisation, samples continually experience an under cooling and, based on the level of supersaturation in the vessel, may recrystallise at a given temperature after a period of time. Thermal crystallisation tends to generate a cumulative number of samples that are produced over time in a fashion approximating a square root function. This means that initially there is a small bolus of "hits", after which the rate of crystallisation tails off over a period of time, typically in days to weeks. This results in a manageable hit rate for analysis, on the order of approximately 10% in aggregate. This mode of solids generation has the lowest throughput rate, typically, because experiments span days to weeks, with system residence times of months being possible.

In contrast, anti-solvent addition, also known as "crash-out" (or "drown out") crystallisation, relies on the fact that an API is soluble to varying degrees in the crystallisation medium, but is largely insoluble in a particular solvent or solvents (e.g., the anti-solvent). As a result, this mode of crystallisation can operate at high-throughput rates, with samples being turned around hourly. When crystallisation vessels containing API in reagent mixtures are exposed to aliquots of anti-solvent, nearly all vessels will contain API that has precipitated out of solution. This creates a challenge to the analytical process, as the near 100% hit rate leads to a large bolus of samples. There are, however, advantages to this mode of solids generation, such as the ability to produce microfine crystallites and amorphous solids, should they be desired.

Lastly, evaporative crystallisation can be carried out on the combinatorial array of samples. This mode of operation relies on gradually increasing the concentration of API in the vessel to achieve supersaturation and to increase the degree of supersaturation (by preferential evaporation) in order to induce crystallisation. Concentration of samples can be achieved either passively or actively by controlled flow of inert gas while maintaining temperature. With evaporative methods, differential rates of solvent loss from mixtures result in unknown composition of the crystallisation medium at the time of crystal nucleation. In addition, the degree of supersaturation changes over the course of the experiment, often resulting in the appearance of multiple crystal forms. The evaporative mode of solids generation typically produces throughput and hit rates intermediate between the thermal and anti-solvent processes.

In appropriately configured HT crystallisation systems, several process modes may be used in series or in parallel. Frequently, the preparation of replicate plates (in some systems "daughter" plates) is necessary for parallel processing by different process modes. Systems may be additionally equipped with the ability to serially process sample arrays using different process modes. This feature is particularly attractive for cases where only small quantities of sample are available, increasing the drive to generate useful information from every sample. Here, samples may be processed by optimal modes first (e.g., thermal crystallisation), then a secondary process step can be applied to maximise the hit rate.

In general, the percentage of wells that yield solids varies, depending on process mode and experimental time scale. For example, evaporative modes usually result in a solid in virtually every vessel, while slow undercooling results in far fewer (on the order of low percents). The differences in hit rates between these process methods arise in part from the differences in the supersaturation attained. For evaporative crystallisation, supersaturation is achieved in all cases as the concentration of the active compound is continuously increased as solvent is evaporated. In contrast, the composition of wells processed by thermal crystallisation is fixed. In some cases, because there is limited data on the precise state of supersaturation for each of the large variety of experimental compositions and potential crystal forms, some wells may remain subsaturated during the process.

For these wells, additional process steps, such as partial evaporation or anti-solvent addition, may be employed to generate supersaturation to yield a solid. In contrast, a fraction of the wells may not go fully into solution at elevated temperatures. In this case, the temperature of the system may be raised to achieve full dissolution, additional solvent may be added to solubilise residual solids or the samples may simply be monitored for slurry conversion over time. Sherry L. Morissette, *et.al*, of TransForm Pharmaceuticals, Inc., 29 Hartwell Avenue, Lexington, conducted a study to address these issues and opportunities. They developed a solubility calculator tool using group contribution theory to estimate the solubility of the reference solid phase at specified temperatures in each solvent composition. These data are then used at the DOE step to define the viable concentrations of the active compound for crystallisation (i.e., minimum concentration required to achieve saturation and maximum solubility limit or concentration) in each solvent mixture. Additionally, the timescale of the experiment has a significant impact on the observed hit rate.

Hit rates will approach 100% for viable crystallisation conditions in the limit of infinite time, but in practice most experiments are conducted over days to weeks, so observed hit rates reflect this temporal influence. In fact, similar behaviour is observed in manual experimentation. Only some HT crystallisation systems are configured to permit selective sampling .of "hits", providing the ability to further incubate un-crystallised samples to monitor for slow growing crystal forms. Solids detection can be achieved by examining each sample using machine vision systems. Samples may be monitored over time to detect precipitation in vessels that were previously devoid of solids. This simple, yet robust process can rapidly and non-destructively determine state changes in the crystallisation vessels and signal when a particular vessel or set of vessels is ready for solid-state analysis.

Depending on the sample array configuration, the signaling of "hits" results in harvesting of samples by one of two approaches. In the "cherry-picking" approach, only those samples that have been flagged as containing solids are selected for further processing. In contrast, using a sacrificial approach the entire plate must be moved forward after a predetermined fraction of the samples in that array have produced precipitates. The latter, of course, can be carried out without an online detection system. Here, samples can be processed in batches, without regard to whether there are actually solids present in a vessel. This simple process approach is effective, but has significant limitations, the primary of which being that samples are destroyed after a fixed amount of time regardless of their state. Hence, it is advantageous to employ an online detection and harvest system so that samples can be differentially and asynchronously processed, with only those vessels containing solids undergoing analysis.

Sample analysis is the final action in execution of the HTcrystallisation process. Depending on the mode of operation and the choice of analytical measurements employed, this process may involve several steps. Most HT crystallisation systems use Raman spectroscopy and/or powder X-ray diffraction (PXRD) for primary analysis of harvested solid-state samples. Both techniques have advantages and disadvantages in terms of their ability to discriminate between forms of a solid (i.e., polymorphs, salt forms, solvates, hydrates). The rate of generation of samples for analysis likely dictates which technique is used for the primary approach. Generally speaking, Raman spectroscopy can be employed in a more rapid fashion than PXRD, since acquisition times for Raman are considerably less dependent on sample size. In addition, plate-based PXRD methods are susceptible to problems with preferred orientation effects, which may prevent accurate classification of samples. As a result, Raman spectroscopy methods are often used as a primary means of characterisation in HT crystallisation systems. Although one disadvantage of the Raman technique is interference due to fluorescent samples, the wavelength of the excitation laser can be changed to the near-IR to reduce fluorescence of problematic samples. Recent advances in PXRD instrumentation, brought on by the increasing demands of HT crystallisation, make it possible to achieve similar analysis timescales with PXRD and Raman, on the order of less than one minute per sample depending on the capabilities of particular instruments used.

Once the primary solid-state characterisation data are collected and stored, samples are generally classified into groups (or bins) that display similar characteristics (e.g., Raman spectra or powder X-ray diffraction patterns) using informatics tools. Avariety of methods can be used to accomplish the binning. For instance, Raman spectra may be compared (based on relevant features or over the entire spectral range) and clustered using calculated similarity measures, such as Tanimoto coefficients. In one method, each Raman spectrum, which represents the contents of an individual well at a given time, is filtered to remove background and to accentuate Raman peaks and shoulders.

Peaks are then located and assigned a wave number using standard derivative methods and the amplitude of each peak is calculated. These data are used to calculate a similarity (or distance) measure related to the Tanimoto coefficient, from which the Raman spectra are binned into groups of similar samples using a classification algorithm such as hierarchical clustering. This method often uses peak positions, rather than amplitudes to discriminate between different patterns in order to reduce the significance of potential preferred orientation effects, which can result in modulation of relative peak intensity for certain crystallographic planes.

The window over which two peaks are considered to be at the same position (e.g., 1 cm^{-1} wave number), as well as a minimum height for a filtered peak to be considered for clustering, can be selected by the user, allowing regions of interest (e.g., spectral ranges) to be explored in greater detail. With appropriate settings, a Raman spectrum that has only one peak or feature in a slightly different location than observed in other patterns can be differentiated and binned as unique, indicating a different or new crystal form. During clustering, each spectrum is assigned an arbitrary number, i.e., a sorted spectrum number, for ease of tracking, and the resultant clusters are graphed , where the red-colored regions repre-sent bins of similar samples.

Alternatively, the results from several analytical methods such as Raman and PXRD can be used to simultaneously classify samples. Regardless of the choice of primary analytical method, and in keeping with traditional methodologies for solid form screening, it is necessary to further characterise the solids generated in HT crystallisation systems to accurately determine their solid form and properties. Most HT systems integrate multiple analytical methods as part of the screening process. These so-called secondary analytical methods often include thermal property measurement (e.g., melting point) and optical microscopy (for crystallinity, habit, etc.).

Depending on how the samples are processed and the degree of computerised support, these techniques may be applied to all samples, or a subset of selected samples. For systems that analyse all samples by secondary techniques, several HT plate-based methods for optical microscopy and melting point determination have been developed. It is important to note that, in this case, all samples are destroyed during characterisation of the melting point. When replicates are retained, the functional properties such as dissolution rate and hygroscopicity can be analysed using either manual or HT methods.

With the aid of informatics tools, the data sets obtained can be used to generate information about the experimental space. Software interfaces that allow access to the data permit classification and regression analysis to be performed. The results are displayed in high-dimensional visualisation tools that can be used to guide further experiments toward optimising processes to make each form. For instance, sample composition and processing information can be linked to the resulting crystal form and morphology. Correlation of trends between experimental factors and the products can lead to hypotheses that can be used to direct the design of follow-up experiments.

While these new methodologies provide unprecedented capabilities for solids form discovery, it is clear that there remains a need for some level of manual processing, particularly in the case of detailed form characterisation such as single crystal structure determination, scale-up of the desired form and understanding the effects of downstream processing on potential form conversion. HT methods provide the landscape of possible forms and their properties and should be used in conjunction with traditional methods to enable rapid, efficient selection of the optimal form for development.

HT technologies offer unprecedented capabilities for form discovery and characterisation. Potential applications range across the entire pharmaceutical value chain, including screening of active molecules in discovery during ELO, form selection for preclinical candidates, final form optimisation for early clinical candidates, process chemistry development of crystallisation processes for bulk drug and intermediates, as well as identification of new or enabling solid forms for product life cycle management. While numerous impact points have been identified, only limited information on the use and performance of HT form screening systems is available in the literature, indicating that the benefits of these new methodologies have just begun to be realised.

Salt Form Preparation

Preparation of salt forms of an active compound is commonly used to modulate physicochemical properties. In most cases, the goal is to increase solubility (or dissolution rate) to improve bioavailability or to enhance the manufacturability of poorly soluble ionisable compounds. Salts may also be employed to increase chemical stability or to reduce the solubility of a given compound for certain applications (e.g., sustained release dosage forms). Thus, it is important to consider the route of administration and dosage form requirements when selecting a salt form for development. Since the choice of counter-ion affects the properties of salt forms, salt selection studies involve the preparation of a number of different salts using a variety of pharmaceutically acceptable acids or bases with differing properties.

The relevant physicochemical properties of each salt are characterised, including degree of crystallinity, hygroscopicity, aqueous solubility, crystal habit, and physical and chemical stability. Based on these properties of the salt forms, their suitability for development can be evaluated. Several strategies for streamlining and optimising salt selection procedures have been reported, including in-situ techniques for ranking the solubility of salts, tiered approaches in which the least time-consuming studies are carried out first and used to remove from consideration salts that are not viable. One issue not readily considered by existing strategies is the polymorphism and solvate forming behaviour of the different salt forms of a compound, which could be used as an additional criterion when more than one salt may be viable, but the degree of polymorphism and solvate formation of each may become a criterion for form selection.

HT crystallisation technologies have been used to more rapidly and comprehensively identify the range of salt forms that may be prepared for a given compound or series of compounds, and characterise their crystal form diversity (polymorphs, solvates, hydrates). However, only a few studies have been published or presented. Several HT salt selection studies on well characterised pharmaceutical compounds have been carried out to demonstrate the power of these technologies in solid form discovery. For example, in a small HT study (i.e., 96 wells) on the antibacterial sulfathiazole, salt formation was explored using varying stoichiometric ratios of pharmaceutically acceptable organic and mineral bases in an array of solvent conditions. The screen resulted in the rapid identification and characterisation of 10 salt forms and showed that the salts exhibited a range of melting points depending on the counter-ion type and stoichiometric ratio. Similar HT salt selection experiments on caffeine and naproxen resulted in the identification of numerous salts of each compound.

In the discovery phase, HT crystallisation has been used to identify soluble salt forms of compounds during ELO to facilitate early animal dosing, thereby providing the ability to uncover underlying chemical and/or biological responses elicited by candidate molecules, including toxicity or efflux. Such information permits rapid identification of problematic compounds or scaffolds, allowing resources to be directed to projects with greater opportunity for success. HT crystallisation can facilitate selection of leads that are more likely to survive preclinical development. HT crystallisation has been used successfully to identify multiple new salt forms and the polymorphs and solvates of each compound belonging to two discovery programmes using less than 200 mg of compound per screen.

Approximately 150–200 experiments were performed on each compound using a library of pharmaceutically acceptable acids or bases with an array of solvent compositions and process conditions. Each screen resulted in discovery of multiple new salt forms, and in some cases polymorphs and solvates. Interestingly, similar salt types were identified for each compound in a given series, where the frequency of occurrence is plotted as a function of counter-ion for each discovery series. Clear trends in the degree of solid form diversity of salt forms, including polymorphism and solvation behaviour, were also evident within each compound series.

These data indicate the potential for identifying salts suitable for most compounds tested in a particular scaffold or series, based on analysis of only a portion of the series, i.e., a platform-based approach to salt selection, provided the chemistry surrounding the ionisable functionality is not significantly altered during further structure–activity relationship (SAR) development. Furthermore, solubility measurements of each salt form in physiologically relevant fluids allowed ranking of salt forms in a given series, and comparison of salts between series was also possible. The average turnaround time per screen was approximately 2 weeks, such that feedback on the physicochemical properties of each compound was provided to the medicinal chemists on a similar time scale as potency, selectivity and metabolism screens.

Salt selection is normally part of the standard preformulation studies carried out during preclinical development, where rapid identification of the possible salts of a compound and their properties can facilitate product development. To further facilitate such studies, a microplate technique capable of investigating an array of conditions has been developed to determine which counter-ion and solvent conditions can be used to prepare crystalline salts of the compound. Each plate is prepared by first depositing approximately 0.5 mg of compound into each well using an appropriate amount of stock solution. The counter-ion type is systematically varied along the rows of the plate and different crystallisation solvents are deposited down the columns of the plate. Crystallisation is monitored by optical microscopy over the course of the evaporative crystallisation, which can be accelerated by flowing a stream of dry nitrogen over the plate.

The microplate approach was demonstrated by Bastin et al. through several examples, however little detail of the specific screening protocol and results was provided. All three of the reported examples are on compounds that are weak bases with pK_a between 4.1 and 5.3. Only a small number of stable, crystalline salts could be prepared for the two very weak bases (i.e., $pK_a < 4.25$), as opposed to the larger variety found for the stronger base. In each case, the salt forms were scaled-up for more detailed analysis and comparison to the respective free base compound to determine the optimal form for development. This approach provides a useful mechanism for preliminary, small-scale salt formation studies. Both the crystallisation media and process modes accessible by the technique are somewhat limited, resulting in a narrow exploration of experimental conditions for salt formation. For example, only solvents compatible with plate materials can be used, there by reducing the probability that a crystalline phase can be identified. In addition, current protocols only provide for evaporative crystallisation, likely due to difficulties with sealing of the plates. In this case, the composition of the crystallisation medium is not well controlled. The utility of HT crystallisation in ELO, although demonstrated by initial reports of feasibility, is less well documented than the use of HT on later stage compounds.

PHARMACEUTICAL POLYMORPHISM

The statement by the late Walter McCrone in 1965 that "the number of forms of a given molecule is proportional to the time, money and experiments spent on that compound" has gained credence in recent years, as illustrated by the significant increase in reported crystal form diversity of pharmaceutical solids. Depending on when alternative solid forms of a compound are identified, the appearance of a novel form may or may not be a welcomed discovery. Occurrence of a new form in research or early development is potentially enabling. At later stages, the appearance of new forms, particularly stable ones that are not bioequivalent or deemed unprocessable, can have catastrophic consequences for product performance as well as regulatory compliance. Additionally, recent rulings on the use of alternative, commercially viable solid forms not protected by patents from innovator companies have opened the market to generic competition. In order to mitigate these risks, and to save time and reduce costs, many pharmaceutical companies have begun to re-evaluate their strategies for solid form screening and are looking to HT crystallisation technologies to address the needs for more rapid and comprehensive exploration.

Polymorphic systems are quite common among many types of organic crystals. Compounds exhibiting more than three polymorphic forms will be classified as being "highly polymorphic". While only a handful of well-known organic compounds are considered for practical purposes to be non-polymorphic, e.g., aspirin, sucrose and naphthalene, it should be stressed that one will never be able to exclude the possibility of polymorphs appearing, even a century after the initial discovery of the compound. So far, no polymorphs of aspirin have been found, despite the proposal by Payne et al. that polymorphic forms may exist.

In contrast, acetaminophen form III was observed by Burger in 1982 using thermal microscopy, but it took another 20 years for a crystal structure to be proposed. Many reports exist on the polymorphic nature of specific drug compounds with one or two alternative packing modes for the same chemical composition. However, literature examples of compounds with more than three packing modes are considerably rarer. The increased number of reports on highly polymorphic compounds in recent years is likely the result of enhanced screening practices and more sensitive characterisation techniques.

Highly polymorphic compounds present several challenges in drug development. First, the generation of different forms is often not a simultaneous event, but rather a gradual evolution of form diversity leading to the branding of a compound as being highly polymorphic. Consequently, once more than one form is identified, concern is raised that additional forms may eventually be discovered. For instance, the 13 polymorphs of phenobarbitone evolved over ca. 13 years, and a fourth polymorph of carbamasepine was reported in 2002, a full two decades after the publication of the structures of the initial three forms. Second, selection of the preferred form of a highly polymorphic compound for development demands a complex set of thermodynamic and kinetic investigations, due to the geometric increase in the number of stability relationships that need to be established. More complexity arises when some polymorphic pairs are enantiotropic, exhibiting a switch in the identity of the stable form as a function of temperature.

Third, concerns over bio-performance and the impact of a large number of polymorphs on processing lead to regulatory issues that need to be addressed. Decision trees have been established to aid scientists in assessing the impact of polymorphic change and have been incorporated into the ICH guidelines. Lastly, the analytical challenge of monitoring polymorph content in the dosage form increases as the number of possible forms grows, particularly with low dose compounds where the concentration of drug in the formulation is small.

In general, pharmaceutical polymorphism is likely to be underreported in the literature, since much of the polymorphism research is carried out in companies. As a result of growing interest in the subject and advances in techniques to study polymorphism, it is expected that reports of extreme form diversity will grow. Conferences on the subject, such as the ACS ProSpectives symposium, reflect the appreciation for the complexities introduced by the appearance of polymorphism in important materials such as pharmaceuticals. Work has recently commenced to understand the opportunities and challenges of using HT technologies in pursuit of rapid identification and characterisation of the large number of forms presented by highly polymorphic compounds.

Form IV of carbamazepine was reportedly discovered as the result of crystallisation trials in the presence of hydroxypropyl cellulose HPC. Subsequent to this publication, Lang et al. published the use of polymers to influence polymorphic form using a 96-well plate system for the screening of polymorphs of carbamazepine and acetaminophen. In all, 84 different polymers were employed to direct nucleation. Form IV of carbamazepine was found to crystallise from methanol in the presence of hydroxypropyl cellulose, poly(4-methylpentene), poly(Rmethylstyrene) or poly (p-phenylene ether-sulfone).

Using the same approach, the monoclinic and orthorhombic forms I and II, respectively, of acetaminophen were also isolated. The strategy of employing polymeric additives is of interest, as it can direct the course of crystallisation and because polymeric impurities may be in contact with a drug substance and/or formulation at various points in development.

Another approach, reported by Anquetil et al., identified selective conditions for the crystallisation of carbamazepine polymorphs forms I and III, as well as the dihydrate, from methanol and/or methanol/water solutions by thermal processing in a microliter cell format. Optical laser trapping was used in situ to target the microcrystals for real-time form analysis using Raman spectroscopy.

The crystallisation process was monitored optically and with Raman spectroscopy as a function of temperature and time. The study revealed the conversion of form I to form III, as evidenced by a change in characteristic crystal habit from needles to prisms. Raman spectroscopy on the solution phase measured the saturation solubility of each crystal form produced. Although only several experiments were carried out in this study, the authors advance the microfluidic cell format as a potentially viable system for HT polymorph screening. A third report details the use of in situ Raman spectroscopy to optimise process conditions. The compound MK-A has four anhydrous polymorphs and several other forms, including two hydrates and numerous solvates.

The study gives an example of the complex thermodynamic relationships (monotropic and enantiotropic pairs) that can exist in highly polymorphic systems and demonstrates the power of in-situ methods for monitoring the crystallisation process. The angiotensin-II antagonist MK-996 is an example of a highly polymorphic compound. The structure of MK-996, contains seven rotatable bonds, the conformations of which could lead to many configurations for crystal packing. HT crystallisation experiments with MK-996 in 96-well arrays comprising over 1500 discrete recrystallisation trials from a set of 21 solvents or solvent mixtures yielded 186 solids, which were harvested over a period of 7 days.

PXRD analysis of these solids suggested the presence of at least 18 distinct forms, some resulting from solvent-mediated recrystallisation. A hydrate (originally named form I), obtained by slurry conversion in the presence of aqueous solvent mixtures in the HT experiments, was the form previously selected for pharmaceutical development. Importantly, a form (form D) reported by the innovator to be a "disappearing polymorph" once form I appeared, was also found in the HT screen. Clearly, sufficient experimentation with rationally selected diverse conditions affords the possibility to regenerate elusive forms.

Sertraline HCl, the active ingredient in the antidepressant ZoloftR, is found in various crystal forms. Information on various solid phases can be found in patent disclosures filed by several companies. Survey of these documents, which published between 1992 and 2001, reveals data for 27 purported crystal forms of Sertraline HCl, including 17 polymorphs, 4 solvates, 6 hydrates and the amorphous solid. Further analysis and comparison of characterisation data for the various forms presented in the patents revealed that mixtures have been mistaken for real polymorphs on at least two occasions, and at least two polymorphs were disclosed more than once (by different workers each time).

In addition, the hydrate forms reported were not readily identified as polymorphic and many of the forms are likely transient, e.g., only identified by variable-temperature and humidity-controlled XRD. With the help of HT crystallisation, the extent of true polymorphism of the HCl salt was estimated at eight forms so far. Two new solvates were also found in the HT studies. Care should be taken in isolation of such forms, particularly at small to intermediate scale, as desolvation of solvates due to aggressive drying during processing may cause one to overlook solvated forms.

Comparing the results of the HT study to the congruence of historical data, one can conclude that HT screening gives rise to relevant forms of the drug in a time frame of weeks rather than years. One metastable form, polymorph IV, remained elusive in the hands of the authors. The lack of observation of form IV may be due to a subtle purity difference between early batches at Pfizer and the materials available for testing in the HT screen. Clearly, impurity effects should be explored further. To date, HT studies on highly polymorphic materials highlight the importance of varying processing conditions to find as many forms as possible. It has been shown that multiple process modes, including HT processing, coupled with detailed follow-up characterisation studies of form stability, facilitate insight into crystal form diversity. Such a multimode strategy becomes valuable in the quest for the most comprehensive dataset possible for a given pharmaceutical material.

Very few cases of latent polymorphism have been reported in the literature. It is likely that many more instances of the phenomenon have occurred, but unless product development was slowed, product performance was impacted, or generic competition was threatened, a spotlight is not usually cast on the issue. As an example of a public polymorph issue, form 2 of ranitidine hydrochloride was discovered 2–3 years into development but it was (and is) the form still marketed by GlaxoSmithKline. Paroxetine hydrochloride hemihydrate, the active ingredient in PaxilR, was discovered during development after only an anhydrate had been known for a number of years. The hemihydrate is the form marketed by the innovator, but recent litigations have occurred between the innovator company and generic competition around the anhydrate form. One of the most recognised cases of latent polymorphism occurred with Abbott Laboratories' NorvirR. Two years after entry into the market, a previously unknown, but thermodynamically more stable, polymorph of the active ingredient (Ritonavir) appeared. This new form (form II) was approximately 50% less soluble in the hydroalcoholic formulation vehicle, resulting in poor dissolution behaviour and eventual withdrawal of the original NorvirR capsule from the market. At some considerable cost, a new formulation of NorvirR using form II was eventually developed and launched. In a recent HT crystallisation study on Ritonavir, a total of five forms were found: both known polymorphs and three previously unknown forms. The HT polymorph screen, which consisted of 2000 experiments was carried out with less than 2 g of the API and used multiple, and sometimes combined, process methods.

The three new forms were described as a metastable polymorph, a crystalline solvate and a non-stoichiometric hydrate. Interestingly, the solvate was easily converted to form I via the hydrate phase using a simple washing procedure, and provided an unusual route to prepare the form I "disappearing polymorph". Since the crystals of form I prepared using this method retained the small needle morphology of the solvate, the authors suggest that the process may offer a potential strategy for particle size and morphology control.

Crystal structure prediction is a challenging area of research. Due to the overwhelming influence of packing forces in determining crystal structure, it remains extremely difficult to predict the structural impact of subtle conformational effects and weak interactions between adjacent molecules in a crystalline arrangement. Although significant progress has been made in the last decade, crystal structures are by and large not reliably predictable from first principles. While this important area of theoretical research is too large a topic to be considered in detail here, a brief overview of the successes and challenges will be presented, and the potential for using HT crystallisation as a validation to aid model development will be highlighted. For a more detailed discussion on polymorph and crystal structure prediction.

Polymorph prediction of pharmaceuticals is thwared by the complexity of active pharmaceutical molecules. The number of degrees of freedom in torsion angles and the molecule count in the unit cell (which can be deduced by such techniques as solid-state NMR) are frequently too great to allow computations on a reasonable time scale. Additionally, predictions are typically carried out one space group at a time. This limitation is mitigated by the fact that over 90% of the organic compounds in the Cambridge Structural Database (CSD) crystallise in only a few space groups.

The prevalence of multicomponents systems, some of which have charge transfer (salts) and many of which exist as hydrates, solvates or mixed hydrate/solvates, essentially limits the usefulness of the prediction methods to neutral compounds. Various other technical issues remain as the science of crystal structure prediction matures. Some of these issues were highlighted in two blind tests that were conducted in recent years to determine the accuracy and robustness of crystal structure prediction. In the latest round, 17 methods were used to predict structure, yielding only three correct predictions. For one of the compounds used in the study, experimental characterisation of a second, more stable, polymorph provided the key to the correct prediction by three participating research groups. The structure could have easily been overlooked, leading to the misinterpretation of the results as an apparent failure of the computational methods. Thus, compounds that are amenable to structure prediction are not always studied experimentally to the extent necessary to ensure that the relevant forms have in fact been discovered and characterised ahead of computational studies.

Despite the challenges, a few methods have been developed that allow structure prediction of small, relatively rigid organic compounds with only a few functional groups in several important space groups. Polymorph Predictork has been implemented within the commercial software Cerius2 (C2 Polymorph by Accelrys). In general, current prediction methods generate large ensembles of different packing arrangements along with calculations of relative energetics. In reality, many of the calculated structures are not observed, giving the appearance of over-prediction of polymorphism. This was apparently the case with acetaminophen (paracetamol). In their study of the drug, Beyer et al. calculated 14 structures, 2 of which were the known monoclinic (stable) and orthorhombic forms.

The remaining 12 structures were considered as candidates for the metastable form III, which had been observed by thermal microscopy methods but for which diffraction data were unavailable. Using calculations of mechanical properties and morphology, Beyer et al. separated the 12 energetically feasible structures into two groups, based on the likelihood of each structure to exist as a stable form. Shortly after the publication of the prediction study, the experimental powder pattern of form III became available. Rietveld refinement and comparison of the experimental diffraction results with the theoretical powder patterns published by Beyer et al. yielded a monoclinic structure solution for form III. This structure is in fact part of the prediction set, but was considered an unlikely contender based on its extreme plate-like morphology.

The potential for complementarity of HT crystallisation and polymorph prediction is evident from these studies. In one sense, polymorph prediction can serve as a yardstick for "risk assessment" when it comes to form diversity, but inevitably one will require experimental data to assess the scope of polymorphism that can be elicited and the precise relative stabilities of different crystalline arrangements. Opportunities do exist for current use of predictions in solid form discovery. For instance, certain hydrogen-bonding motifs or molecular layer types may be observed in predicted structures. Such information can be used to aid the design of crystallisation experiments. It might be desirable to employ a particular type of interaction with salt selection or co-crystal formation by the strategic selection of crystallisation conditions, solvents, additives and processing methods.

Chapter 3

Study of Pro-drugs

A prodrug is a pharmacological substance (drug) which is administered in an inactive (or significantly less active) form. Once administered, the prodrug is metabolised in vivo into the active compound. The rationale behind the use of a prodrug is generally for Absorption, Distribution, Metabolism, and Excretion (ADME) optimization. Prodrugs are usually designed to improve oral bioavailability, with poor absorption from the gastrointestinal tract usually being the limiting factor, often due to the chemical properties of the drug.

Additionally, the use of a prodrug strategy increases the selectivity of the drug for its intended target. An example of this can be seen in many chemotherapy treatments, in which the reduction of adverse effects is always of paramount importance. Drugs used to target hypoxic cancer cells, through the use of redox-activation, utilise the large quantities of reductase enzyme present in the hypoxic cell to convert the drug into its cytotoxic form, essentially activating it. As the prodrug has low cytotoxicity prior to this activation, there is a markedly lower chance of it "attacking" healthy, non-cancerous cells which reduces the side-effects associated with these chemotherapeutic agents.

In rational drug design, the knowledge of chemical properties likely to improve absorption and the major metabolic pathways in the body allows the modification of the structure of new chemical entities for improved bioavailability. However, sometimes the use of a prodrug is unintentional, especially in the case of serendipitous drug discoveries, and the drug is only identified as a prodrug after extensive drug metabolism studies. Some prodrugs, such as Codeine and Psilocybin, also occur naturally.

It is well documented that till recent times drugs derived from plants were used to relieve patients from suffering. But at the turn of the last century, with the improvement in purification methods using chromatographic techniques, single compounds with well-defined structure became available for testing and treatment. Simultaneously, progress in organic synthesis allowed the synthesis of a plethora of pure compounds some of which became readily available for use as drugs. In fact today more than half of the drugs used in practice are of synthetic origin. A drug can be defined as a chemical used for treating, curing or preventing disease in human beings or in animals. In the process of treatment, drugs are also used for medical diagnosis and for restoring, correcting, or modifying physiological functions. Conventional drugs suffer from many drawbacks in their performance.

Site Specificity

Most of the drugs do not specifically attack the affected parts of the body. Orally or intravenously administered drugs need to necessarily travel through blood stream to the site of requirement. In the process, they may cause toxic side effects. For example almost all the presently available anticancer chemotherapeutic agents are cytotoxic in nature i.e., they attack growing cells. Since cancer cells grow at a faster rate than the normal cells, the anticancer drugs act as chemotherapeutic agents. However, they are not target specific, and therefore are also toxic to normal cells.

Permeability

Orally administered drugs must cross the cell membrane barrier twice. When a drug is taken, it must initially cross the cell membrane barrier to get into the blood stream for transportation. After reaching the affected part of the body, it must cross the cell membrane again, this time of the affected cell. Naturally, drugs cannot be effective if their permeability properties into or out of the specific cells do not meet the desired levels. Resistance: The drugs must be resistant to degradation from different body parts and fluids. It is also desirable to retain the drug molecule in the specific parts of the body for a longer duration so that its effective activity profile is completely realized.

Albert and his coworkers were the first ones to suggest the concept of prodrug approach for increasing the efficiency of drugs in 1950. They described prodrugs as pharmacologically inactive chemical derivatives that could be used to alter the physicochemical properties of drugs, in a temporary manner, to increase their usefulness and/or to decrease associated toxicity. Subsequently such drug-derivatives have also been called 'latentiated drugs', 'bioreversible derivatives', and 'congeners', but 'prodrug' is now the most commonly accepted term. Thus, prodrug can be defined as a drug derivative that undergoes biotransformation enzymatically or nonenzymatically, inside the body before exhibiting its therapeutic effect. Ideally, the prodrug is converted to the original drug as soon as the derivative reaches the site of action, followed by rapid elimination of the released derivatizing group without causing side effects in the process. The definition of the prodrug indicates that the derivatizing group is covalently linked to the drug molecule. However, the term prodrug has also been used for salts formed by the drug molecules.

Characteristics of a Prodrug

In recent years numerous prodrugs have been designed and developed to overcome barriers to drug utilization, such as low oral absorption properties, lack of site specificity, chemical instability, toxicity, bad taste, odour, pain at application site, etc. It has been suggested that the following characteristics of a prodrug must be improved for site-specific drug delivery.

1. The prodrug must be readily transported to the site of action.
2. The prodrug must be selectively cleaved to the active drug utilizing special enzymatic profile of the site.

3. Once the prodrug is selectively generated at the site of action, the tissue must retain the active drug without further degradation.

Development of Prodrugs

Prodrugs, which were developed by taking specific administration properties into consideration, are discussed here.

To improve membrane transport: Barbiturates (Figure 1) are a group of compounds responsible for profound sedative-hypnotic effect. They are weakly acidic in nature and are converted to the corresponding sodium salt in aqueous sodium hydroxide.

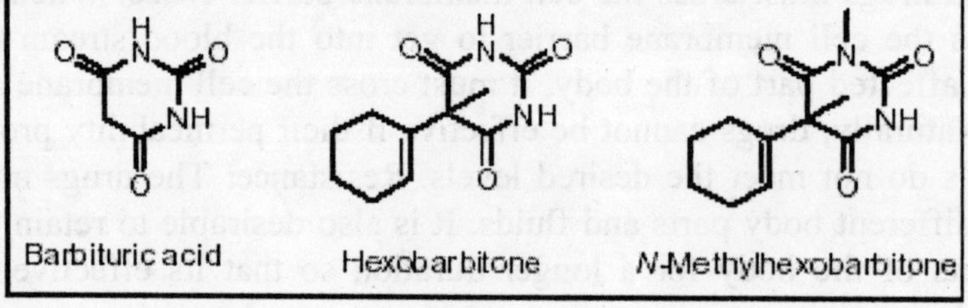

Barbituric acid Hexobarbitone *N*-Methylhexobarbitone

Figure 1. Hypnotic and sedative agents.

The sodium salt is extensively employed for intravenous anaesthetic properties. Barbituric acid is the parent member of this group of compounds. Various barbiturates differ in the time required for the onset of sleep and in the duration of their effect. Hexobarbitone was found to be an effective drug but its membrane permeability was found to be low. However N-methylhexobarbitone a simple derivative of the parent drug was found to have better permeability characteristics. After intake, the N-methyl group is cleaved in the liver to release the physiologically active drug. Similarly, membrane transportation characteristics of the neurotransmitter dopamine (Figure 2) used for the treatment of Parkinson's disease can be improved by administering its prodrug L-3,4-dihydroxyphenylalanine.

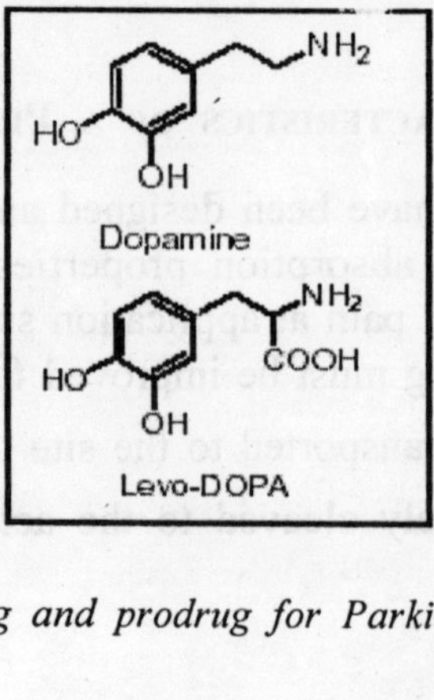

Dopamine

Levo-DOPA

Figure 2: Drug and prodrug for Parkinson's disease

This derivative has better blood-brain permeation characteristics since it uses amino acid channels for transportation.

Prolonged Activity

Nordazapam (Figure 3) is a drug used for sedation, particularly as an anxiolytic. It is also used as a muscle relaxant. However, it loses activity too quickly due to metabolism and excretion. A prodrug introduced to improve the retention characteristics is valium (Figure 3). Due to presence of N-methyl group the prodrug resists quick degradation. Slow release of the nordazapam in the liver by demethylation prolongs body retention characteristics.

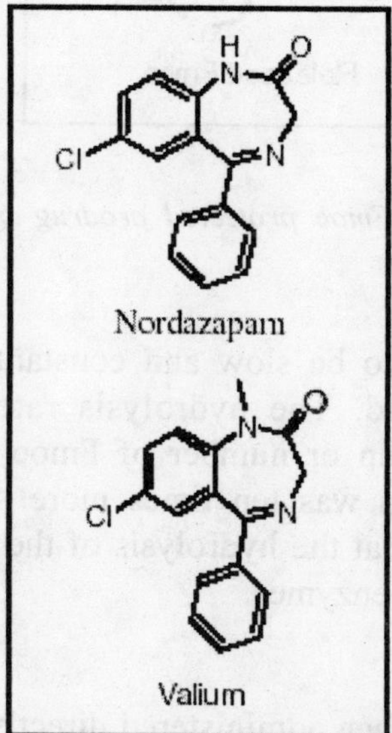

Figure 3. Anxiolytic and muscle relaxing agents

Decreased or lack of secretion of the enzyme insulin in pancreas leads to diabetes. Insulin is responsible for degradation of carbohydrate molecules to smaller units and is important in the catabolic process. Chronic diabetic patients take bovine insulin supplement through intravenous injections. Retention time of insulin in the blood is about six hours. So, patients need to administer required dose of insulin frequently. It is desirable to increase the retention characteristics of the enzyme so to make it effective for prolonged periods. It was found that 9-fluorenylmethoxycarbonyl (Fmoc) protection (Figure 4) of the hydroxy/amino groups of the enzyme makes it inactive and also increase its retention in blood for prolonged periods. The Fmoc group binds to the enzyme covalently and in the process makes it inactive as well as reduces its rapid degradation by natural body process. However, at the pH of about 7.4 prevalent in the blood serum the protected enzyme gets hydrolyzed slowly and irrevers-ibly back to the enzyme and Fmoc protecting group.

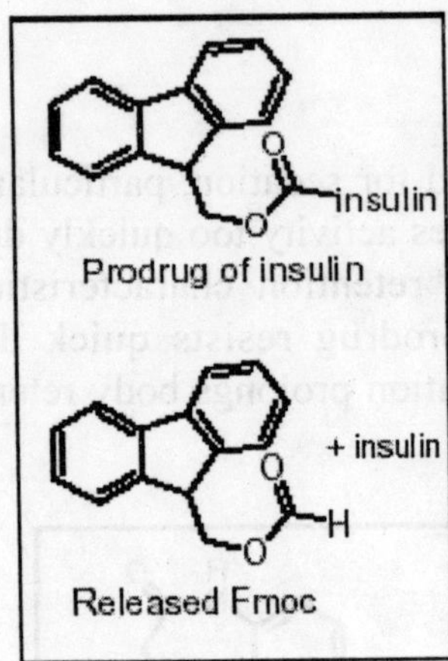

Figure 4. Fmoc protected prodrug of insulin.

The hydrolysis process was found to be slow and constant, which means that the release of enzyme is also slow and regulated. The hydrolysis rate can be fine tuned by selecting derivatives of Fmoc protecting group or number of Fmoc groups. It was shown that insulin having two Fmoc protecting groups was ten times more stable and more effective than the parent enzyme. It should be noted that the hydrolysis of the protecting group takes place in the blood without mediation from other enzymes.

Masking from other Enzymes

Sometimes drugs are highly toxic when administered directly. Suitable modification of the drug molecule to an inactive agent reduces toxicity. For example propiolaldehyde (Figure 5) is used in the aversion therapy on patients addicted to alcohol. However, it is a highly irritating chemical and causes allergic reactions. As an alternative, closely related compound, pargylene (Figure 5), which is converted to propiolaldehyde by oxidative enzymes only in liver, is used for alcohol deaddiction.

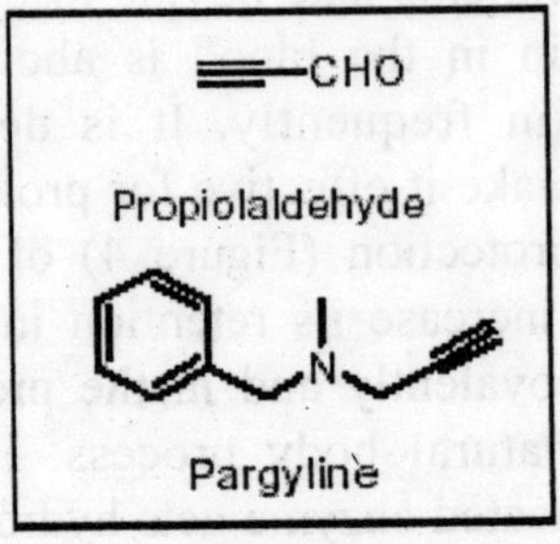

Figure 5. Prodrug for antialcoholic addiction

Tissue Specific Prodrug Design

In this approach of prodrug design the site-specific drug delivery can be achieved by the tissue activation, which is the result of an enzyme unique to the tissue or present in higher concentration. For example glycosidase enzymes are present in much higher concentration in bacteria associated with colon. This aspect can be utilized in the design of colon specific drug delivery. Glycosides are hydrophilic in nature and are poorly absorbed in small intestine. Once they reach the colon, bacterial glycosides release the free drug to be absorbed in that region. Dexamethasone and prednisolone (Figure 6) are corticosteroids used for anti-inflammatory properties. They are steroid drugs and are hydrophobic in nature. They are absorbed efficiently in intestinal tract and as such do not reach colon area for treatment.

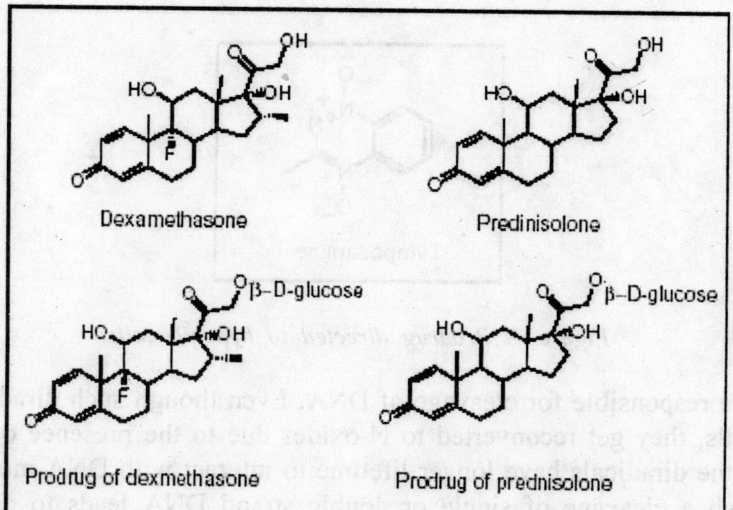

Dexamethasone

Predinisolone

Prodrug of dexmethasone

Prodrug of prednisolone

Figure 6. Antiinflammatory corticosteroid drugs and their prodrug derivatives.

However, when produgs dexamethasone-21- ß-glucoside and prednisolone-21- ß-glucoside were used they were absorbed in colon more efficiently compared to their parent drugs. The prodrugs are hydrophilic in nature and therefore are absorbed poorly in intestine. The glucosidase enzymes present in the bacteria located in colon release the parent hydrophobic drugs for absorption in the area.

Prodrug Design Based on Site-specific Conditions

A variety of conditions such as pH, oxygen content, which are site specific and are different from other parts of the body, can be effectively utilized for prodrug design. This aspect is an important feature in the research on prodrugs targeted at cancer cells. The cancer cells grow at a much faster rate than normal cells. Tumor cells associated with cancer can be differentiated from normal cells. The blood vessels in the tumor tissue often lack regularity and systematic connectivity leaving unvascularized zones, especially in the interior areas leading to unstable blood flow. Cells that do not have blood supply die as a result of lack of oxygen supply and also the intermediate regions get deficient supply of oxygen. This area is called hypoxial region.

Lack of oxygen in hypoxia cells or the bio-reductive conditions prevalent in them can be utilized for specific prodrug development wherein the active drug can be selectively released under bio-reductive conditions. The bio-reductive enzymes present in the cell perform one electron reduction. In normal cells oxygen reverses this reduction process. However, in hypoxia cells, due to near absence of oxygen, further reduction takes place to generate drug from prodrug moiety. For example, Tyrapazamine (Figure 7) has been developed as a cytotoxic agent. It has two N-oxide moieties, which on one electron reduction twice gets converted to highly reactive diradicals.

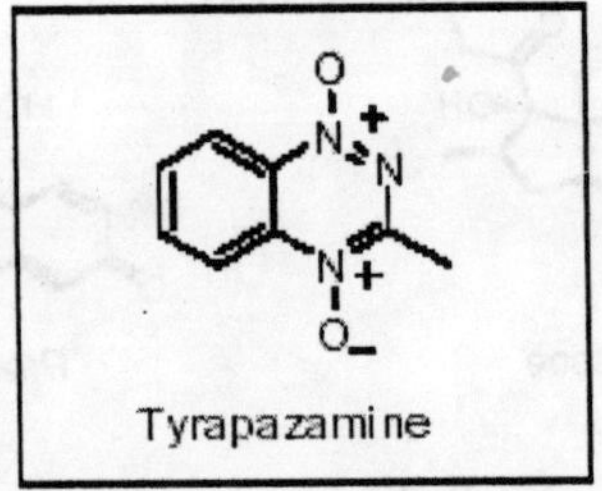

Figure 7. Prodrug directed to hypoxia cells.

The diradicals are responsible for cleavage of DNA. Even though such diradicals are generated in the normal cells, they get reconverted to N-oxides due to the presence of oxygen. Whereas in hypoxia cells the diradicals have longer lifetime to interact with DNA molecules and further cleave them. Such a cleavage of single or double strand DNA leads to destruction of cells. Thus, the N-oxide prodrug was found to be highly effective in hypoxia cells.

Enzyme Specific Prodrug Design

As described previously certain enzymes express predominantly at the affected parts. Prodrug development can take advantage of this aspect so that the over expressed enzymes at the affected parts of the body can be induced to release the drug at the site. This condition is of particular importance in targeting cancer cells. Due to differing physiological conditions enzyme groups such as glucuronidases, proteases2, receptors show activity in excess in cancer cells compared to normal cells. Several prodrugs have been developed taking advantage the excessive activity of the above enzymes in tumor tissues.

Scheeren and his group clearly demonstrated that the cytotoxic activity of important antitumor drugs could be enhanced and restricted to tumor-affected tissues by making peptide derivatives. They prepared derivatives of doxorubicin (Figure 8) and paclitaxel (Figure 9) wherein active sites are blocked by strategically attaching suitable polypeptide to the drug but separated by spacer. The spacer was used to expose the polypeptide chain open for plasmin activity. Both the prodrugs were found to be inactive and stable under biological pH conditions but they were readily cleaved with the release of parent drugs in the presence of plasmin enzymes present in tumor cells. The prodrugs were synthesized by blocking important functional group in the molecule with a polypeptide-capping agent to make them inactive. The spacer group was designed to self eliminate after hydrolysis of the polypeptide chain by the enzyme.

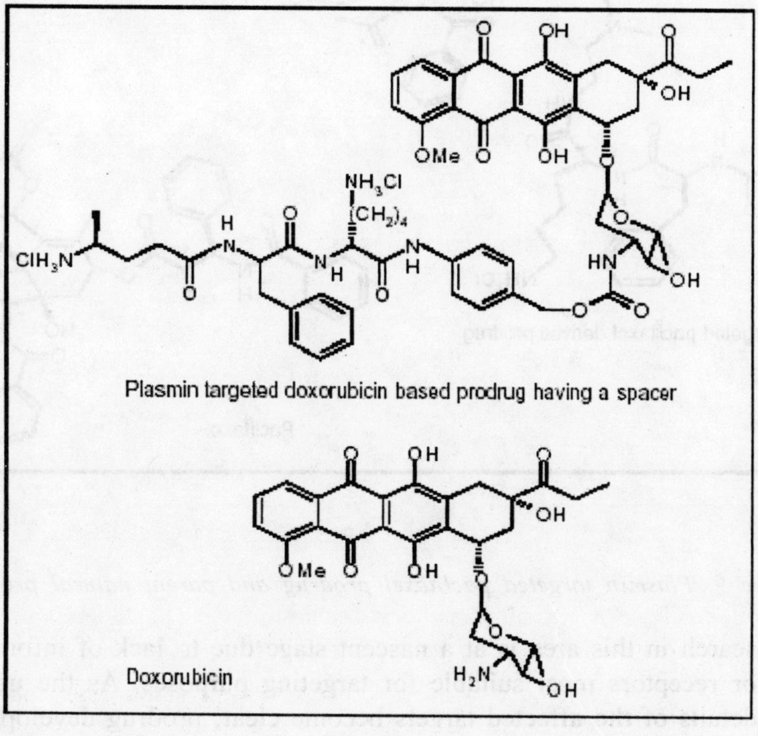

Plasmin targeted doxorubicin based prodrug having a spacer

Doxorubicin

Figure 8. Plasmin targeted anticancer prodrug and its parent drug.

It is clear from the foregoing, that the development of prodrugs promises to be a very effective method for treatment of diseases in the future. This approach has several advantages over conventional drug administration. Site specificity is central to the prodrug development strategy. Even though at present prodrugs are not prevalent in clinical use, in future there will be prodrugs for every known drug to make them effective in treatment. Drug discovery and prodrug development appear to be complementary for the generation of target specific medicines of future.

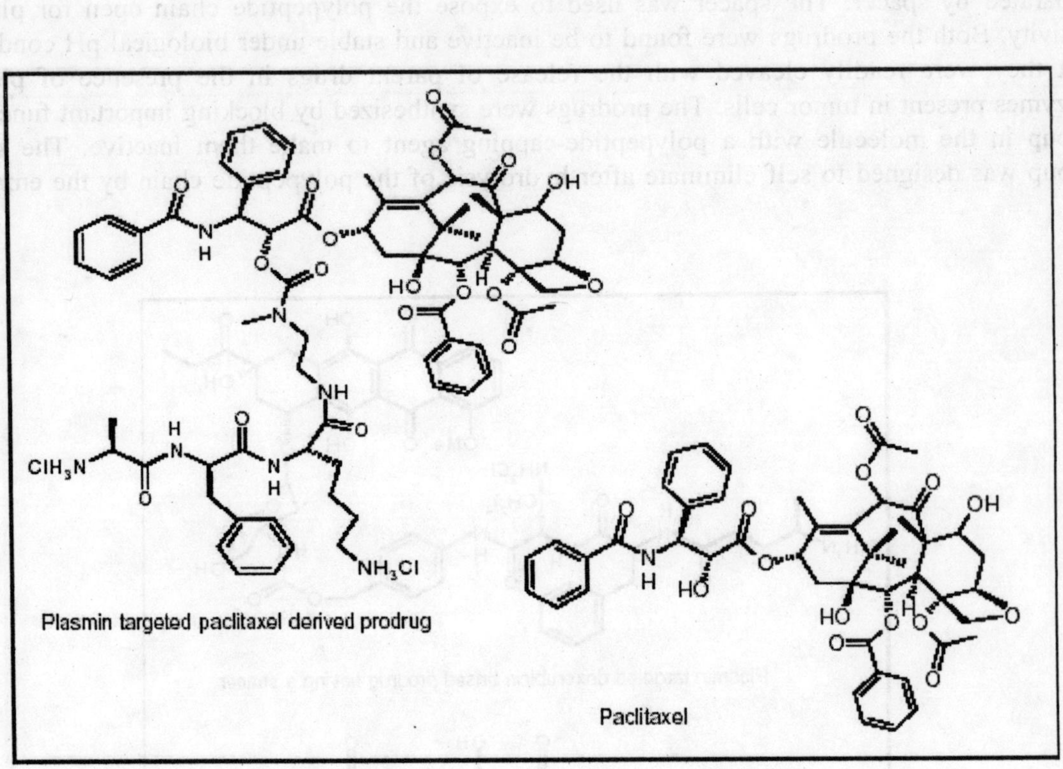

Plasmin targeted paclitaxel derived prodrug

Paclitaxel

Figure 9. Plasmin targeted paclitaxel prodrug and parent natural product

At present the research in this area is at a nascent stage due to lack of information regarding all the enzymes or receptors most suitable for targeting purposes. As the unravelling of the micro-biological details of the affected targets become clear, prodrug development will surely decrease side/toxic effects of drugs and also trigger development of more potent primary drugs.

Chapter 4

Drug Discovery Process

Historically, screening for new drug leads has involved primarily studies in animals and isolated tissues. Recently, cultured cells as well as isolated enzyme preparations and receptor-binding preparations have been used for assays. Screening in animals has the advantage of most relevant feedback. If a reasonable animal model can be used to demonstrate the desired effect, it provides a largely proven bioavailability and biological effect. This type of screening is so successful that Beyer has noted that in the search for novel diuretic agents in the 1950s while many laboratories searched for carbonic anhydrase inhibitors and synthesized very potent agents, his group, which relied on screening in animals, synthesized and developed a new class of diuretic agents, the thiazides.

However, there are several drawbacks to the use of animals in screening. The use of animals tends to be slow and requires large quantities of experimental compounds. The use of animals is also very labour intensive, and together these disadvantages make such screening an expensive proposition. In addition, if the animal model is not chosen carefully, nonspecificity may result. For example, if inflammatory reactions are initiated in animals, then, if the animal becomes ill with the experimental agent, the inflammatory reaction generally will not occur.

Screening in isolated tissues or cultured cells generally requires less compound than in animals and often is less labour intensive. In addition, screening at this level of complexity allows the determination of whether an agent is an agonist or an antagonist. As with animals, inhibition of a response may reflect toxicity rather than efficacy.

The use of receptor binding requires the least amount of compound. In many laboratories, a single disbursement of 1 mg of compound may be sufficient to perform screening in as many as a dozen assays in different receptors.

Receptor binding is also rapid. In the author's small laboratory, as many as 1,000 compounds often are screened per day in a given receptor assay. In receptor-binding assays, specificity often may be readily determined by assaying the compound in preparations of several different receptors. However, receptor assay screening gives little or no clue of bioavailability and ultimate efficacy in an animal. In addition, it is impossible to determine from a single receptor assay whether a compound will be toxic to an animal.

The theory of ligand-binding assays is quite simple. A preparation of the receptor is prepared using either tissue homogenates or intact cells and incubates replicate tubes with a radiolabeled ligand. Certain tubes contain saturating concentrations of unlabelled ligand to allow the determination of nonspecific binding (figure 1). It is possible to determine potency of a competitor by adding various concentrations of competitor to different tubes and determining the amount of ligand bound. Then, one can either determine percent inhibition of binding or the IC50. value for inhibition of binding by the competitor. In mass ligand-binding screening, a single concentration of competitor is often chosen for testing. Any compounds that inhibit binding a certain specified percentage are further evaluated to determine IC50. This approach dramatically speeds the process because very few compounds will generally be shown to be active.

Ideal Receptor-binding Assay

Optimization of a receptor-binding assay requires attention to two primary components, the tissue and the ligand. The goal is to achieve the highest signal-to-noise ratio possible, that is, to maximise specific binding and minimise nonspecific binding. The ideal tissue will have a high density of binding sites, Often, there are 10,000 to 50,000 binding sites per cell in a tissue. Tissues with only a few hundred binding sites per cell tend to have very low signal-to-noise ratios. In addition, the tissues should express a pure receptor subtype.

For example, to simply homogenise brain and then attempt to perform dopamine binding, it is necessary to deal with distinguishing among binding to dopamine D1, D2, D3, D4, D5, and D6 subtypes. With currently available ligands, this would be impossible. Evaluating compounds against one of these dopamine receptor subtypes would require the identification of a tissue that expresses only one subtype or would require access to a cell line that stably expresses a cloned subtype. Stably transfected cell lines expressing only a single receptor subtype are becoming more common and will probably be the norm within the next few years. Finally, an ideal tissue must be readily obtained in quantity.

A ligand must be highly specific for its receptor. Norepinephrine, for example, would make a poor candidate for a binding ligand because it binds to virtually all subtypes of -and -adrenergic receptors. When novel receptor subtypes are screened, a specific ligand rarely will be available. Generally, the goal of the screening exercise will be to discover such ligands. Thus, in practice the option is to choose a tissue that expresses only a single subtype of receptor to achieve this specificity.

In addition, a ligand must be of as high specific activity as possible to evaluate binding. 125l-labeled ligands are preferable to tritiated ligands because, after completion of the binding experiment, processing of samples is minimised. Tritiated ligands may require solubilisation in liquid scintillation cocktail, which greatly increases the labour involved in a binding assay because of filling and capping vials. However, because 125I has a relatively short half-life, in practice tritiated ligands tend to be more stable and easy to use.

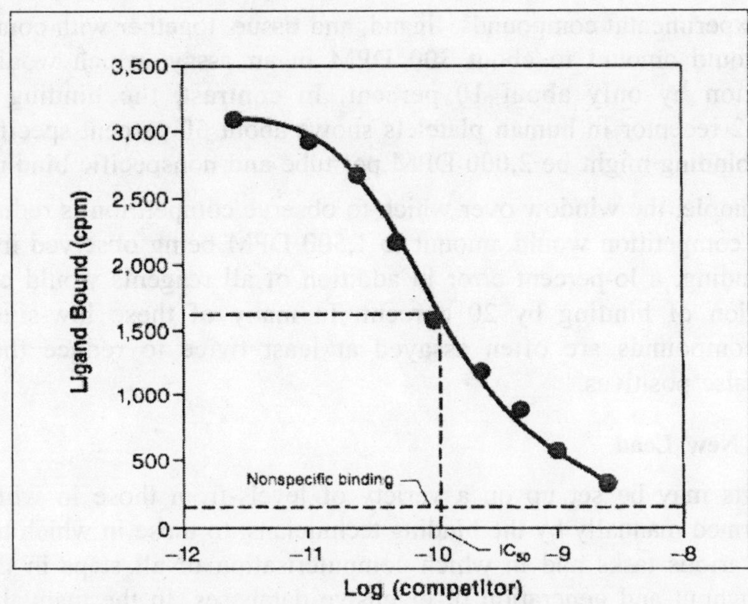

Figure 1. Theory of ligand-binding assays

In choosing a ligand, an antagonist is often better than an agonist. In particular, affinity shifts for agonists in G protein-coupled receptors in response to ions make for increased nonspecificity when dealing with unknown competitors.

Of course, for the reasons mentioned above, an agonist may have to be used because discovery of an antagonist is often the goal of the exercise. Receptors for many biogenic amines and many peptide hormones are expressed at 10,000 to 50,000 per cell. This translates to about 10 12 sites per gram of tissue wet weight and allows the evaluation of 200 to 300 experimental tubes per gram of tissue. In contrast, many cytokines are expressed at 200 to 3,000 sites per cell. This often necessitates the use of 106 cells per tube or more for experimental assays. For those receptors that are expressed in the least abundance, as few as 2 to 5 tubes may be assayed using a 10 cm^2 dish for contact-dependent cells or perhaps only 10 to 20 tubes per T-75 flask for contact-independent cells. Increased receptor densities may often be obtained in transfected cell lines expressing cloned receptors in which the expression is commonly as high as 50,000 to 100,000 receptors per cell. Alternatively, transformed cells may overexpress certain receptors. For example, certain leukemia cell lines express as many as 50,000 to 100,000 interleukin-1 (IL-1) receptors per cell compared with 200 per cell in nontransformed lines.

Assays with high signal-to-noise ratios make screening a much simpler process. For example, binding of bradykinin to B2, receptors in guinea pig ileum exhibits about 95-percent specific binding. If in a given tube total binding is 3,000 disintegrations per minute (DPM), then nonspecific binding is about 150 DPM, leaving a window of 2,850 DPM over which to observe competition. Fifty-percent competition at this site would result in observing 1,575 DPM. If errors in addition of experimental compounds, ligand, and tissue, together with counting error, total 10 percent, this would amount to about 300 DPM in an assay, which would change apparent percent inhibition by only about 10 percent. In contrast, the binding of ligands to the thromboxane A2 receptor in human platelets shows about 50-percent specific binding. In such an assay, total binding might be 2,000 DPM per tube and nonspecific binding 1,000 DPM.

In this example, the window over which to observe competition is reduced to 1,000 DPM, and 50-percent competition would amount to 1,500 DPM being observed in a tube. With such low specific binding, a lo-percent error in addition of all reagents would change the apparent percent inhibition of binding by 20 percent. In many of these low-signal assays, all the experimental compounds are often assayed at least twice to reduce the number of false negatives and false positives.

Discovery of a New Lead

Screening efforts may be set up on a variety of levels-from those in which all parts of the assay are performed manually by the binding technicians, to those in which teams of technicians subdivide the various tasks and in which computerisation of all steps in the process leads to very high throughput and generation of extensive databases. In the manual approach, a single technician harvests and prepares the tissues, sets up and terminates the assays, calculates results, and places them into a database. Using this type of system, it is often not possible to perform assays more than 2 days in a given week.

In such a system, a single technician should be able on a given day to set up and assay twelve 48-tube racks or six 96-tube racks. This amounts to 576 tubes. Each rack has duplicate total and nonspecific binding tubes, and a standard compound is run each day. Therefore, about 520 tubes are available for test compounds. In this scenario, a single technician disburses compounds. Each disbursement technician can weigh and solubilise about 250 compounds per day. Thus, in a given week, somewhat more than 1,000 compounds may be solubilised and assayed by these two people. If such an approach is used to screen a library of 10,000 compounds, then about 10 weeks, or 20 technician-weeks, would be required.

Considerable time and cost benefits can accrue using a high-throughput approach. In this scenario, two disbursement technicians are required for each binding technician. Each binding technician performs an assay each day. Therefore, about 2,500 compounds are assayed per week. The disbursement technicians weigh bar-coded compounds, and the computer attached to the balance notes how much diluent to add to each vial. Scintillation counters also are accessed by the computer, which calculates percent inhibition by the test compounds. Before commitment of data to a database, the binding technician quickly calls up the assay for examination to determine that total and nonspecific counts are within normal values and that the standard compound inhibited with the expected potency. Using this kind of approach, the 10,000-compound library can be screened through one receptor assay in about 4 weeks, requiring only about 12 technician-weeks.

This high-throughput approach can be extended to other receptor assays with minimal cost. If a single batch of compound is disbursed, it may be stored in a cold room in dimethyl sulfoxide or other appropriate solution and used for up to several dozen different assays. Low signal-to-noise assays require more time because each compound is assayed multiple times.

Definition of Success

Depending on the definition of an active compound or a "hit," success may be great or little. Certain assays tend to have many apparent hits (false positives), whereas others have very low hit rates. Receptor-binding assays for excitatory amino acids tend to have hit rates of 10 to 20 percent in libraries of "random" compounds, when hit is defined as 50-percent inhibition at a concentration of 10 µm. In contrast, in the IL-1 receptor-binding assay in fibroblasts in the author's laboratory, the hit rate is less than 1 in 5,000 using the same criteria. Given these examples, to avoid being swamped following up false positives, inclusion criteria must be strict. Of course, if criteria are too restrictive, then promising leads may be missed.

In the author and colleagues' work, an example of the weakest compound in a bradykinin receptor-binding assay that can be shown to be an antagonist in a functional assay is NPC 361, which has a Ki, of 400 nm. The prototype cholecystokinin antagonist, asperlicin, had a Ki of 600 nm in a binding assay. For either of these examples, even our relatively strict inclusion criteria of 50-percent inhibition of binding at a concentration of 10 µm would have tagged these compounds as active. However, Wong and colleagues' angiotensin II antagonist lead had a Ki, of 40,000 nm in their assay. Such a compound would have been excluded in any of the assays in the author's laboratory as inactive.

If such weakly active compounds are included as hits, then 50-percent inhibition at 100 µm would be required. Unless the assay is very "clean" (as described above for IL-l), a method is required to make certain that most nonspecific (false positive) compounds are weeded out quickly. This is done by running the compounds in several different binding assays and excluding those that are hits in multiple assays. In situations in which compounds are routinely screened at only a single site, all apparent hits are collected and run in additional binding assays. Thus, a "receptor profile" or a "cross-selectivity report" is obtained.

In the cross-selectivity mode, an attempt is made to determine Ki, values in each assay. Concentrations to be evaluated are chosen by noting the apparent Ki, in the assay of interest, then bracketing that value. In these studies, two compounds are evaluated per 48-tube rack (11 duplicate concentrations of each test compound plus duplicate total count and nonspecific count tubes). Each binding technician can perform determinations for 24 compounds per day. For the specialised laboratory that performs screening in only its target of interest, Ki, determinations in multiple assays may be contracted commercially with several companies.

Functional Screening

Functional screening is the vital next step after a hit is identified in a binding assay. The functional screen is necessary to determine whether a given compound is an agonist or antagonist. Functional screens also serve to provide an idea of selectivity or, at times, toxicity. When determining whether a compound has agonist activity, one must always evaluate the compound in an assay alone, even if the antagonist assay suggests that the compound does reduce the activity of an agonist. It must be remembered that a partial agonist will appear to be an antagonist when assessed in an antagonist assay.

The first choice in deciding on a functional screen is whether to use an isolated tissue response (e.g., smooth-muscle contraction) or a second-messenger assay (e.g., increase in intracellular inositol phosphates [IP3] or cyclic AMP [CAMP]). The second-messenger assays often lend themselves to very high throughput. For example, using a radioreceptor assay for IP3, the author's laboratory cultures fibroblasts in 24-well plates. Cells are then stimulated with bradykinin to determine whether test compounds inhibit bradykinin-induced IP3 accumulation. This assay also lends itself to determination of affinity by determining Kb, or pA2 values. Such assays may be used to assess selectivity of test compounds. In the assay just cited, the cells also express receptors for angiotensin II, vasopressin, a,-adrenegic agonists, and bombesin, all of which increase the accumulation of IP3. Similarly, the cells express -adrenergic and adenosine receptors, whose activation increases the accumulation of CAMP. These, too, can be used to assess selectivity and may be preferred, because assessing the effect of a compound on a second transduction system adds an additional chance to detect nonspecific effects.

The utility of a functional screen is increased if it measures a "positive activity" rather than a "negative activity." In a negative-activity assay, an attempt is made to block the ability of an agonist to elicit a response in a resting cell or tissue. This type of assay often is used and represents the common agonist-induced muscle contraction or agonist-induced IP3 accumulation. Here, the test compound is assessed for its ability to inhibit the response. A problem that often arises when assessing unknown compounds is that, if the compound nearly kills the cell, usually an agonist will not cause increased IP3, accumulation, appearing to confirm activity of the test compound as an antagonist. Thus, the negative-activity assay may be prone to generating false negatives.

In the positive-activity assay, the agonist does something to decrease the function of the cell or tissue, and an antagonist restores a normal state. For example, tumour necrosis factor (TNF) induces cytotoxicity in many cell types. If a test compound blocks this effect, then the cell, rather than dying in response to exposure to TNF, continues to act normally. In this type of assay, a toxic compound tends to augment the ability of TNF to kill the cell rather than make the cell function more normally. Thus, nonspecifically toxic compounds will tend not to appear as active receptor antagonists.

Process Technology

Process technology refers to throughput methodologies. Many laboratories spend extraordinary amounts of money and time on automation of assays. In my laboratory I find automation largely wasteful. Given hand-held automatic pipetting devices, multiple-sample filtration manifolds, and dry scintillant pads, my laboratory always outperforms automated laboratories. Often, a library of compounds may be screened in the time it takes to reprogram all the automation devices. The only situation in which automation may be arguably worth the bother and expense is when a library of many thousands of compounds will be screened.

ANTIBODY AND PEPTIDE STRUCTURE-BASED DRUG DESIGN

For more than a century, the search for new drugs has been rooted in an organic chemistry-driven technology based on the synthesis and biological evaluation of large numbers of candidate compounds. Highlighting the inefficiency of this process is the fact that US. pharmaceutical companies were estimated to have spent $7.3 billion on domestic research and development in 1991 to achieve U.S. approval of only 11 new chemicals.

Hoping to improve the success rate in drug discovery, today most major pharmaceutical companies and several startup companies have organised efforts in rational drug design. Several distinct strategies are employed, including approaches based on computer modeling of data obtained from binding assays and enzyme crystallography as well as methods depending on bioorganic chemistry. These applications of rational drug design thus require at least the purification and sometimes the crystallisation of targets that are central to each disease process. Yet many prospective drug targets are membrane-bound macromolecules that cannot readily be crystallised or even identified. For example, in a recent inhibitor design study involving the crystal structure of the RNase H domain of human immunodeficiency virus-1 reverse transcriptase, only an inactive RNase H fragment could be obtained as diffraction quality crystals.

Antibody and peptide structure drug design is aimed at avoiding these pitfalls. In the antibody approach, the remarkable power of the mammalian immune system is first harnessed to access the threedimensional (3-D) structural information contained in pharmacological receptors, enzymes, and viruses without the need for special purification or isolation efforts.

Then, the pharmacophoric information embedded in the resulting monoclonal antibody is read out by one of several methods. From the data obtained, peptide agents are produced whose structure is used as the basis for the computerassisted design of orally active nonpeptide peptidomimetic drugs with receptor subtype specificity for many therapeutic applications. In those cases where thestructure of a lead peptide, such as a natural mediator, is known, the process can begin without the creation of the antibody, which serves only as an informational intermediate. These steps are considered briefly in the next sections.

ANTIBODY TECHNOLOGY

Antibody-directed drug design begins with the selection of a drug target, which can be a pharmacological receptor, an enzyme, or a virus. Through monoclonal technology, idiotypic antibodies (Ab-1) to key drug action sites in such receptors, enzymes, and viruses can be selected and produced in any desired amount without the need to isolate the target. The production and selection of antibodies to drug targets represents a screening of a repertoire of several billion different antibody structures generated by the immune system and a fine tuning of these structures through somatic cell mutation.

Antibody-directed drug design requires the antibodies to the drug target to have functional (druglike) activity. Clearly, an antibody that binds to a nonfunctional area of the target, or one that binds in some nonfunctional manner, will be useless as a prototype for drug design. A list of functional antibodies that have been obtained to targets such as peptide hormone receptors, autocoid receptors, and enzymes is given in table 1 and is an impressive array of the potential of this technology.

The idiotypic antibody is a mirror image of the target site, both in a spatial and an electronic sense. For example, Conti-Tronconi and colleagues have mapped the binding site of the nicotinic acetylcholine receptor a-subunit with several monoclonal antibodies raised against native Torpedo receptor. The binding of these antibodies to the receptor is inhibited by all cholinergic ligands, and it was found that the antibodies bound to specific amino acid clusters positioned discontinuously within the receptor sequence 181-200.

By using the idiotypic antibody as an antigen, an anti-idiotypic antibody (Ab-2) can be produced as a positive image of the target site. Again, selection criteria exist for anti-idiotypic antibodies that are faithful internal images of the original antigen.

Screening of Compound Libraries

Idiotypic antibodies have high affinity both for the antigens that were used to raise them as well as their corresponding anti-idiotypic antibodies. Because the interaction of these pairs can be observed conveniently using conventional or sandwich enzyme-linked immunosorbent assay (ELISA) methodology, it is possible readily to screen large numbers of compounds (compound libraries) for their ability to inhibit this interaction. In this way, potentially useful compounds that bind to either receptors or their anti-idiotypic images can be identified.

X-Ray Crystallography

Important drug design information is obtained from antibodies, their fragments, and complexes and from peptides by crystallisation using conventional protein crystallisation techniques. After x-ray diffraction data are collected, the crystal structure is solved using the conventional multiple isomorphous replacement technique requiring heavy atom derivatisation of the crystals. An alternative approach is molecular replacement, which depends on some degree of knowledge of the structure of the antibody, the antigen, or both.

. A closeup view shows the spatial and electronic complementarity of the interacting surfaces of lysozome residues 41-46 and light chain residues 55-59 that contribute to the hydrophobic, electrostatic, and hydrogen bonding accounting for the nanomolar affinity of the two ligands.

The specific interactions between antibody and antigen demonstrate dramatically the potential of the approach for directed drug design. Such analyses provide an unequalled structural basis for the creation of synthetic molecules, peptides, or peptidomimetics that share with the idiotypic antibody the ability to interact with the antigen. Related information can be deduced for anti-idiotypic antibodies that are replicas of receptors or other inaccessible macromolecules.

Through the use of molecular graphics algorithms, the interacting residues in the antibody may be excised from the rest of the structure as a "virtual peptide". The virtual peptide is a computer construct of the interacting residues in their constrained conformation, although this conformation would not be maintained if the peptide were synthesized free of the rest of the antibody molecule. The virtual peptide is used as the pattern for the synthesis of constrained peptidomimetic drugs as outlined in a later section.

Information Extraction

In addition to x-ray crystallography, three other techniques are used to read out structural information from the embedded pharmacophore in the antibody or from the anti-idiotypic antibody.

First, if specific leader sequences are used in the polymerase chain reaction, the amino acid sequence of the hypervariable loops of the antibodies can be determined. With the knowledge of these sequences and of the x-ray crystal structure of representative antibodies, a combined knowledge-based and ab initio algorithm can be applied to model the structure of the hypervariable loops. In this way, structural information similar to that which can be obtained from x-ray crystallography is at hand without the need to resort to the crystallographic methodology.

Second, peptides that are complementary to the surface of anti-idiotypic receptor surrogates can be selected from libraries of filamentous phage clones, each displaying one peptide sequence on the virion surface. A properly selected peptide that is complementary to a receptor surrogate results in a receptor antagonist.

Last, evidence for the location of key amino acid sequences in the hypervariable loops of anti-idiotypic antibodies can be adduced from their homology with sequences in the initial antigen.

Derivatives of these peptide sequences, chemically constrained to preserve their spatial characteristics, have been evaluated as drugs in their own right. For example, a synthetic mimetic derived from an omega loop structure that mimics a prominent, exposed series of eight residues in interleukin-1 (IL-1) was evaluated for its ability to bind to IL-1 receptors.

Peptidomimetic Drug Synthesis

The use of peptides as design templates for peptidomimetic drugs is the key step in the implementation of antibody- and peptide structure-based drug design, In the preceding process, the end product is the design of a peptide drug that may be an enzyme inhibitor, a receptor antagonist (or sometimes an agonist), or an antiviral. Alternatively, the end product may be an antibody containing the embedded pharmacophore for any of these activities. Because both peptides and antibodies typically have short biological half-lives and poor oral bioavailability, it remains to synthesize a peptidomimetic based on the peptide structure to afford a bioavailable, orally active drug.

The design of peptidomimetics requires two different applications of computer-assisted drug design techniques. First, an estimate of the bioactive conformation of the peptide must be obtained from x-ray or nuclear magnetic resonance results and from modified data obtained from primary sequence information through the application of computational chemistry algorithms such as those of V.N. Balaji and U.C. Singh. This information is used to interpret the structure-function studies on the molecule. For example, it has been shown that the fragment Phe7-Trp8-Lys9-Thr10 is essential for growth hormone release inhibitory activity by somatostatin and that a ß II-type turn and a ß-sheet are also required for activity.

Based on the predicted or observed 3-D spatial and electronic characteristics of the peptide, a database and an algorithm of peptidomimetic surrogate elements are used to design candidate drugs for synthesis. A measure of conformational flexibility is required in these compounds to allow for the conformational changes that occur on binding to the target. Docking routines may be used to optimize complementarity in those cases where the 3-D structure of the receptor surrogate has been obtained.

A recent example of this approach involved the synthesis of a synthetic p-loop structure that mimics the second complementarity-determining region of a monoclonal antibody, which recognises the cell surface receptor for reovirus type 3 (Reo3R). The synthetic organic mimetic, termed the 87.1 mimetic, is a water-soluble, 10-membered macrocycle containing amide bonds. Evidence was obtained that indicates the 87.1 mimetic binds efficiently to Reo3R.

Antibody- and peptide structure-based drug design offers wholly new insights and approaches in the design and optimization of new lead compounds for therapeutic application, and risk is minimised by the multiplicity of available strategies. As these methods are developed further, even greater savings in time and effort will be at hand in the search for new drugs.

Cloned Human Receptors for Drug Design

The availability of sets of transfected human receptors makes it possible to target drugs to single human proteins from the inception of a drug design project. A critical requirement of this technology is that human genes must express a human pharmacology when expressed in the host cell line chosen for transfection. Studies on the human serotonin 5-HT2, and 5-HT1D/ 5-HT1B receptors demonstrate that the gene sequence appears to determine the expressed receptor's pharmacological properties, with only a minor role played by the cellular environment in which the receptor is expressed.

The cloning and characterisation of the 5-HT1B receptor also demonstrate another emerging principle of molecular pharmacology: the equivalent G protein-coupled receptor gene in different species can encode proteins with strikingly different pharmacological properties. Another important issue is the relationship between agonist and antagonist binding sites.

Studies comparing agonist-1-(2,5-dimethoxy-4-methylphenyl)-2-aminopropane (DOM)-and antagonist binding sites of the human 5-HT2 receptor demonstrate the strong differences exhibited by these two binding states of the same receptor protein, Finally, the fact that receptors of the G protein-coupled or 7TM (7 transmembrane) receptor superfamily exhibit many properties in common allows receptor homologies to be used to predict certain drug-binding properties. Examples from the serotonergic and adrenergic receptor families are presented.

MOLECULAR PHARMACOLOGY

Cloned human receptors, conveniently expressed in transfected mammalian cell lines, now make it possible to approach drug design from a truly molecular perspective. In the past several years, the amino acid sequences of many receptor genes have been determined. Most of these cloned receptors are members of a closely related superfamily of genes known as the G proteincoupled receptors (or 7TM receptors), because of their characteristic singlesubunit structure with 7TM-spanning segments. Similar cloning successes are now being reported for multisubunit ligand-gated ion channels, including the GABAA receptor, the 5-HT3 receptor, and the N-methyl-D-aspartate receptor. Molecular pharmacologists are beginning to integrate this new information into their views of physiological and pharmacological processes and are introducing cloned human receptors into the drug development process, often from the very start of a drug design effort.

Expression of cloned human receptors in mammalian cell lines allows pharmacologists to develop assay systems that individually express each receptor subtype important to a drug design project. Host cell lines can be chosen that are devoid of any related receptor sites, producing clean, unambiguous assay systems. These subtype-specific human receptor assays will allow medicinal chemists to design drugs with high affinity for the desired site of action and low affinity for those receptor subtypes that may induce side effects.

In many cases, this design strategy can be expected to produce more potent medications with fewer side effects because of an improved molecular targeting of the drug. Even in cases where a blended drug possessing a spectrum of receptor activities may be the desired endpoint, pure human subtype assays provide a drug design team with an important advantage: unambiguous assays of the affinity of the drug candidate at each human receptor site of interest.

The second advantage of the cloned receptor approach is that low abundance sites, which have been difficult to study in tissue preparations (e.g., autoreceptors), can now be isolated and expressed at high density for use in ligand screening and basic science investigations. The third, and perhaps'most important, advantage is the fact that many new receptor subtypes have been and continue to be discovered by receptor cloning efforts, which are providing a rapid increase in the number of potential drug target sites and can be expected to lead to several new medications in the future.

Species Differences in Receptors

The pharmacological binding properties of receptors are often similar for the same receptor subtype in different species, although many exceptions do occur. When species differences do exist, they dictate that great care be used in the choice of receptor assays for the purpose of human drug design. The best situation is found when human receptors can be used to screen for drug activity and selectivity.

Cloned human receptors are making human receptor screening possible. These clones are commonly expressed in mammalian or sometimes in bacterial expression systems for use in drug-binding assays. This leads to the important question of what influence the cell-line will have on the pharmacological properties of the human receptors that they express, For the purpose of drug screening, host cell lines must be chosen so that cloned human receptors will properly reproduce the binding properties of native human tissues.

The influence of the cell-line host on the pharmacological binding properties of cloned human receptor subtypes has been studied in some detail. The binding properties of the serotonin 5-HT2, receptor have been known to differ in different species, especially for certain ergot compounds. For example, mesulergine exhibits approximately thirtyfold higher affinity for rat cortical membranes than for comparable human tissue. Transfection of a cDNA clone encoding the human 5-HT2, receptor subtype into mouse fibroblast cells leads to expression of a serotonin receptor whose binding properties match that of human rather than rat cortical membranes.

The largest drug-binding differences are seen for mesulergine, which binds to both the transfected human receptor and to human cortical membranes with an apparent affinity of approximately 150 nM, thirtyfold weaker than its affinity for the rat cortex 5-HT2, receptor. This species difference also is seen for ritanserin, which belongs to an entirely different chemical class. In both cases, the transfected human receptor exhibits binding affinities in close agreement with human cortical tissue, even though the human gene has been expressed in a rodent, nonneuronal cell line. Together, these observations suggest that it is the amino acid sequence of the receptor (nature), rather than the cellular environment in which the receptor gene is expressed and processed (nurture), that determines the species-specific pharmacological properties of the receptor.

Further studies are needed to determine whether this will prove to be a general property of neurotransmitter receptors. For most cases examined so far, it appears that transfection of a human 7TM receptor gene into mammalian cell lines has produced ligand-binding properties in good agreement with previous binding assays in human brain tissue preparations. Furthermore, the use of different cell lines as transfection hosts was not found to substantially affect the pharmacological binding properties of a series of human G protein-coupled receptors that the author and colleagues at Synaptic Pharmaceuticals have been investigating. This information provides a welcome degree of freedom in the choice of host cells for transfection, which can then be chosen based on ease of transfection, complement of native G proteins, or other desirable criteria.

A similar result was observed in the case of the serotonin 5-HT1D receptor, which illustrates an extreme case of the variations that can occur in the pharmacological properties of homologous genes in different species. The 5-HT1D receptor is not present in rat cortical membranes: however, the rat brain contains a homologous receptor that exhibits such different pharmacological properties that it has been named a separate serotonin receptor subtype (5-HT1B). Recently, a gene encoding the rat 5-HT1B receptor was isolated and shown to be highly homologous to the human 5-HT1D receptor gene. This demonstrates that a previous suggestion that the 5-HT1B and 5-HT1D receptors are essentially the same receptor subtype was correct. This suggestion was based on the fact that both receptor subtypes show similar distribution in the basal ganglia, similar coupling to adenylate cyclase inhibition, and similar roles as terminal autoreceptors on raphe neurons.

When a human 5-HT1D receptor clone was expressed in the same mouse fibroblast cell line used to express the 5-HT1B receptor, this human receptor exhibited the binding properties appropriate for the human origin of its gene, rather than the mouse origin of its cell host. It appears that no counter example has been described where the host cell line dictates the pharmacological binding properties of a transfected gene. Protein processing and glycosylation patterns will differ from cell to cell, which may influence receptor kinetics, desensitisation phenomena, receptor turnover, and the membrane compartment distribution of the receptor. Nevertheless, it appears that the pharmacological binding properties of 7TM receptors are determined primarily by their gene sequences with a much smaller role (if any) played by their cellular environments.

Agonist and Antagonist Binding Sites

G protein-coupled receptors cycle through a complex series of G protein- and ligand-binding affinities. These binding states induce different affinity states for agonist ligands. The availability of transfected cell lines expressing single receptor subtypes now makes it possible to examine these binding states in much greater detail. Two recent studies have resolved a long-standing controversy in the serotonin receptor field, namely, whether the serotonergic binding site for the agonist 4-bromo-2,5-dimethoxyphenylisopropylamine (DOB) and other related compounds is the high affinity agonist binding state of the 5-HT2 receptor, which binds antagonist ligands such as ketanserin, or is a separate, closely related receptor subtype.

Both interpretations have been advanced but the existing data now appear to strongly support the two-site rather than the two-receptor interpretation, as two studies utilising transfected human and rat 5-HT2 receptor clones have shown. Both studies reached the same conclusion: Transfection of a single cDNA clone into host mammalian cells produced two distinct binding sites (distinct [3H]DOB and [3H]ketanserin binding sites). Addition of guanine nucleotides to these systems reduced the number of agonist high-affinity binding sites with no change, or a slight increase, in the number of antagonist binding sites. Thus, it appears that [3 H]DOB and [3H]ketanserin binding sites are distinct ligand-affinity states that exist at different times on the same 5-HT2 receptor protein.

The scientific community's increasing molecular understanding of this ligand affinity cycle needs to be better integrated into investigations of receptor function and into drug design programmes. Because a complex interaction cycle involving two separate proteins and several forms of guanine nucleotides is involved in agonist binding, the model systems used as templates for drug design must be carefully chosen and carefully adjusted. They must properly mimic the natural processes occurring in those regions of native human brain that are chosen as a target for drug design. Because the types of G proteins, the relative receptor excess (spare receptors), and the amounts of intracellular guanosine diphosphate (GDP) and guanosine triphosphate (GTP) may vary widely in different brain regions, this complexity should be dealt with from the start of a drug design effort.

Fortunately, the great freedom of choice of cell hosts and transfection densities that is possible when using cloned human receptors allows just the type of experimental freedom needed to address these issues. It also must be kept in mind that two distinct, but partially overlapping, sets of conformational states are involved in antagonist and agonist binding, and it is important to be sure that the proper mix of the proper states is present in biological screening models.

Amino Acid and Pharmacological Homologies Between Receptors

Receptor researchers have traditionally organised their research groups around a specific neurotransmitter or hormone that activates a set of closely related receptors. For example, serotonin clubs and histamine meetings tend to segregate away from neurokinin researchers, even though all three of these biological mediators activate a group of 7TM receptors with many properties in common. Recent advances in molecular understanding of receptor structures suggest that this approach should change. Receptors of the 7TM superfamily are much more closely related in amino acid sequence and function than had been recognised previously. In addition, Hartig and colleagues have found that 7TM receptors of the same family (e.g., serotonin receptors) are often less closely related to each other than they are to other 7TM receptors.

For example, the serotonin 5-HT1A and 5-HT1D receptors are both more homologous to several adrenergic receptors than they are to either the serotonin 5-HT2 or 5-HT1C receptors. Interestingly, this relationship is also reflected in the pharmacological binding properties of these clones. Many compounds that are classically recognised as adrenergic compounds exhibit moderate-to-high affinity for the 5-HT1A receptor, and a similar relationship holds for the 5-HT1D receptor. For example, yohimbine, which is a classic antagonist, exhibits a 25-nM affinity for the 5-HT1D receptor. This value is only sixfold weaker than its affinity at the site.

These molecular homologies have implications that extend beyond nucleotide sequence comparisons into the field of pharmacology. As is true for all proteins, the form of a neurotransmitter receptor determines its function. As a consequence, the pharmacological binding properties of 7TM receptors often cross family lines in ways that are reflected in the amino acid sequences of these receptors.

In general, neurotransmitter receptors that display significant amino acid sequence homologies often display some overlap in the chemical structures that they will bind. Thus, the existence of greater than 50-percent transmembrane amino acid sequence homology should alert researchers to the possibility that receptors from different families may be more closely related in their binding properties than had been previously appreciated. Increased attention to these similarities in sequence and pharmacology could greatly aid the medicinal chemist in efforts to find high-affinity compounds for each receptor subtype and will help establish a much more directed approach to drug design.

Concept of Frament-based Drug Discovery

Fragment-based drug discovery builds drugs from small molecular pieces. It combines the empiricism of random screening with the rationality of structure-based design. Though the concept was articulated decades ago, the approach has become practical only recently.

Historically, most drugs have been discovered by one of two methods. The first of these was famously summarised by Nobel Laureate Sir James Black, who noted that the best way to find a new drug is to start with an existing one. Indeed, any successful drug spawns a surge of similar molecules, as illustrated by the number of chemically similar COX-2 inhibitors or HIV protease inhibitors on the market and in development. Though often disparaged as "me-too" or "patent-busting", such efforts are productive. The first drug to market is rarely the best; one need only consider the state of HIV medication now compared to a decade ago to appreciate this fact. Even the search for new drugs often begins with known starting points in the form of natural ligands such as substrates, co-factors or inhibitors.

For diseases and targets where no drug or other starting point exists, the second major route of drug discovery, random screening, is essential. This approach to drug discovery is perhaps the oldest and most venerable but requires serendipity. Indeed, it was a serendipitous observation of bacterial killing by fungus that led Alexander Fleming to the discovery of the natural product penicillin. Many highly successful drugs, from cyclosporine to paclitaxel, have been discovered by screening collections of compounds. With each medicinal chemistry program, more chemical compounds and their analogs are added to corporate screening libraries.

The invention of combinatorial chemistry in the late 1980s and early 1990s vastly expanded the number of compounds in chemical collections, just as the development of sophisticated automation equipment and miniaturisation of biological assays led to the advent of high-throughput screening, or HTS. Today, most major pharmaceutical companies and many biotechnology companies have inhouse collections of hundreds of thousands or even millions of molecules.

In parallel to HTS, more rational routes for drug discovery have been sought. Structure-based drug design attempts to design inhibitors *in silico* on the basis of the three-dimensional structure of the target protein. Among the latest developments in drug discovery is a concept called fragmentbased drug design, or fragment-based screening (FBS). In contrast to conventional HTS, where fully built, "drug-sized" chemical compounds are screened for activity, FBS identifies very small chemical structures ("fragments") that may only exhibit weak binding affinity. Follow-up strategies are then applied to increase affinity by elaborating these minimal binding elements. Fragment-based drug design thus attempts to build a ligand piece-by-piece, in a modular fashion. Structural information plays a central role in most follow-up strategies. Therefore, fragmentbased drug design can be viewed as the synthesis of random screening and structure-based design.

Features of Fragment-based Ligand Design

Fragment-based screening promises to have a great impact on drug discovery because of several advantages, which are summarised in the following sections.

FBS Samples Higher Chemical Diversity

Typical chemical libraries used for HTS contain 10^5 to 10^6 individual compounds. Though a million-compound library sounds vast, it covers only a very small portion of "drug space", the theoretical set of possible small, drug-like molecules. In fact, a widely quoted estimate places this number at 1063 molecules, a number beyond the comprehension of anyone except perhaps astrophysicists.

A recent estimate of the total number of molecules available for screening in all the commercial and academic institutions on the Earth is around 100 million, or 10^8, so even a planet-wide screening effort would not even scratch the surface of diversity space. This will never change in any meaningful way. To understand why, imagine assembling a library of 10^{63} molecules. Even if miniaturisation advances to the point where we need only 1 pmol of each molecule (about 0.5 ng for a 500-Da molecule), this would still require gathering 5×10^{47} tons of material, roughly 26 orders of magnitude larger than the mass of our planet. Clearly, libraries screened in HTS will always explore only a tiny fraction of drug space.

The explored fraction of diversity space swells when working with smaller molecules ("fragments"), because there are fewer possible small molecules than possible large molecules. If we screen small molecular fragments, rather than drug-sized molecules, we can cover exponentially larger swaths of diversity space with much smaller collections of molecules. To illustrate, imagine two sets of compounds, each consisting of 1000 fragments. If we were to exhaustively make all binary combinations with a single asymmetric linker, this would yield (1000 molecules) × (1000 molecules) = 1 000 000 molecules to synthesize and screen, a daunting task. In contrast, if we could identify the five best fragments in each set and only combine and screen those, we would only need to synthesize and test [(1000 molecules) + (1000 molecules)] + [(5 molecules) × (5 molecules)] = 2025 molecules. This number is clearly much more manageable, and still covers the same chemical diversity space.

A first-principles computational analysis suggests that there are roughly 13.9×10^6 stable, synthetically feasible small molecules with a molecular weight less than or equal to 160 Da (44×10^6 once stereoisomers are considered, although the approach excludes compounds containing three- and four-membered rings and elements other than carbon, hydrogen, oxygen, nitrogen, and halogens). This is still a large number, but it is at least a comprehensible number, especially compared with 10^{63}. It shows that, with fragment-based screening, a higher (although still very small) proportion of diverse drug space can be covered. From a technical standpoint as well, focusing on these smaller fragments could simplify many aspects of the drug discovery process, from compound acquisition and synthesis through data management.

FBS Leads to Higher Hit Rates

Imagine a small fragment with high but imperfect complementarity to a target protein. Now imagine adding a methyl group at exactly the right spot to increase complementarity even further: rendering the fragment more complex in the right manner leads to slightly increased affinity to the target protein. But imagine adding the methyl group at any other spot, so that it protrudes from this fragment towards the receptor such that the modified fragment can no longer bind to the target: rendering the fragment more complex in the "wrong" manner ablates affinity for the receptor. Notably, there are many more ways to increase complexity in the "wrong" manner, and doing so often leads to a decrease of binding affinity by several orders of magnitude, whereas in the lucky case of increasing complexity in the "right" manner, binding is generally only enhanced by one or two orders of magnitude. This simple example makes sense intuitively, and a more rigorous theoretical analysis comes to the same conclusion: as molecules become more complex, additional chemical groups are much more likely to ablate binding than to enhance it. The probability of binding (the "hit rate" in screening) thus decreases with increasing ligand complexity. Libraries containing smaller compounds ("fragments") are expected to exhibit higher hit rates, although the resulting affinities are generally weak and so require sensitive detection methods.

FBS Leads to Higher Ligand Efficiency

Screening drug-sized molecules is thought to favor ligands with several sub-optimal binding interactions, rather than those with a few optimal interactions. This is schematically shown in Fig. 2: the drug-sized molecule on the left side is identified by HTS since it binds to the receptor. However, none of the binding interactions are optimal, since establishing one optimal interaction would disrupt another interaction. All binding interactions are thus compromised and do not retain the full strength they would have without the molecular strain. Relative to their molecular size, fragments can thus show more favorable binding energies than drug-sized molecules. The binding energy, normalised by the number of heavy atoms in the ligand, is referred to by the term ligand efficiency. Smaller fragments can have higher ligand efficiency, leading to smaller drugs with better chances for favorable pharmacokinetics. This concept is also being applied to conventional HTS with the advent of "lead-like", instead of "drug-like," compound libraries.

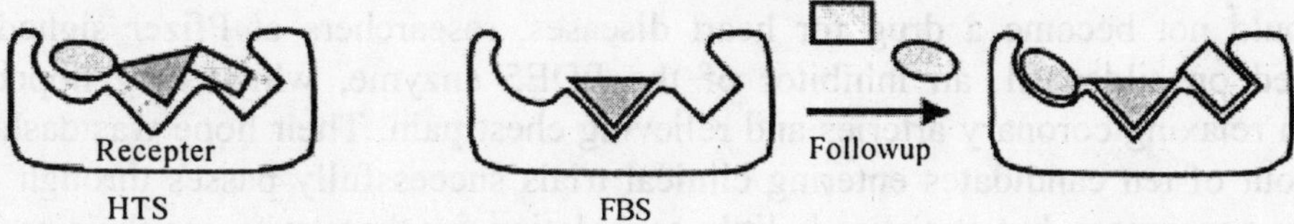

Figure 2. Potential drawback of HTS (left), and principle and advantages of FBS (right): In HTS, fully assembled, "drug-sized" ligands are identified, but with multiple compromised, non-optimal binding interactions.

Historical Development

The basic concept of fragment-based drug discovery was developed about 25 years ago by William Jencks, who wrote in 1981 that the affinities of whole molecules could be understood as a function of the affinities of separate parts:

"It can be useful to describe the Gibbs free energy changes for the binding to a protein of a molecule, A–B, and of its component parts, A and B, in terms of the "intrinsic binding energies" of A and B (ΔG_A^{i} and ΔG_B^{i}) and a "connection Gibbs energy" (ΔG^s) that is derived largely from changes in translational and rotational entropy."

Despite these developments, Jencks' formulation did not immediately have an impact on drug discovery. The practical implementation of the theoretical promise required overcoming two difficult barriers: finding fragments and linking them. Finding weakly binding fragments is inherently difficult because the binding interactions are easily disrupted. Moreover, there are hidden hazards in looking for weak binders: apparent hits could be "false positives". For example, compounds forming aggregates at low to mid-micromolar concentrations can inhibit biochemical functional assays without specifically interacting with the target.

But even if a true weak hit was identified, what could be done with it? Jencks provided an elegant theoretical framework for combining two weakly binding fragments into a single molecule, but enormous practical difficulties remained: First, one had to find a suitable fragment. One then had to find a second fragment; and that second fragment had to bind in close proximity to the first. Finally, one had to figure out how to link these two fragments while not distorting the binding mode of either. It was no wonder that the field remained largely theoretical and computational for well over a decade.

Prepared Mind in Drug Discovery

Chance and accidents play important roles in scientific discoveries, but they are not blind luck. Serendipity is not merely stumbling on things unsought for, it is the ability to see significances and find values in the things stumbled upon. As Pasteur observed: "Chance favors the prepared mind." What are the characteristics of a prepared mind in science? How do chance and serendipity work in scientific research in general and drug discovery in particular?

It would not become a drug for heart diseases, researchers at Pfizer sighed. For years they worked on sildenafil, an inhibitor of the PDE5 enzyme, which they hoped would be effective in relaxing coronary arteries and relieving chest pain. Their hope was dashed by 1992. Only one out of ten candidates entering clinical trials successfully passes through the gauntlet and reaches consumers, but statistics is little consolation for those who see their projects falling on the heap of nine.

Gloomily, the researchers terminated the trial and asked participants to return the unused drug. Many men refused, clutching to the drug as if it was gold. Idiosyncrasies being present in all clinical tests, researchers gave the objection little thought until they heard rumors about the drug's side effects on sex life and, more important, read a paper on the role of PDE5 in the chemical pathway of erection. Gloom evaporated in the excitement that sildenafil may be a blockbuster after all. This time, their expectation was confirmed by new clinical tests on impotent men. They stumbled on an effective drug for erectile dysfunction Pfizer would market as Viagra.

The accidental origin of Viagra is closer to the rule than the exception in drug discovery. Here serendipity – the knack of finding things not sought for – has won many trophies: sulphur drugs, penicillin, chloroform, vitamins, tranquiliser, and cancer drugs. Often several serendipitous discoveries contribute to the establishment of a major therapy. Take for example insulin for diabetes. Chance observation of flies attracted to the sugar-rich urine of experimental dogs with pancreas removed led to the discovery that the pancreas is causally related to diabetes.

Since that discovery in 1889, many scientists tried to extract the pancreas' secretion and use it as a remedy for diabetes. Some almost made it; others failed, but not necessarily because they were more ignorant. When Frederick Banting, Charles Best, and John Macleod succeeded to extract insulin and demonstrate its therapeutic efficacy in 1921, they designed their crucial experiment on a wrong conception. Microbiologist and historian Alexander Kohn observed: "Nearly all the great discoveries in chemotherapy have been made as a result of a false hypothesis or due to a so-called chance observation."

Chance, accidents, and serendipity extend beyond drug discovery to scientific discovery at large. Scientific research delves into the unknown. Like all frontiers, the scientific frontier is not a thin line separating light and darkness. It is a broad zone ranging from pockets of puzzles in mostly settled areas to virgin wilderness penetrated only by a few pioneers. The prevalence of chance correspondingly varies.

For matured topics with well-established principles from which specific results can be deduced, accidents happen but are relatively rare. For example, chance had little to do with the discovery of the planet Neptune. Astronomers noticed that the observed orbit of Uranus deviated from theoretical prediction, attributed the persistent deviation to the gravitational effect of an unknown planet, calculated its trajectory and, knowing when and where in the vast sky to look, found Neptune in 1846. Such process of discovery is a glory of science, but should not be made into the stereotype of scientific discovery.

The possession of theories such as Newtonian mechanics capable of such precise predictions is not a rule in science, especially in sciences dealing with complex phenomena. Furthermore, powerful deductive theories are not omnipotent. Compared to things such as the living body, the solar system is rather simple. Even so, 159 years separated the discovery of Neptune from Newton's Principia, years of hard work engaging the best scientific and mathematical minds. It would take another 84 years for planet Pluto to be observed along its predicted trajectory. A third round, whether a tenth planet exists as theory suggests, still awaits an answer.

Where the frontier of knowledge is wide open, where causes of phenomena mostly hide in the dark, where many scientists deem research most challenging and exhilarating, chance and serendipity play bigger roles. Alexander Becquerel mistakenly developed an unexposed photographic film that sat beneath some uranium salts, saw the salts' image on the film, and discovered radioactivity. Some chance observations led to new sciences or industries. The synthetic dyes industry, one of the forerunners of the modern pharmaceutical industry, traced its origin to the discovery of aniline dye when William Perkin, while washing away some black junk from his failed synthesis of quinine, noticed that the water and washcloth turned purple.

Biochemistry, a backbone of biotechnology and biomedicine, was born in 1897, when chemist Eduard Buchner helped in his brother's microbiology laboratory. He added sugar to some juice extract from yeast cells, just as people did to preserve jams and fruits. Instead of being preserved, the juice started to bubble. Surprised, he investigated and found that the chemical process in fermentation, which had been identified with living beings, also occurs outside the living body in cell-free media. This discovery enabled chemists to study biological processes in test tubes and petri dishes, and the field of biochemistry emerged rapidly. Accounts of these and other serendipitous discoveries in science fill books.

Scientific research proceeds with an infinite variety in the availability of data, the maturity of conceptions, and the mix of conviction and uncertainty. Often a major discovery is the culmination of a process with numerous blunders, wrong turns, false hypotheses, missed opportunities, persistent hard work, lucky breaks, rational arguments, insightful conjectures, and accumulating knowledge over decades. Along this tortuous path fogged by ignorance, chance plays on many occasions.

Scientistfic Treat to Chance

From birth into a certain family and culture, fate accompanies us to our graves. Acknowledging luck tacitly renounces merit. It has a psychological leveling effect on social inequalities, as in the familiar remark about the downtrodden: There but for the grace of God go I. Many people contrast chance with logic. Detractors often use chance discoveries to denigrate science as accidental, irrational, arbitrary, and just another myth. They make at least three mistakes. First, they confuse a step in the research process with the whole process consisting of many steps, sidesteps, and backtracks. Second, they confuse the process of research with the result of research. Third, they confuse rationality with absolute certainty. Uncertainty is a human condition, and rational ways exist to reckon with chance, for instance the probability theory.

The scientific community is mainly meritocratic and rational. However, scientists relish at stories of serendipitous discoveries. Even straight-faced textbooks, which usually contain only technical contents and not their paths of discovery, sometimes cannot resist these stories. Scientists are not shy to admit the role of chance in research because they know that fate does not imply fatalism; chance leaves ample room for determination, effort, and sound judgment. Chance happenings in the process of research do not imply that the results of research are irrational, because accidents must pass many further tests before they are justified as scientific results, if they make it at all. Rationality lies in how one handles chance happenings.

A *eureka* moment, when one realises the solution to a significant problem in a flash of insight, is among the most dramatic of serendipitous discoveries. The eureka idea can be internal or external, depending on whether it happens purely "inside one's head," so to speak, or is triggered by some external events. Sometimes an idea pops up in one's mind, unbidden, under unlikely circumstances. Mathematician Henri Poincaré found a series of Fuchsian functions, for which he had toiled in van for weeks, during a geological excursion. Molecular biologists Kary Mullis told how he invented polymerase chain reaction, which kicked biotechnology into high gear: "The revelation came to me one Friday night in April, 1983, as I gripped the steering wheel of my car and snaked along a moonlit mountain road into northern California's redwood country." In these cases, the idea occurred without external prompting to a mind engaged elsewhere.

The original eureka moment, however, was triggered by the observation of an external event. Legend had it that Archimedes tried hard to find a way to measure the volume of the king's crown, but to no avail. One day when he slipped into a public bath, he noticed that the water spilled over, upon which he jumped out and ran home, dripping wet and crying: Eureka – I have found it. In the chance observation, he realised that he could measure the volume of an irregular object by measuring the volume of the water it displaces.

More often chance encounters trigger not solutions but inspirations, not aha but why. A glass broken but not shattered or a chicken living after a lethal injection presented not answers but intriguing questions. People bump into puzzles all the time, but most simply ignore them, rushing on in their daily businesses. Credits go to the scientists who stop and ponder about the puzzles they stumble upon, recognise their significances, and make effort to pursue the leads to significant discoveries.

"Chance favors the prepared mind," remarked Louis Pasteur, a founder of microbiology who had made several serendipitous discoveries himself. Fruitful ideas do not come in an intellectual vacuum. They may pop up at a bus stop or a mountain road, but Poincaré and Mullis had thought long and hard about their problems. Most accidents that led to discoveries occurred in laboratories, which were themselves designed for explorations. Experiments are different from passive experiences, they are active inquires. An experiment is a question by which scientists try to wrestle answers from nature. The answers may be unexpected, but in setting up experiments, scientists have already primed their minds to pounce on surprises.

We explore the characteristics of a prepared mind in three cases. In the cases of scientists getting their ideas in dreams, we examine the cognitive psychology of thinking and problem solving. The second case we take is one of the most famous serendipitous drug discoveries, that of penicillin. Here we examine how the ability and inability to "connect the dots" facilitated and limited Fleming's contribution to the development of the antibiotic medicine. Many people would consider our third case, drug screening, to be the antithesis of serendipity. Sure, instead of running into something unintentionally, screening set out with the intention to find something. However, it is also fraught with ignorance and depends on sagacity to pick the gems out from the dirt. In screening, the mind is prepared to take chance systematically.

Cognitive Psychology of Serendipitous Discovery

Stories abound about how a scientist got an idea not while working on the problem at issue but while working on something unrelated, relaxing, or even sleeping. For instance, according to the report of his daughter, physiologist Otto Loewi told his the family about a dream in which he got the idea that would later win him a Nobel Price: nerve impulses are transmitted by chemicals.

Many historians, especially those of sociological bend, are skeptical if not hostile to such accounts. Inspirations are private experiences, for which the only evidence are the scientists' own reports. Moreover, they do not fit into the dogma that science is a social construction. Sociological accounts of science often ignore the intellectual dimension of science and treat scientists as mindless things on the same status as scallops and electrons, all being "actants" in the "actant-network model." Inspirations have no place in such models, which prefer to interpret the scientists' reports as fictions fabricated for credit grabbing, self aggrandizement, and other power motives.

Some skepticism is healthy. For example, August Kelulé's discovery of benzene's hexagonal ring structure. The benzene ring is a cornerstone of the structural theory of compounds, which is foundational to organic chemistry and instrumental to the dyes and pharmaceutical industries. Probably Kelulé was prone to dozing off and dreaming. He reported that he had illuminating dreams in two separate occasions during the years when he struggled to work out the structural theory. In the second case, he fell asleep while writing a textbook and had a dreamy image of a chain of twisting atoms bending on itself, a snake biting its tail. Awaken, he dropped the textbook and turned enthusiastically to work out the consequences of the hypothesis that the atoms of benzene form a ring.

Was Kelulé's inspirational dream fact or fiction? He talked about it twenty-eight years after its alleged occurrence, during which no account of it can be found. Amassing circumstantial evidence, some historians conclude that he made it up on ulterior motive. Others disagree. In any case, the dream story continues to circulate widely, especially among chemists. Perhaps many people find Kelulé's dream story plausible because they too have experienced getting ideas in dreams or dozes, although their ideas may not be price winning. Perhaps the persistent circulation reveals something akin to Aristotle's remark that poetry is more philosophical and serious than history because whereas the historian speaks of particulars, things that have happened, the poet speaks of universals, kinds of thing that can happen. Perhaps more important than whether someone did dream is the common psychology of learning and discovery expressed by Kelulé's dream story.

In the state between sleep and awakening, when we have those dreams that we remember, ideas and images occur to us. Most of them are silly, but not necessarily all. It is not impossible that some ideas are answers to questions that worry us. In our daily life, we sometimes encounter something that makes no sense despite our wrecking our brains on it, only to become obvious later and make us wonder in retrospect: How could I be so stupid? Understanding, the transformation from opacity to clarity, involves much effort and is often a prolonged process of knowledge accumulation, but it is often not continuously conscious. "Let me sleep on it" is a common response to a puzzle. We may put it away or have forgotten about it. The answer may emerge gradually or quite abruptly. Sometimes, perhaps prompted by a tiny cue, perhaps as a surprise, the solution pops out. Such phenomena are expressed in common idioms: it strikes me, it dawns on me, it occurs to me. Our newly gained insight may be trivial or an old hat to others. However, our experiences in gaining them make us resonate with scientists' accounts of understanding something new or making unexpected discoveries, perhaps in unexpected circumstances.

The skeptics' strongest argument is that two years before Kelulé's 1856 paper, benzene had already been depicted as a hexagon in a book by French chemist A. Laurent, which Kelulé knew and proposed to translate into German. Did the depiction undermine Kelulé's claim to originality? Apparently not. In line drawings, a circle can mean either a disc or a ring; the ambiguity can only be resolved by context. Laurent used the hexagon in the same page to represent benzene, benzoyl chloride, and ammonia, whose structure was a pyramid. Accompanying explanations suggested that his hexagon depicted not a ring structure but was simply the artist's rendition of a molecule as a chunk capable to bind with other chunks.

A hexagon with "Bz" on it printed in a chemistry book was a suggestive image. Why did it fail to inspire Laurent himself of the benzene ring structure? Why did it fail to inspire Kelulé on the spot? Why did he have to wait for his snake dream? No one can answer this question, but one can venture some guesses. Perhaps his research was not advanced enough. Cognitive psychologists have found that what one sees is at once more and less than what strikes the eyes, being influenced by the meaning one anticipates or attributes to it. Some experiments on vision find that when reading, we see the meanings and not the shapes of the words. Readers of Laurent's diagram may simply see a chunk and never see the alternative interpretation of a ring. This is not unusual. Serendipitous discoveries often involve a phenomenon that many people have encountered before one person sees it in a new light and recognises its significance.

Skeptics claimed that Kelulé got the benzene-ring idea from Laurent's diagram and invented the dream story to avoid giving credit to the French, whom the German loathed in that time of rampant nationalism. Such accounts of "the social construction of science" are now popular. They are not impossible, but not more probable than the dream story. Let us assume for argument's sake that Kelulé did get a mental jolt from Laurent's diagram. Does this imply that he stole credit on a sociological motive? Or could he have honestly forgotten the origin of his inspiration? Again cognitive psychology can help. Whatever jolt Kelulé got could not be strong, because he took more than a year to publish the benzene theory. During this time the source of the hexagonal image may have faded from memory.

Memory researchers have found that attributing an idea or a piece of information to a wrong source is very common. Many people misremembered how they got the news even for such memorable events as the Kennedy assassination or space shuttle Challenger explosion. With no intention whatsoever to lie, eyewitnesses sometimes mistake what they heard afterwards for what they saw on the crime scene. Misattribution is a weakness for memory per se. However, cognitive psychologists argue that it has evolved because it can also be beneficial to a person as a whole. Human memory capacity is limited. Most although not all sources are quite irrelevant to the contents of information, and forgetting them spares scare mental resources for tasks more important for survival. The cognitive psychology of memory provides an alternative explanation to nationalism-motivated lying: Kelulé did not refer to Laurent because he had a lapse in source memory. They also help us to understand the unending credit disputes in the scientific community. In a culture where people freely exchange ideas and tidbits thereof, many halfbaked, it is not surprising that a scientist has an idea and, not remembering where it came from, claims it his own.

The role of the unconscious in scientific creativity is emphasized by cognitive psychologists and reflective scientists. One cognitive psychological model roughly divides a discovery process into four stages. During the familiarisation stage, the scientist toils consciously to acquire relevant knowledge and solve the problem. This is followed by an incubation stage, when consciousness turns to something else but the unconscious mind continues to dwell on the problem. Unconscious processes may lead to a eureka moment with an illuminating insight. The eureka moment, however, is not the moment of truth; for more often than not, the eureka turns out to be a blah. In the final stage, the scientist deliberately scrutinises the insight and, if it is valid, develops it into a solution of the problem.

Unconscious incubation of ideas sounds vague. However, it has received certain substantiation from cognitive science. In the past several decades, cognitive psychologists and neuroscientists have uncovered vast infrastructures that underlie our conscious mind. Our vision is not like a camera taking in whole pictures. Our memory is not like a stamp on a wax tablet or a file on a computer hard disc, stored and retrieved in one piece. They are far more complex and rightly so; we understand what we see and remember, the camera and computer do not. Simply seeing a balloon or recalling a birthday party involves an incredibly large amount of processing that shape our conscious experience, because it is their end product. We are unaware of these processing, which occur in split seconds and faster. Some of these unconscious processes constitute implicit learning and implicit memory, currently hot topics in cognitive psychology.

Suppose you are reading a paper. Processing starts as soon as light hits your retina, and information does not simply flow one way from the eyes up to the brain. Stored concepts and knowledge are activated by your anticipation and meaning of the previous sentence. Partly under their influence, the current visual input is analyzed into various aspects, processed further, and its gist extracted and partially combined into facets of meaningful objects or concepts. The processing facilitates categorization and understanding at the price of leaving out many details in the input.

The result of visual processing goes through the hippocampus, the brain's memory center. Then its various facets split to be stored in various parts of the brain, leaving a kind of index in the hippocampus to facilitate retrieval. Recollection of an event involves retrieving its bits and pieces and combining them into a memory. Retrieval mechanisms are mainly associative; the word "bank" associatively activates "money" or "river," depending on context. Because association can vary with the cue or strategy of remembering, the activated memory can also vary.

Associative processes are also responsible for false recognition, in which people recognise things that they did not encounter or recall imagined events as experienced. A memory can be distorted by repeated retrieval under various conditions, as some associations are strengthened and some weakened. The weakest links eventually drop out, resulting in things forgotten. All these memory processing proceed without our awareness. They are implicit, as cognitive psychologists say.

Analytic processing, gist extraction, and associative activation are information processing mechanisms hardwired into our brains. Without our awareness, they work for the most ordinary of our daily experiences. Their peculiarities are also favorable to scientific and other creativity. False recognition and memory distortion are flaws. However, the associative processes responsible for false recognition can also generate valuable novel links among ideas. The distortion of repetitive memory retrieval can also facilitate selective winnowing of unimportant factors. Connecting ideas and selective forgetting are two processes scientists identify to be crucial to the unconscious incubation that give birth to illuminating insights and serendipitous discoveries.

Connecting the Dots

The person who stumbles on an event, recognises its novelty, and publishes a factual description of it, makes a discovery. However, the rudimentary discovery has little impact if it is not connected to other phenomena, for only in connections are causality explained and significances fully revealed. Making connections, which develops and exploits a discovery, often requires much more knowledge, insight, and effort than the initial description of event. It can lead to a much bigger discovery.

Serendipitous connection of dots led to the discovery that vaccination is a general method for preventing infectious diseases. It occurred during Pasteur's struggle to establish the germ theory of disease, specifically in the case of chicken cholera. To demonstrate that chicken cholera was caused by germs and not some toxins in the blood, it was important to isolate germs from toxins, which was very difficult in those early days. To purify germs, Pasteur extracted them from diseased chickens, grew them in cultures outside the body, and injected the culture into healthy chickens, which would become sick and a new source of germs, hopefully less contaminated with toxins. An autumn day in 1879, he injected a culture into some chickens and found them to be hardly affected. Later, because of a mix up or shortage of supply, the "used" chickens were recycled, together with some new chickens, in experiments to test a fresh virulent culture. This time the new chickens all died but the lucky recycled chickens remained unscathed. A colleague recalled that when Pasteur heard of this surprising development, he "remained silent for a minute, then exclaimed as if he had seen a vision: 'Don't you see that these animals have been vaccinated!'"

Pasteur accidentally obtained the stale culture, according to the traditional account. This account is disputed by historians. However, the dispute changes neither the crux of the discovery nor its serendipitous nature. The major accident in the story was reusing the chickens for a second injection. It led to the serendipitous discovery, which resided less in the source of the stale culture than in the recognition of its effectiveness as a vaccine and the general applicability of vaccination.

Vaccination itself was not new. Chinese and Indians since the eleventh century had been inoculating scabs of smallpox pustules to prevent smallpox infection. The practice passed through Constantinople into Europe around 1700. It was popular there in 1798 when physician Edward Jenner, based on the observation that English cow maids exposed to cowpox were immune to smallpox, introduced "vaccine" derived from cowpox. Smallpox vaccination was accepted strictly based on empirical success, and as such it did not point to the possibility of vaccines for other diseases.

Jenner, perhaps inspired by inoculation, discovered the factual connection between dots: cowpox vaccine and smallpox prevention. Pasteur discovered the theoretical connection between three groups of dot, each represented by a concept. His discovery turned vaccination from a peculiar procedure for a particular disease to a theory connecting germs, vaccines, and disease prevention in general. One no longer needs to wait for a lucky observation to suggest a vaccine for a specific disease. The fruitful idea that a vaccine for a disease can be developed by tinkering on the germs that caused it unleashed a flood of experiments designed to develop vaccines for various infectious diseases.

The first success was Pasteur's vaccine for anthrax, which is discussed in the following chapter. He justifiably asserted: "to look at things solely from the scientific point of view, the discovery of these anthrax vaccines constitutes a considerable advance over the Jennerian vaccine against smallpox, for the latter has never been obtained experimentally." Experiments are not passive observations; they are actively planned according to some conception to look for something.

Prepared and Open Mind

Chance unlocks a door. Most people just walk pass. A few with prepared mind open door and look inside the room. However, without an open mind ready to exploit new possibilities and connect the dots, one may not discover that the room hides more doors that lead to even greater treasures. An interesting case of luck without open mind is the discovery of penicillin, not only as a bacteria-killing mould but also as an antibiotic drug.

The mould story is well known. Alexander Fleming inoculated several dishes with the bacteria staphylococcus, forgot to cover them up, and left for a vacation in the summer of 1928. When he returned, one of the dishes was contaminated by a patch of mould. Observing that the bacteria around the mold were all dead, he had the mould identified as Penicillium, extracted its juice, determined its antibacterial effect, and named it penicillin. Luck graced the incidence in many places. The mould that landed on Fleming's bacteria was not ordinary Penicillium; if it were it would not have produced enough penicillin to have visible effects. It was a rare strand extraordinarily productive in antibacterial substance. The substance is effective only when bacterial colonies are quite young.

Bacteria grow quickly in summer heat. However, London that summer had a string of nine exceptionally cool days that slowed bacteria growth for the mould's effectiveness. Right mould at the right place at the right time, fortune did smile on Fleming. However, his discovery was not a mere chance; no scientific discovery is. A person with unprepared mind would wash out the penicillin with the dirty dish. In contrast, Fleming tried various ways to concentrate it, classified it as a slow-acting antiseptic, and promoted it as a laboratory reagent to differentiate and select microbes.

Fleming was not the first to come across Penicillium. Joseph Lister, the father of antiseptic, noticed the antiseptic effect of Penicillium and used it topically to treat a wound in 1884. Fleming went beyond Lister in two important ways. He published a paper on penicillin and gave out samples of his mould to several microbiologists. One of these samples, cultivated as laboratory reagent over a decade in Oxford University, would take part in experiments to realise penicillin's therapeutic value. Serendipitous discoveries often involve a phenomenon that many people have encountered before one person sees it in a new light and recognises its significance.

The major significance of penicillin is its efficacy as an internal medicine against infectious diseases. This significance neither Lister nor Fleming saw; both stopped at its potential as a topical antiseptic. Penicillin's therapeutic property was discovered by Howard Florey, Ernest Chain, and their Oxford team in 1940, around the time when the British expeditionary force in Dunkirk barely escaped annihilation by German panzers. The property was developed by a huge effort, mostly in the United States, which turned penicillin into an antibiotic drug by the time the Allies invaded Normandy to begin the end of Hitler's reign.

Capitalising on people's gratitude for the miracle drug that saved countless lives, the popular media constructed a sensational but misinformed image of all glory to Fleming the heroic genius. When the 1945 Nobel Prize for penicillin was awarded, however, it was equally divided among Chain, Fleming, and Florey. Since then a puzzle persists and incites arguments from many colleagues, biographers, and historians: After he discovered the wonder mould, Fleming could have pressed on to discover the wonder drug, thus saving many lives during the years when the mould sat on the shelf. Why didn't he? It was not that he tried in vain to explore penicillin's therapeutic property; all historical evidence showed that he hardly even tried. What stopped him?

Chain suggested that Fleming did not perform the simple experiment of injecting penicillin into infected mice to test its therapeutic effect not because he was unable to but "because he did not think it was worth while trying." If so, Fleming made not a value but a technical judgment. Antibiotic medicines were very worthwhile to him. He wrote in 1918, moved by the sight of soldiers dying of infection: "I was consumed by the desire to discover . . . something which would kill these microbes, something like salvarsan." He was among the first Britons to test salvarsan, a drug for syphilis and other infections. However, later when penicillin into his lap, all he proffered were data on its instability and nontoxicity and a few trials to apply it topically on shallow wounds. How did his consuming desire for antibiotic drugs reconcile with his indifference to the golden opportunity of developing one – if he realized it was an the opportunity?

One reason for failing to connect the dots of penicillin and antibiotic therapy, attested by Fleming himself, was that he was a microbiologist and lacked the chemical expertise to perform the requisite experiments. Relevant knowledge is essential for scientific investigation, not the least for therapeutic properties, which are subtle and difficult to ascertain. Here Chain, a biochemist, and Florey, a pathologist with chemical training, had definite advantages. Their expertise enabled them to probe penicillin in a deeper level to reveal its therapeutic potentials. "Penicillin" for Fleming referred to the crude extract, which was just the filtered broth in which the mould was grown. After Florey and Chain, "penicillin" refers to the purified chemical compound that is the active principle of Fleming's mould juice. The latter meaning facilitated precise measurement, experimentation, scientific understanding, and practical manipulation. In this regard, Fleming was disadvantaged in expertise.

Nevertheless, Fleming's the disadvantage was not debilitating. As Chain pointed out, many animal experiments required little chemical expertise and were completely within Fleming's repertoire. Furthermore, it is not unusual for a scientist to lack competence for solving a particular problem, for scientists are mostly specialists and interesting problems often involve factors in widely disparate domains. Under such situations, common practices are to seek collaborators or hire assistants to complement one's own resource. Fleming did it too. He consulted a fungi expert to identify the godsend mould as Penicillium. His two young assistants were not ignorant of biochemistry. They made significant progress in concentrating the mould juice and performing biochemical experiments. Despite their eagerness, Fleming gave them little support, assigned them elsewhere after a few months, and threw their results into a drawer, unpublished.

Proponents of the lonely-hero image blamed people for ignoring Fleming's claim on penicillin antiseptic, as if he had worked to generate interest. Attention is a scarce commodity that one must fight to attract, and one must fight harder to win support and collaboration. Interesting problems abound and everyone is busy. It is incumbent on scientists to make effort in bringing out the importance of their own discoveries to drum up enthusiasm. Where Fleming tried, he succeeded. His paper "On the antibacterial action of cultures of a Penicillium with special reference to their use in the isolation of B. Influenz" emphasized the use of penicillin as a laboratory reagent. For this use he had interested several microbiologists. It was very different with medicinal potentials. Only at the very end did the paper state briefly: "It is suggested that it [penicillin] may be an efficient antiseptic for application to, or injection into, areas infected with penicillin-sensitive microbes." In the many papers he wrote during following twelve years, only one mentioned penicillin's medical future, that it would be likely to be "used in the treatment of septic wounds."

These were Fleming's strongest medical claim for penicillin. They suggested only topical treatment of wounds. Even as antiseptic, his claim remained speculative; he gave up finding empirical supports after a few unsuccessful trials. When the author considers his own claim not worth the effort to substantiate, the reader can hardly be blamed for shrugging. Some sociologists suggest that people were indifferent because Fleming was a poor speaker.

Social skills are important for anyone, scientists including, but scientific persuasion should not be confused with snake-oil salesmanship. In rational arguments, solid data and sound reasons are more eloquent than flowery rhetoric. Anyone can say, this stuff here will make a good drug, but the conjecture is empty without evidence that the stuff can satisfy stringent conditions of efficacy and safety. Evidence for the stuff's therapeutic properties is laborious to gather. Florey and Chain made the effort that Fleming spared. Their paper "Penicillin as a chemotherapeutic agent" generated more enthusiasm than Fleming's paper not because their prose was better;

Fleming wrote well and clearly. Their claim of antibiotic therapy was more significant than Fleming's suggestion of antiseptic. More important, they backed up their claim with substantial data on a series of controlled animal experiments. Lack of evidence, not lack of words, was what harmed Fleming's case most. Fleming was enthusiastic about Florey and Chain's paper.

The adversity is more cultural than administrative. Fleming, as professor and assistant director of the department, had considerable freedom to choose his research, which he exercised in studying salvarsan and sulfanilamide. However, probably his choices were biased by his department's communal belief that vaccination was the only way to fight infectious diseases and internal medicine was hopeless. The paralysing pessimism on antibiotic medicine was local to Fleming's community.

Drug therapy was difficult and had suffered many setbacks, but its failure was far from total. Salvarsan, the syphilis drug Fleming once earned to emulate, was ineffective for some cases and difficult to administer, but at least it offered some hope for some patients. The scientific community at large had not despaired of improvements. Several months before Fleming discovered penicillin, Gerhard Domagk at Bayer quietly started a painstaking screening program that would result in the discovery of the first effective antibacterial drug, sulfanilamide.

Both scientists had access to the literature, but they made diametrically opposite technical judgments about the feasibility of antibacterial medicine. Scientific research is always risky and fraught with setbacks, therapeutic research especially so. Domagk judged the risk worthwhile and his optimistic commitment sustained him through countless failures for almost four years. He might not have won the Nobel Prize had Fleming proceeded to develop penicillin that, being superior to sulfanilamide, would have preempted his result. Fortunately for him although not for victims of infection, Fleming gave up at the tiniest negative result, imbued with the pessimism of his local communal belief. Citing Fleming's predicament, Chain said it was "a good example of how preconceived ideas in science can stifle imagination and impede progress."

Preconceived ideas are not themselves bad; in fact, they are necessary for any inquiry. Without some hunch that it might be significant, Fleming would have simply washed the Penicillium with the dirty dish. Albert Einstein asked: "If the researcher went about his work without any preconceived opinion, how should he be able at all to select out those facts from the immense abundance of the most complex experience, and just those which are simple enough to permit lawful connections to become evident?" To investigate the unknown, one must make some initial conjectures; otherwise, one cannot even decide what direction to look. However, scientists must be ready to criticise and modify their preconceived ideas. Examples abound of research born on wrong conjectures leading to important results. Here the disparate responses of Fleming and the Oxford team to similar evidence are illuminating. Neither party was initially interested in therapy.

Difficulties for internal medicine were well known. The worst was toxicity: substances powerful enough to kill germs in the body were thought likely to be too toxic for the patient. Fleming and the Oxford team both injected some penicillin into mice and found it nontoxic. These initial nontoxicity results were not definitive, because the dosages were not certain, and in medicine, dosage makes the poison. Nevertheless, they were first shots directed at the Achilles heel of any preconceived idea about the impossibility of drug therapy. Chain considered their nontoxicity result the most important data that turned the team toward penicillin as chemotherapy and motivated subsequent experiments. Fleming reported his result and did nothing more. Science is impeded not by preconceived ideas but by the failure to challenge them in light of evidence.

A blank mind is an impotent mind, not a prepared mind. A prepared mind has preconceived ideas but is simultaneously eager to seek alternatives and ready to change. Dale, Nobel laureate for discovering neurotransmitters, had also reflected on the nature of scientific research. He wrote that chance favors "him who, while continuously busy with the work of research, does not close his attention from matters outside his principal aims and immediate objective but keeps it alert to what unexpected observation they may have to offer."

Several conditions make chance prominent in drug discovery. Animal bodies, medicines, and their interactions are so complex as to defy complete understanding despite tremendous scientific advancement. For a long time they stayed in almost total darkness. Ignorance, however, did not quell people's craving for something to relieve sickness and suffering. In desperation they leveraged what little knowledge they possessed to the fullest and took risk to try new things.

Memories of the errors they made and the prices they paid linger in the word "pharmacy," the Greek pharmakos meant both remedy and poison. Fortunately not all accidents were fatal; some led to valuable solutions. By trial and empiricism, our ancestors in various cultures accumulated knowledge on diagnostics, prognostics, and medicines. Many folk remedies are placebos, many are effective, and many are still in use. Their increasing popularity in western countries as alternative medicine irritates some mainstream physicians.

A drug is a chemical that is effective and safe in treating a disease or its symptoms, hence drug therapy is also known as chemotherapy, as distinct from surgery, radiotherapy, or physical therapy. The first drugs were chemicals isolated from herbs of known effectiveness, for instance the painkiller morphine from opium and the malarial drug quinine from cinchona bark. The apothecaries that produced them capitalised on the fruits of eons of chance discoveries to become a cornerstone of the pharmaceutical industry. Besides nature, drugs have a second source in chemical laboratories that combine atoms and molecules to synthesize novel compounds.

Manufacturers of fine chemicals, especially dyes, became another cornerstone of the pharmaceutical industry. Nature offers millions of herbs and organisms, chemists can synthesize as many compounds. How to find in this haystack of substances the few with therapeutic potentials? Four Gs –Geduld, Geschick, Glück, and Geld (patience, skill, luck, and money) – were the answers offered by Paul Ehrlich, commonly acknowledged to be the father of chemotherapy. Based on the observation that different dyes stuck specifically to different kinds of cell, he developed around the turn of the twentieth century a "receptor theory" of specific chemicals binding to specific receptor sites on cells. A drug molecule, especially a toxin, could bind to a bacterium and kill it.

The receptor theory, which would become a foundation of pharmacology half a century later, was speculative in his time. Nevertheless, it encouraged him to synthesize hundreds of arsenic compounds and test them against bacteria that cause syphilis, a major scourge of his time. Working together with Sahachiro Hata, they discovered in 1909 the drug salvarsan. The systematic way in which Ehrlich screened and explored the biological activities of a class of chemicals to target a specific disease set the paradigm of drug discovery in industry. A similar screening program would lead Domagk to discover the precursor of sulfanilamide in 1932. Dumb and dull at first blush, screening appears to be the opposite of serendipity. Yet of the three elements of serendipity – chance, sagacity, and inadvertency – it lacks only the third. Luck is crucial; both salvarsan and sulfanilamide were near misses.

The screening approach is a deliberate attempt to make chance discoveries. Acknowledging that the inability to predict compound actions makes one dependent on chance to find effective drugs, scientists increase their chance of success by effort. Screening efforts are laborious but not blind; scientists employ whatever knowledge they have to design effective search strategies. It is like trawling for fish, the chance of a catch increases if one has the sagacity to refine the net and find a good place to cast it. Nature is a vast repository.

Soil microbiologist Selman Waksman started in 1939 to screen soil microbes for activities against pathogenic bacteria. Over the years his group isolated and tested some 10,000 cultures, from which came 10 drugs. The most important was streptomycin for tuberculosis, for which he won the Nobel Prize. This was only the beginning of massive screening programs. Sponsored by pharmaceutical firms, government agencies, and universities, bioprospectors combed every corner of Earth to collect samples from the land, air, and sea, sometimes guided by the wisdom of folk medicines.

From nature's cornucopia came the leads to most antibiotics, immunosuppressants, anticancer substances, and over a hundred of the most important drugs. Then in the 1970s, the number of new substances plummeted. After screening literally millions of soil microorganisms, new tests kept turning up the same old stuff. Nature is bountiful but exhaustible. The pendulum swung back to the other source of drugs, synthetic chemicals. Medicinal chemists had synthesized many drug-like compounds over the decades. Their productivity was boosted since the late 1980s by combinatorial chemistry, which can generate new compounds a thousand times faster at lower costs.

Libraries of millions of chemical compounds are amassed in industrial and academic laboratories. Computers, robotics, miniaturisation, and other technologies of automation enable researches to process them efficiently. High throughput screening can handle 100,000 compounds a day. Massive screening is not necessarily blind screening. Arbitrary searches through the greatest libraries had been tried with dismal results. Much more productive is focused screening, which is guided by scientific knowledge to concentrate on smaller libraries with relevant themes. Chance needs the help of knowledge in drug discovery.

Drug therapy involves the interaction between therapeutic chemicals and living bodies. So far, we have looked only at the chemical side. Equally important is the biological side, the body and its functions and malfunctions. Knowledge from the life sciences, especially microbiology, biochemistry, and molecular biology, become increasingly important in pharmacology. Ehrlich likened a potent drug to a magic bullet.

A bullet can work its magic only if aimed at the proper target. The targets for infectious diseases are apparent after the establishment of the germ theory in late nineteenth century. They are alien bacteria tracked down by microbe hunters and cultured in laboratory dishes so convenient for target practice. But where do the magic bullets aim in diseases such as cancer or ulcer? The question cannot be answered without some knowledge of disease mechanisms. Without such knowledge, drug discovery relies on mere empiricism, finding things that work without knowing why they work.

The body is a huge chemical factory with myriad biochemical pathways – chains of biochemical reactions – that maintain the normal physiology of life. Sometimes, an errant link in the chain causes a pathway to malfunction, resulting in a disease. Then a cure may lie in repairing the link and recovering the pathway's normal function. Errant links in biochemical pathways present targets for drugs. To identify them require detail knowledge about the pathways, which come from biochemistry.

Since Buchner demonstrated fermentation outside of the living body in 1896, biochemistry progressed fast. By the 1970s it was matured enough to step into the center stage of pharmacology. Biochemists identify many macromolecules that control strategic links in the body's biochemical pathways. Pharmacologists choose as drug targets those macromolecules whose mechanisms are susceptible to intervention by small chemical molecules. Drug therapy currently works on about 500 targets.

About a quarter of known drug target are enzymes that facilitate crucial chemical reactions. An example is the COX2 enzyme, which aspirin blocks to relieve pain and inflammation, as we saw in the preceding chapter. About one-half of drug targets are receptors on cells, as Ehrlich predicted half a century ago. Receptors are macromolecules that sit on the surface of a cell and are crucial to the normal functions of healthy bodies. A specific kind of receptor receives specific chemical messengers from other parts of the body that regulate a specific process in the cell. If that process goes wrong in sickness, a drug can hopefully set it right by binding to its regulating receptors. Genes can also be drug targets, although their numbers are rather small at present. The impact of genetics in pharmacology is increasing dramatically since the 1990s.

Genomics, which has sequenced the human genome, and proteomics, which aims to catalog and unravel all human proteins, hold out promises for 5,000 or more potential drug targets. Practical therapeutic exploitation of these targets, however, requires much more research into their physiological roles and interactions with drug-like chemicals. Disease mechanisms, targeted remedial actions, and other scientific concepts turn drug discovery from mere empiricism to rational empiricism. Previously, people tried anything without any prior idea whether it would work. Trial and error still plays a major role, but now it is guided by partial knowledge of drug targets. Knowledge of a target's structure gives pharmacologists some idea of what the new drug should be like.

Drug discovery takes on a sense of rational design. It costs around $800 million and 10 to 15 years to develop a new drug and bring it to market. With so much money and patience are at stake, people make utmost effort to complement luck. Suppose after considering medical, financial, social, and technical factors, the decision is made to find a drug for a specific disease. A typical process begins with identifying the potential targets and confirming that the chosen targets are indeed critical to the disease mechanisms. Target selection and validation draw on knowledge in pharmacology, biochemistry, and increasingly molecular biology.

A drug target is a macromolecule and is often compared to a lock. Given a target, the next step is to find a key for it and for it alone; a key that fits also into other locks would generate unwanted side effects. Researchers usually, although not necessarily, begin with screening the appropriate chemical libraries to search for leads – chemicals that roughly fit the target. Leads are like appropriate blanks for a lock. To cut the blanks into a key, researchers must optimise the lead chemicals. They synthesize hundreds of chemicals that vary on a lead's basic structure and test them in animal models.

Besides therapeutic effectiveness and toxicity, they also look for variants that are better absorbed, metabolised, distributed, and excreted. After many iterations of tinkering and testing, they find a candidate ready to be tried in human beings. This preclinical phase of drug development consumes on the average about five years and a third of the costs. The clinical trials, which come in three phase, each engaging ten times more subjects than the preceding one, take another five or six years and about half of the costs. They knock out ninety percent of the candidates; what work in mice do not necessarily work in humans. Finally, the triumphant few obtain approval from government regulators to go to physicians and patients. Drug design guided by knowledge of targets has produced an abundance of diverse drugs. Familiar ones are ulcer drugs (Tagamet) and statins that reduce cholesterol (Lipitor and Zocor).

Less familiar ones are the leukemia drug Gleevec and several drugs for HIV/AIDS. Development of HIV drugs reveals how much drug targets have been refined since Fleming's days. Microbe hunters pinned down the Human Immunodeficiency Virus as the culprit of Acquired Immunodeficiency Syndrome in 1983. Antibiotics kill germs but not viruses. A virus, being less than a cell, cannot reproduce on its own.

To reproduce, it must sneak into a cell, merge into its DNA, and commandeer its facilities. This viral reproductive process is susceptible to attack at several points. Investigation of HIV's life cycle identified three targets. They led to three types of drug, now making up the expensive therapeutic cocktails that, although short of a cure, enable many AIDS patients in the developed world to lead a normal life for a long time. The first drug target is an enzyme that enables the HIV virus to incorporate its genetic material into the human DNA.

Inhibiting this enzyme is the job of AZT and other drugs. The second target is an enzyme that produces the protein essential for the HIV to replicate. Drugs such as Viracept are designed to suppress this enzyme. The third and newest class of drugs targets a receptor through which the HIV makes its way into a human cell, thereby denying entry to the virus. These drugs were developed by methods ranging from empiricism to computer-aided design. AZT resulted from an extensive screening of natural products, which found a lead in a substance derived from salmon sperm. Viracept is an outstanding case for designing a drug almost from scratch using computer modeling, based on knowledge of the structure of the target enzyme and the mechanisms of interaction between the target and potential drug chemicals.

Designing from scratch remains an ideal that boasts only a few successes besides HIV drugs. Most drug development projects employ a rational mix of empiricism and theory: focused screening yields leads, which are optimised by computer modeling. It is estimated that for each marketable drug, hundreds of thousands of compounds are screened or synthesized. The rejects are not total wastes, however. Some of them have been extensively scrutinised before they are discarded, and knowledge about them remains and can be exploited for other drugs. This is a source of serendipity in drug discovery. A substance intended for one disease sometimes turns out to be efficacious for another instead. The chemical active in AZT was originally developed for cancer therapy, and that in Viagra was for heart ailment. Screening for antibiotics turned up substances with surprising uses, for instance in drugs that suppress the body's immune system and prevent it from attacking alien organs, thus revolutionising organ transplantation. The unexpected values of failed chemicals would be missed by the one-track minded. To recognise them, as in all chance discoveries, researchers must be open to areas sometimes quite distant from their core expertise.

Productivity for drug discovery declines recently. Increases in research funding are not matched by increases in the number of new drugs. Perhaps this is a manifestation of what economists call the law of diminishing return. Perhaps most "soft targets" have already fallen, leaving chronic diseases such as cancer, which are much more difficult to treat. Molecular biology, biotechnology, and genomics create waves of optimism, but spectacular scientific successes have so far led only to modest therapeutic successes. Of course researchers should be prepared to criticise and modify their approaches. To blame science for "the fall of modern medicine," however, is unfair. Perhaps the case of biotechnology is similar to that of information technology.

Computers proliferated in the 1970s. Although they were supposed to make people work more efficiently, productivity of the national economy was anemic for two decades. As late as the early 1990s, a Nobel laureate economist quipped that one saw information technology everywhere, except in productivity. Then productivity perked up in the late 1990s, grew with a vengeance and did not subside during the subsequent recession. Economists attribute most of the growth to information technology, which finally bears fruit after climbing a steep learning curve. Chance favors a prepared mind. Success favors an open and persevering mind.

Technology in Drug Discovery

Many disease states still remain untreated or are currently treated by agents whose side-effect profile leaves significant cause for concern. The aging of the population, partly a result of the availability of more effective medications, has presented additional challenges in therapeutic agent development, with an urgent need for drugs to treat arthritis, cancer, neurodegeneration, and cognition impairment. However, the process of drug discovery is complex and costly, and innovative science is especially so. But drug discovery is more than the application of basic research knowledge and technologies; it involves many facets of project management and focus.

To precisely define the drug discovery process and the parameters crucial to success is a difficult task. For each successful drug there are many accounts, both corporate and scientific, as to the process and the visionaries and facilitators involved in bringing the compound to the marketplace. Overviews of the drug research and development (R&D) processes have been complemented by insightful case studies for several important drugs. Given the proprietary nature of the drug discovery process, the failures, the blind alleys, and the persistence that are such an important part of the drug discovery environment and that can account for up to 80 percent of the corporate research effort are rarely documented. Thus, the database from which to derive lessons that may aid in the implementation of new projects is limited.

The commercial focus of the drug discovery process equates the success of a project with a product and rarely with the successful testing of a hypothesis that results in the advancement of scientific knowledge. Given that discovery is a process of "learning things not already known", success is equally tenable when a project is terminated for technical or competitive reasons, resulting in the avoidance of further "sunk costs".

A uniform strategy for the drug discovery process has remained elusive despite considerable analysis. Like the science on which the drug discovery process is based, the approach to a problem involves many paths, with considerable trial and error. Strategies for drug discovery are dependent on interrelated factors that include:

— Corporate, research, and marketing department cultures
— Individual scientists working within a company
— Synergies among various research disciplines
— Morale and quality of research management
— R&D leadership
— Individual and corporate experience
— Extent to which the management of a company is accustomed to risk
— Serendipity
— A particular company's market franchise (the therapeutic areas in which it markets drugs)

Inevitably, many drugs are described in terms of the individuals who were associated with championing the research effort, often against considerable scientific and corporate odds. Although making for interesting (and often exciting) reading, drug discovery is inevitably a team effort requiring constant iteration based on experimental findings, planning, and synergies across many different scientific, development, and marketing disciplines.

The drug discovery and development process can be divided into distinct steps that interface with each other. The first step involves deciding on a given therapeutic target, which entails an iterative process involving the current state of the understanding of disease etiology, scientific knowledge and available technology, unmet medical need, and commercial opportunity.

In diseases such as hypertension, for which there are many effective medications already in the marketplace, new programmes directed at this target must focus on significant additional benefits. For agents being developed for diseases such as Alzheimer's disease (AD) or cancer, for which there are currently no effective or safe treatments, the decision to target the disease state is an easier one to justify even though the science involved represents a significantly greater risk.

Once a decision has been made to target a particular therapeutic area, diseases within the given area can be evaluated and prioritised based on the existence of potential molecular targets, existing technologies (both in-house and external) and scientific expertise, competitive aspects of the marketplace, project maturity (and time to market), unmet need, ease of clinical trials, and so on. After this prioritisation has been done, the process of drug discovery can begin. From a historical perspective, drug discovery as a distinct scientific discipline is very much a 20th century endeavour that has undergone continuous evolution as the scientific skill bases that support the process have increased in sophistication.

Through the early 1940s, much of the process of drug discovery was dependent on plant sources and serendipity. The technology base was synthetic chemistry, often based on dyes, with qualitative testing of compounds as anti-infective agents, in whole animals, with microbiology and limited biochemistry to support compound evaluation. Among the drugs from this era were the fungal antibiotics. A second phase of drug discovery emerged with advances in enzymology and protein biochemistry. Many of the biological pathways and processes were identified as enzymologists and pharmacologists defined new enzymes, receptor ligands, and their functions. As a result, although serendipity was still a major factor, drugs were now directed toward distinct molecular targets, The evolution of this phase was rapid, with increased Federal support of the biomedical sciences, growing sophistication in computational processing, and the availability of the personal computer.

The third phase of drug discovery is one represented by the popular vision of computer-driven discovery and development of compounds that not only treat the symptoms of the disease but also lead to its cure. The potential for the Intellectually rigorous targeting of therapeutic agents to molecular targets whose genetics, structure, function, and pathophysiology are well understood is a noble goal. Unfortunately, this somewhat naive view of several promising yet still emerging technologies presumes more than biomedical science has learned to date. Although there are superior medications to treat hypertension, asthma, schizophrenia, and anxiety, for example, their etiology remains unknown, leading to a major dependence on hypothesis testing.

Interestingly, the drug discovery wheel has come full circle as fermentation, plant, marine, and invertebrate sources have again emerged as important sources of novel therapeutic entities. Among the compounds identified in the past decade from such sources are the cholecystokinin antagonist asperlicin and the immunosuppressant FK 506.

Once a disease has been targeted and the appropriate test protocols have been assembled, it is still uncertain whether a particular approach will result in a drug. When little is known about the disease, to the extent that molecular targets are unknown or sufficiently ill addressed by the available compounds, test procedures usually depend on animal models. Such models are usually empirical, relying on either the inducement of disease-like symptoms via the use of exogenous agents or surgical procedures or on the expression of behaviours that have been defined for compounds known to be clinically efficacious.

In the former instance, asthma can be induced by allergens in guinea pig and new compounds used to relieve the symptoms. However, this process does not define the causative factors for asthma in humans but does address the symptoms. Similarly, anxiolytic drugs are currently tested in several variations of a passive avoidance situation. In such a paradigm, an animal is taught to perform a behaviour for a reward. It is then exposed to aversive stimuli so that it does not perform the behaviour. When given a compound with antianxiety actions, disinhibition of the aversion behaviour occurs so that the animal will seek rewards in spite of the aversive stimuli. Although the benzodiazepines and N-methyl-D-aspartate antagonists are active in this paradigm, its relationship to human anxiety is empirical.

Identification of compounds in such paradigms is a useful indication of potential human activity, When a molecular target can be selected, there is still uncertainty as to whether stimulation or inhibition of that target will be effective in a given disease state. Thus, to a major extent, the design, synthesis, and testing of new molecular entities selective for a given target frequently provide the tools by which a hypothesis can be evaluated. If the hypothesis proves to be in error, information is added to the scientific literature but no drug is found. This is the working approach to drug discovery that is frequently unappreciated and unreported. If drug targets and the design of their ligands were as simple as the application of new technologies, more than 20 percent of the effort in drug discovery would reach fruition in the identification of clinical candidates. As it stands, 80 percent of the effort is valuable, if ultimately nonproductive, hypothesis testing.

As noted, a major target in the drug discovery process is to develop a high degree of "rationality." This would represent an intellectually rigorous approach incorporating computer-assisted molecular design (CAMD), limited but sophisticated chemical synthetic effort, and highly focused biological assays. To many, rational drug design suggests that it is now possible, with the knowledge of the three-dimensional (3-D) structure and sequence of various drug targets, to design new compounds, by iteration, on a computer. Thus, the drug design process may become significantly less of a risk and quantally more resource efficient.

However, many of the enabling technologies that support the rational design approach are still in the emergent stage; that is, they have theoretical promise usually based on their use in the retrospective analysis of known compounds. With the exception of the enzyme thymidylate synthase, molecular modelling techniques have yet to be generally used in a predictive manner.

It is important to recognise that individual technologies, however sophisticated, may become self-limiting if there is insufficient vision in their appropriate application and integration into the mainstream drug discovery effort. A goal-oriented discipline such as drug discovery is dependent on the coherent, focused, and resource-efficient use of necessary technology rather than technology for technology's sake.

Using a building as an analogy, the architect represents the individual who provides the global vision of the final product. In the process of building, he or she makes use of various technologies provided by experts such as carpenters, electricians, stonemasons, and plumbers in a highly integrated and focused manner. To allow the electrician, the artesan of what was high technology in the late 19th century, to drive the building process based solely on what electrical wiring could do would not be considered a particularly wise approach to completing the building project. To continue the analogy, the architect of the drug discovery process is by necessity the pharmacologist, who, because of training in a hierarchical systems approach, orchestrates the biological testing technologies to the desired endpoint.

Receptor binding-the use of radiolabeled ligands to "tag" drug targets, receptors, and enzymes-has revolutionised the ability to determine compound structure-activity relationship (SAR) in a rapid, cost-effective manner. This technology resulted from early work on characterising the insulin receptor by Roth and Cuatrecasas. In its present form (and diversity), receptor binding was driven by the work of Snyder and coworkers such that binding assays for nearly 100 receptors or enzymes have been developed. The technology has also been used in the identification of new receptors and recepto subtypes.

Advantages of the technology include a direct analysis of the interaction of a ligand with a receptor (or substrate with an enzyme), the use of small amounts of material, and rapid throughput, Thus, as little as 3 mg of compound (sufficiently little to permit the analysis of intermediates from a synthetic pathway) can be run in 30 to 40 assays in 2 to 3 weeks at an estimated cost per assay of approximately $200. This allows for a binding profile to be developed, which can then be used as a potential predictor of diverse activity in a compound.

The binding approach can be contrasted with more classical functional assays where as much as 2 g of material was used and 3 to 4 weeks elapsed before data on a compound were available. Although the cost in this instance was typically in the range of $1,500 to $3,000, such assays also provided information on whether a compound was an agonist or an antagonist at the receptor target. Using binding as prescreen, researchers can reduce the number of compounds put into more complex and time-consuming functional assays. Targeted screening involves the use of the receptor-binding technique to evaluate large numbers of compounds- 20,000 to 50,000 per year-in multiple assays to identify new pharmacophores.

Compound sources include herbal, marine, and bacterial fermentations as well as chemical compound libraries, The latter include dissimilar pharmacophores from chemical companies, compounds synthesized as part of a directed chemical effort, and novel structures with no known biological activity. Targeted screening is an iterative process dependent on a finite availability of compounds and binding assays. Ideally, as newer targets are identified and assay systems for them are developed, compounds should be re-evaluated in a continuous manner.

Molecular modelling, or CAMD, is an emerging technology that makes use of knowledge of the steric and electronic aspects of the receptor/ligand, enzyme/substrate interaction to identify pharmacophores or aid in their design or both. The target/ligand interaction can be studied from three vantage points:

(1) knowledge of the SAR within a series and among series of pharmacophores, in effect approaching the receptor or enzyme from the drug perspective;

(2) knowledge of the structure of the receptor or enzyme, approaching the problem from the receptor viewpoint; and

(3) information regarding the receptor/ligand, enzyme/substrate interaction derived by 2- or 3-D nuclear magnetic resonance (NMR), x-ray crystallographic, or other structural protein analysis methods.

Each of these approaches has inherent limitations. The compound SAR approach is limited in that the protein target (receptor or enzyme) is normally configured on a computer database in a minimal energy configuration with an approximation of water content. This approach has traditionally assumed that the protein and ligand have limited degrees of flexibility, a constraint that reflected the computational power available.

With supercomputers such as the Cray 2, the protein/ligand interaction can now be assayed in real time with increased flexibility in the programming assumptions. It recently was noted that the receptor/ligand interaction can involve more than a single step and that receptors can induce changes in ligand conformation features that had been known for enzymes for a number of years. These facets of the receptor/ligand interaction present additional dimensions to the CAMD process.

Knowledge of the structure and 3-D conformation of the protein target provides an opportunity to identify the amino acid sequences and conformations that are responsible for ligand recognition and efficacy. These can be derived by knowledge of the primary sequence and, for a receptor, knowledge of which transmembrane helices are involved in ligand recognition. The interaction of various pharmacophores and compounds within a pharmacophore series can be used to identify the critical amino acids, When molecular biology is used to change these critical amino acids as point mutations, their importance in defining the ligand recognition parameters can be assessed.

Additional information regarding the biophysical aspects of the protein/ligand interaction in real time using NMR can then be used to hierarchically integrate information from the previous two approaches to gain a more concise understanding of those properties of a molecule that impart selectivity, activity, and efficacy at a given protein.

CAMD is frequently a visually attractive technology based on colourful and complex computer images. From a theoretical perspective, it has the potential to significantly enhance the drug design process, As a technology, it is limited by several necessary assumptions already noted and by limitations in database construction. Information from biological assays cannot yet be downloaded into CAMD programmes while knowledge on protein structure is currently being built. In addition, the CAMD process is limited because few biological data are available.

Activity and efficacy represent two compound properties that are amenable to existing technology. Bioavailability and metabolism have yet to be addressed by this important technology. Consequently, to assume that CAMD is presently at a stage where it can be used to design, iterate, and select new chemical structures independently of biological testing and intuition is to devalue the technology by overstating its present-day capabilities.

Molecular biology is the use of recombinant DNA (rDNA) technology to express biologically important proteins and peptides in prokaryotic and eukaryotic cell systems. Although the phrase "molecular biology," or "biotechnology," has become a broad descriptor for many facets of modern biology, including molecular biology, biochemistry, and immunology, it also includes the venture capital-driven revolution in biomedical research, which is discussed further below. Included in the technique of molecular biology are gene cloning, splicing, and expression and polymerase chain and ligase chain technologies.

The drugs produced by molecular biology, proteins or peptides known as biologics, were initially considered as replacements for the small molecules produced by synthetic chemistry. Because biologics were "natural" drugs, they were considered, in the absence of data, to be essentially free of the side-effect profiles of more traditional drugs. Although this has not proven to be the case, many useful therapeutic agents such as insulin, insulinotropin, human growth hormone, tissue plasminogen activator, erythropoietin (EPO); various cytokines, including interleukin 2 and colony stimulating factors; and other growth factors and interferons, monoclonal antibodies, vaccines, and blood products have proven the usefulness of biologics as therapeutics.

The majority of biologics are systemically active replacement therapies for hormones and other blood-borne autacoids. Their effectiveness is then a function of their being administered systemically and acting at sites proximal to the blood supply. Although useful in certain circumstances, biologics in their present forms cannot replace traditional drugs, which cover a broader spectrum of activity and tissue specificity and have superior pharmacokinetic properties.

The role of molecular biology in the drug discovery process has been increasingly enhanced as a tool that, when properly integrated, can offer major benefits to the drug hunter. The cloning, transfection, and expression of receptor and enzyme genes can be used to prepare mammalian cell lines specific for a given drug target, These cell lines can then be used instead of animals to evaluate the activity and efficacy of new compounds free of the complexity of cells derived from animal sources, Deliberate alterations in the genetic material can be used to develop point mutations in amino acid sequences to assess the importance of various substitutions in the expressed protein as well as to prepare chimeric receptors that aid in the understanding of receptor recognition and the transduction processes. Complementary DNA technology can be used to identify new proteins and, using tissues from patient populations, to determine the genetic bases of various diseases.

Such information can then be used to transfect laboratory animals to make transgenic animals that have the genetic code for human diseases. These animals can be used to study the etiology of the disease and the effects of new compounds on disease progress. Transgenic models of various cancers, AD, and diabetes are being developed. In addition, the transgenic approach is being used to produce biologics in cow's milk.

In the AD area, models of cognitive impairment involve either chemical lesions of the basal forebrain cholinergic system or the use of aged rats or primates. In both instances, the experimental paradigms are artificial. Although it is known that the cholinergic system undergoes degeneration in AD, there are major deficits in other neurotransmitter systems as well as plaque and tangle formation associated with amyloid deposition.

Although ablation of forebrain cholinergic systems is an approach to an animal model of AD, it does not reflect the nuances of the human disease state. Similarly, in aged animals, the cognitive impairment is not necessarily reflective of AD. A primary focus in the past year by at least four groups has been to transfect rodents with various amyloid precursor protein constructs with the expectation that overexpression of amyloid protein will lead to AD pathophysiology. To date, the results of these transgenic studies remain controversial.

Peptide combinatorial library technology is an emerging technology that involves the production of many millions of different peptide sequences to enhance the discovery of pharmacophores for peptide receptor targets. The technology exists in varying forms as exemplified by the Affymax, Selectide, and Iterex/Houghten Pharmaceuticals approaches. Given the attractiveness of peptide receptors, adhesion molecules, and so forth as drug targets and the paucity of agonist pharmacophores identified by conventional peptide chemistry approaches, the peptide library approach represents an important new tool for drug discovery.

Antisense technology encompasses the use of synthetic oligonucleotides as potential drugs. This technology has been a primary focus in venture capital companies and has been somewhat modestly described as the "first revolution in drug discovery since the discovery of the receptor". Proponents of the approach view traditional drugs as molecules acting on cellular proteins (enzymes and receptors). These are the product of mRNA expression, By selectively blocking events at the ribosomal or nuclear levels, antisense ligands can potentially prevent the expression of aberrant proteins at a much earlier stage "downstream" and theoretically may be more precise drugs than those blocking the function of the expressed protein. The technology involves oligonucleotides of 15 to 18 bases that act at three levels:

(1) as agents that bind to mRNA to selectively prevent protein synthesis,

(2) as triple helix (triplex) agents that block DNA promoter regions, and

(3) as aptamers, randomly coiled oligonucleotides that interact with conventional protein targets (receptors and enzymes).

Limitations to this technology are bioavailability and selectivity. How does an antisense drug make its way, not only through the gut and liver, but also inside the cell to reach the nucleus? And if this transition can be attained, how is selectivity implied?

Intracellular receptors or hormone-responsive elements (HREs) represent newer drug targets. These entities, nuclear receptors for the steroid receptor superfamily, are present on DNA and act as transcription factors that modulate promoter activity to stimulate or inhibit gene expression. Several putative receptors belonging to the steroid receptor family have no known ligands and have been designated as orphan receptors whose activity may be modulated by phosphorylation in the absence of ligand.

One such orphan receptor, the chick ovalbumin upstream promoter transcription factor, is activated by dopamine, providing an unusual example of an intracellular HRE that is responsive to an extracellular ligand. The HRE technology has been commercialised by Ligand Pharmaceuticals and is being used by a number of companies on a contract basis as a targeted screening approach for their in-house chemical libraries.

Technology Acquisition

The acquisition and incorporation of new technologies into a research organisation can be an expensive, continuous, and, frequently, incremental process. Maintaining a competitive edge requires "technological literacy" whereby a research organisation has a complete and viable repertoire of techniques necessary for the advancement of drug discovery projects within the organisation.

Keeping up with new technologies requires the addition of new staff with expertise in the necessary disciplines or the retraining of existing personnel. The delay in the latter can be 1 or 2 years and may represent a self-defeating catchup process. No sooner do existing staff members become proficient in the new technology than the needs become redefined. In addition, the transitional nature of the retraining process creates a negative impact on the ongoing research effort, inasmuch as those individuals being retrained are no longer able to perform their previous duties. Although the addition of new staff requires incremental head count, the technology acquired is typically available within 3 to 6 months of recruitment and does not involve the transfer of staff from ongoing research efforts. Nonetheless, the issue of redundant technology is not addressed, although retraining can occur when a newer technology replaces an existing one.

Another approach to technology acquisition is contract research. A pharmaceutical company can pay a university laboratory to evaluate a compound or series of compounds in a test procedure ongoing in that laboratory. Similarly, a commercial screening laboratory can also be used to "hire" technology without the need for in-house retraining or increasing head count.

As technologies have become increasingly sophisticated and proprietary via the formation of biopharmaceutical startups, research collaborations have become the means to acquire cutting-edge technology in a highly focused and cost-effective manner. By investing in smaller, high-tech companies, the larger pharmaceutical companies are able to acquire "turnkey" technology in an area without the necessary commitment of increasing staff in-house. This investment can provide a short- to medium-term solution to recruiting, which may be limited by staff, space, and capital equipment availability, at the same time allowing feasibility assessments of new technologies or research areas.

A company could provide seed money to four or five biopharmaceutical companies involved in different technologies or approaches to a therapeutic area and follow the relevant research activities over a 2- to 3-year period before investing heavily in one particular approach. This strategy can provide the means to enhance the amount of exploratory research a company can fund, while avoiding the problem of investing in such research in a new technology or area only to find that it is not relevant or practical and then having to find alternative projects for the staff members who were hired.

Organisational Aspects

The establishment of the project team necessary to integrate the various complex technologies involved in the drug discovery process is highly dependent on the structure of the discovery organisation. Three main types of organisation exist within the pharmaceutical industry.

The functional or technical line organisation (figure 3) is made up of distinct, technologically based departments such as chemistry, biochemistry, and pharmacology. Support groups for these major drug discovery disciplines would include structural biology, CAMD, formulation, drug metabolism, and so on. A project would function across these line organisations, with individuals from each of the major disciplines involved in the ongoing project. Reporting responsibilities would be through the technical directors, who typically would work together to allocate and prioritise resources.

The advantage of this type of organisation is that it permits technological specialisation with an emphasis on "cutting-edge" science. In addition, resource prioritisation is highly flexible in that head count can be moved to higher priority projects as necessary. In addition, there is a central vision as to where the organisation is directing its efforts. The disadvantages are that the individual projects are superimposed onto the technical line organisation and that the directors of each of the technologies (or the research director) decide on priorities. This situation can often lead to friction between different projects and the technical department.

The aggregate resources requested are viewed by the technical director as in excess of his or her resources, whereas the project members view resources used in maintaining cutting-edge technology as negatively affecting their project. Another disadvantage is a perceived diffuseness in the responsibility for project goals because most individuals will be working on two or more projects.

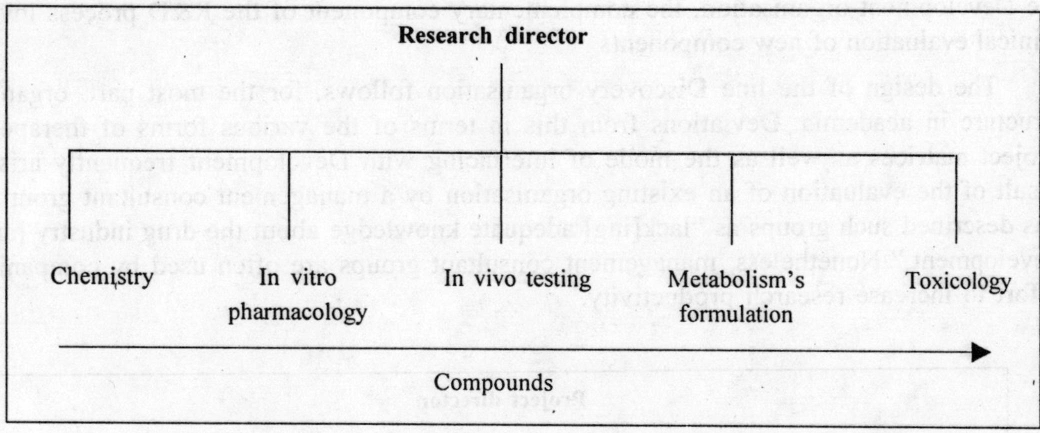

Figure 3. Functional line organisation

The second type of organisation is that of the dedicated project team. In this type of organisation, the technical disciplines necessary for drug discovery are contained within a single unit. Thus, a group of chemists and biologists focus their efforts exclusively on the project. The reporting relationship is to a project leader. The major advantages of this system relate to the focus on a single project with shared therapeutic commitment and a lack of conflicting pressures. The disadvantages are a lack of flexibility, which makes it difficult to effectively reallocate resources without major changes in global priorities; a diminished focus on enabling technology development; and a narrow focus on the project, which has the potential to overlook scientific advances outside the needs of the project.

The third type of organisation is that of the project matrix (figure 4). This is a mixture of the previous two types and involves a basic functional line organisation involving technical specialties with a project team cutting across the organisation. Individuals have line reporting relationships to a technical director but are also responsible to a project leader. The advantages of this system reflect the best of the previous two as well as an accentuation of the negative.

Thus, the matrix is flexible and technology is current, but reporting priorities are complex. Unless there are sufficient resources, technical directors perform a balancing act between the needs of the various projects while providing time for their reports to maintain their technical skill base. The matrix organisation can on the one hand be very dynamic and creative and on the other the source of considerable friction.

Variations on these three major themes abound. Some organisations have line organisations based on therapeutic areas, and others superimpose a therapeutic matrix on a line organisation, Flexibility in some companies is achieved by having chemistry "swat teams." These function independently of the mainstream and are used by the organisation to push projects forward rapidly by injecting a bolus of chemical resources. Such entities are extremely valuable when the project is highly competitive and lead structures among several companies are similar. Discovery organisations may undergo further modification via the nature of their interface with the Development organisation, the complementary component of the R&D process involved in clinical evaluation of new components.

The design of the line Discovery organisation follows, for the most part, organisational structure in academia. Deviations from this in terms of the various forms of therapeutic and project matrices as well as the mode of interfacing with Development frequently arise as the result of the evaluation of an existing organisation by a management consultant group. Spilker has described such groups as "lack[ing] adequate knowledge about the drug industry [and] drug development." Nonetheless, management consultant groups are often used by companies in an effort to increase research productivity.

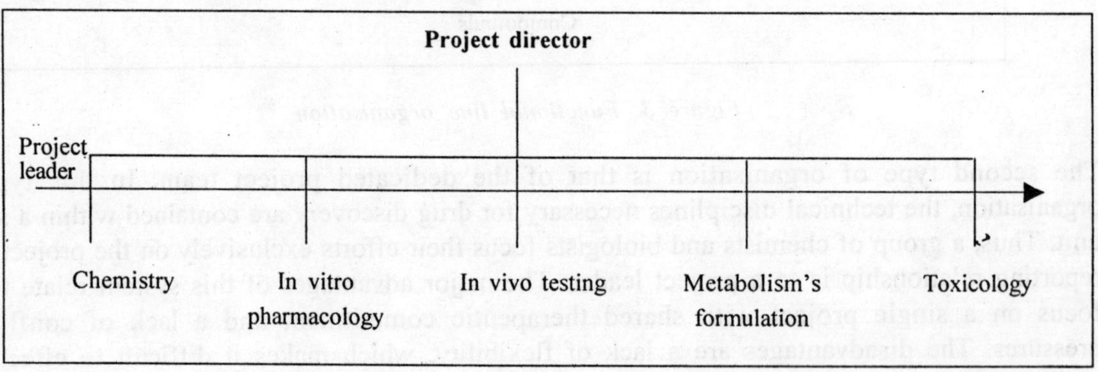

Figure 4. Project matrix organisation

This effort usually results in a reorganisation of the research department, either functionally or from a personnel perspective. For many in the industry, this reorganisation has become a seemingly continuous process that in itself is an effective barrier to productivity. On the positive side, constant reorganisation does provide gainful employment for management consultant groups.

Project management represents an important adjunct discipline to the project team approach. Inevitably, irrespective of the type of project team or the organisational backdrop, there is a need for the objective prioritisation of resources to meet project needs. A typical midsize pharmaceutical company will have 12 to 25 research projects all with their own constituency and resourcing needs that probably exceed those of the organisation by at least twofold. For the research director, the ability to prioritise the project needs via a project management team that is independent of the individual projects with a prime focus on compound flow can be a major benefit.

Scientific Skills

Organisations dedicated to the discovery of new therapeutic entities are multidisciplinary in nature, involving chemistry, biology, and computational and physical sciences. Many subspecialties exist within the major disciplines, reflecting the complexity of the drug process and the specialisation of modernday science. Because an individual is unlikely to have more than passing familiarity with these various disciplines, the drug discovery process has become increasingly dependent on the team approach.

Included in the discipline of chemistry are organic, medicinal, physical, process, theoretical, and computational chemists, each of whom represents a subspecialty of chemical synthesis with different experiences and techniques. As an example, the chemical goals involved in the novel synthesis of milligram quantities of a new compound are very different from those involved in bulk drug manufacturing for commercial sale.

In the first case, the synthetic pathway is developed to reach a new molecule as rapidly and easily as possible. There is little consideration for economies of scale, cost of starting materials, number of steps, yield, timeframe, or synthesis. As a result, synthetic costs per gram of compound at this stage can be as much as $50,000. At the stage of bulk drug manufacturing, synthesis is carried out in line with the U.S. Food and Drug Administration's (FDA) Good Manufacturing Practices conditions. The focus is on cost reduction, ease of synthesis, yield, and quantity of material. Consequently, there is a very different focus on how the compound is made. When kilogram quantities are made, the cost per gram moves progressively downward from about $1,000 to $5.

Although the discipline of chemistry is primarily involved with compound synthesis (deStevens 1991), there is a recent trend toward training "hybrid" chemists with skills encompassing both compound synthesis and molecular biology. Although one benefit from melding the two disciplines has been to more effectively understand the interactions between compounds and their protein targets, it has also augmented an increasing shortage in chemistry graduates with interest and experience in organic synthesis.

Biological disciplines are considerably more diverse and encompass biochemistry (including enzymology); pharmacology (including both in vitro and in vivo aspects of cell, tissue, and whole animal function); molecular biology; cell biology; pharmacokinetics; drug delivery; and drug formulations. It is probably a truism that the biological sciences involved in the drug discovery process are considerably more dynamic than the chemistry skill bases, because change occurs much more rapidly in the biological disciplines and at an ever-increasing pace.

Computational, physical, and organisational disciplines affecting the drug discovery process should not be overlooked. These include CAMD, NMR, and x-ray crystallography, which have already been discussed. Underlying these disciplines are support services, such as research computing, that provide a great deal of programming skill and assistance to benefit computers and the other sophisticated instrumentation that drive these technologies forward.

Information scientists make a major contribution by providing the mechanisms to maintain currency with the scientific literature as well as by designing and supporting laboratory information management systems and databases. Tracking compounds, their activities, and archival storage is an underestimated technology that has a major impact as organisations mature and their information bases expand. Patent activities, an increasingly complex facet of the biomedical research arena, can also be included under this aspect.

However, drug discovery should not be viewed as a technology-driven process, a trend that unfortunately has emerged throughout the industry in the past decade but, rather, as a technology-facilitated one. Technologies represent the tools by which to move the discovery process forward. However, they are fragmented parts of a whole and need a unifying discipline and vision to integrate their contributions and drive the process toward goals that are more global.

The discipline that provides this focus is pharmacology. As a technology, pharmacology has had a major role in establishing the pharmaceutical industry; as a discipline, it seeks the technologies necessary to discover and characterise new drugs rather than abstract uses for the technologies themselves. Although pharmacology is not as widely practiced a discipline as it was 20 years ago and is not widely taught within the U.S. university system, its rightful reemergence as the driving force for drug discovery is reflected in the increasing numbers of pharmacologists from European universities being hired by US. drug companies,

Project Team

Ideally, a project team should include the necessary skill bases, resources, and decisionmaking authority to ensure that the project proceeds in an expeditious, timely, and resource-effective manner. The project team should be viewed as a dynamic organisation driven by goals rather than technology. Thus, the project team process can be viewed in distinct stages

The initiatory stage involves the validation of the concept, which may be taken from existing work from the literature and require internal repetition or may involve an original idea that has to go through the same process of systematic evaluation as any scientific project. In either event, other than the chemistry required for small amounts of reference compounds, this stage of the project would involve a nucleus of biological disciplines.

The staff needs of such a project have been estimated at between 8 and 12 scientists, Once the concept has been validated and accepted by research management, additional resources would be added and the project would then move to a planning stage. This would involve the development of the appropriate screening procedures and their validation in regard to compound flow; the sequence would be incorporated as the project flowchart. At this point, dedicated chemical effort would be added to begin the search for lead compounds. Project resources would increase to about 16 scientists. Once a lead series had been identified, the chemical effort would be enhanced to effect a realised project-the fully resourced effort involving chemistry and biology with appropriate milestones, compound target dates, and corperate society.

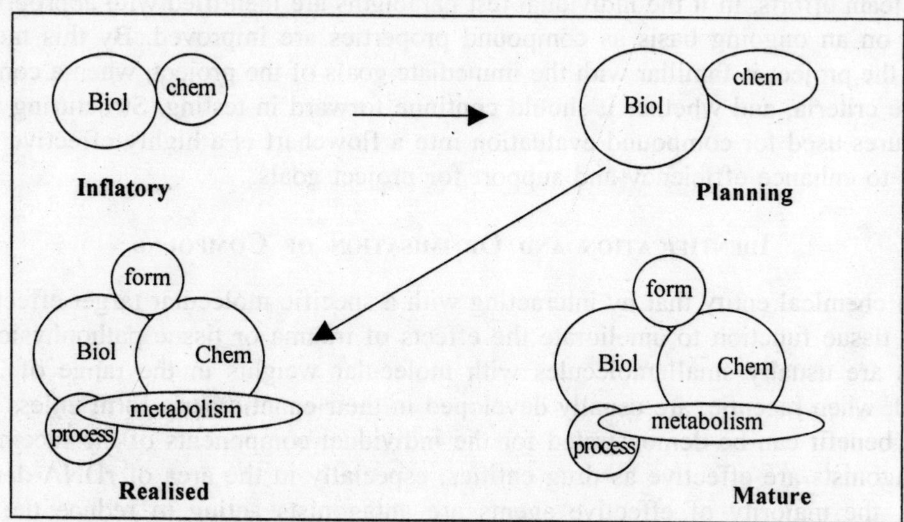

Figure 5. Schematic of the stages of a Discovery project KEY: Biol.=biology; Chem.=chemistry; Form.=formulation; Process=process chemistry

The size of the project at this point would be about 25 people, with additional support in terms of formulation, drug delivery, and process chemistry to begin planning for the scaleup of synthesis of the compound to the larger quantities required for toxicology and clinical testing. With the emergence of a compound candidate for toxicological evaluation and the identification of a backup compound, the project can be reduced in size, releasing resources for new initiatory efforts. At this stage the project would be termed mature and, although still involving formulation, drug delivery, and process chemistry, would be reduced in size.

The timing for termination of effort on a given project has been the topic of considerable debate. One school of thought would argue that a lead compound and a backup compound distinguished by a different chemical structure with related properties would be sufficient. Given that the time when a compound is identified to its progress to marketing approval is in the range of 5 to 8 years, others have argued that a gatekeeping effort should be maintained until the compound reaches the marketplace. If unexpected problems occur, the project then can be revived relatively easily to continue the search for a better compound.

The number of individuals on a project obviously affects the rate of progress toward lead compound status. Clearly, increasing resources, to a point, can facilitate the objectives of the project. Inevitably, irrespective of the organisational structure, there is considerable competition for both finite and incremental resources.

Some projects in larger pharmaceutical companies have been rumored to have 100 to 150 people working on them to accelerate the pace toward compound identification. Some companies use chemistry "swat teams" to move resources from one project to another to ensure critical mass at crucial points. The compound flowchart offers a convenient focal point for project team efforts. In it the individual test paradigms are identified with appropriate criteria established on an ongoing basis as compound properties are improved. By this means, every member of the project is familiar with the immediate goals of the project, when a compound has satisfied the criteria, and whether it should continue forward in testing. Structuring the various test procedures used for compound evaluation into a flowchart is a highly effective facilitatory mechanism to enhance efficiency and support for project goals.

IDENTIFICATION AND OPTIMISATION OF COMPOUND

A drug is a chemical entity that by interacting with a specific molecular target effects a change in cell and tissue function to ameliorate the effects of trauma or tissue pathophysiology. Such compounds are usually small molecules with molecular weights in the range of 250 to 700 daltons and, when racemic, are usually developed in their enantiomeric form unless additive or synergistic benefit can be demonstrated for the individual components of the racemic mixture. Although agonists are effective as drug entities, especially in the area of rDNA-derived drugs (biologics), the majority of effective agents are antagonists acting to reduce the actions of endogenous agonists that contribute to the disease state. Optimal characteristics of a drug are that it be

(1) pure, preferably as a single enantiomer if chiral;

(2) efficacious on repeated administration;

(3) safe in terms of its beneficial actions;

(4) affordable within the context of patient use and cost of discovery and development; and

(5) from a commercial viewpoint, patentable, either by composition of matter or by use.

Safety issues are highly dependent on the disease or condition being targeted. For example, for an appetite suppressant for use on a daily basis for reducing food intake, the safety margins in terms of unwanted side effects would have to be extremely high. For an agent to be used in the acute treatment of stroke, safety issues, although present, are balanced against the brain damage resulting from the reduction in blood flow to the brain.

Once an active lead compound is found, it is refined by further synthetic effort to develop an SAR for a number of properties of the molecule, including:

— *Activity:* a measure of the interaction of a ligand with its molecular target, expressed as a Ki (inhibitory constant) for a ligand-receptor interaction or Km (Michaelis-Menten constant) for an enzyme.

— *Efficacy:* the ability of a ligand once bound to effect a change in cell and tissue function. This refers to whether a compound is an agonist or an antagonist at a receptor or a substrate or an inhibitor for an enzyme. For a receptor ligand, intrinsic efficacy is the relative ability of a ligand to produce a functional effect, biochemical and/or physiological, compared with a reference agonist. A full agonist has an intrinsic efficacy of unity, whereas an antagonist, which lacks efficacy, has no agonist activity and has an intrinsic efficacy of zero.

— *Selectivity:* a measure of the ability of a ligand to interact predominantly with a single molecular target. The concept of selectivity often involves considerable semantic issues. Thus, selectivity may be anywhere between a 10-fold and a 1,000-fold delineation between the activity or efficacy at the desired target compared with its ability to interact with other targets, In vivo, selectivity-as defined by the ability of a compound to produce a preclinical action thought to reflect the therapeutic action of an agent compared with unwanted side effects-is the therapeutic index.

— *Bioavailability and pharmacokinetics:* crucial, yet frequently elusive, properties of a compound series. The susceptibility of a compound to glucuronidation, sulfation, and so forth, and its ability to cross the gut and blood-brain barrier are difficult parameters to define. In vivo estimates are compounded by a multiplicity of factors contributing to the pharmacodynamic actions of the compound. These include the enzymic modification of the compound, especially when given orally; its lipophilicity, plasma levels, and half-life; and in the case of central nervous system (CNS)-active agents, the relationship between plasma and brain concentrations and the retention of the compound in the brain.

Spècies differences in metabolism, rat vs. primate vs. human, become a major confounding feature of bioavailability and pharmacokinetic studies. Compounds may be 90-percent bioavailable in one species and less than 10 percent in another. Predicting what the situation might be in humans becomes very difficult. Extensive efforts in defining such properties using in vitro study approaches (e.g., human liver slices) have yet to prove predictive.

Compound Status

As seen in the flowchart, the establishment of project norms for identifying compounds of interest can greatly enhance communication within a project and avoid misunderstandings as to the priority of a compound. With an extensive synthetic effort, many hundreds of compounds may be made in a year. Although each of these is a well-known entity to the chemist who made it, the biologist, especially one working in a tunctional line organisation where he or she is involved in several projects, needs additional descriptors for the compounds beyond their company numbers.

A system used by companies is a list of new compounds according to their biological activity and evaluation status. One such system involves designating compounds by a numerical system. A category 4 compound is one that has reached a predetermined cutoff point for activity in the primary assays of the flowchart. When selectivity and function have been established, the compound becomes a category 3 compound. With further evaluation in whole animal tests, bioavailability and half-life determination, and preliminary toxicological evaluation, a compound would achieve category 2 status and high visibility within the R&D organisation. At this time it would undergo full review as a potential drug candidate and further workup in terms of formulation as a toxicological candidate. This would lead to the synthesis of a sufficient amount of compound for toxicological as well as stability testing.

On entering toxicology, the compound would be designated as category 1. On completion of the toxicology required for the Notice of Claimed Investigational Exemption for a New Drug (IND) submission, the compound shifts into a similar prioritisation system within Development. The advantage of such a scheme is that each compound, when of sufficient interest to a project team to be elevated to a given status, achieves instant recognition within the organisation so that it can be appropriately prioritised.

Compound Value

The lifeblood of any drug company is reflected in the proprietary compounds it has patented. Patents are of two major types: composition of matter patents, which cover the molecules synthesized, and use patents, which cover specific uses for these entities. Typically, within a drug company both composition of matter and use are contained within a single patent series. In some instances, however, where unexpected data regarding the biological activity of a compound have been derived, a use patent can be obtained. This can extend the proprietary life of a compound beyond that of the initial patent. This strategy is useful when the patent applicant in both instances is the same but can become complex when a second party has a use patent on a compound owned by another party.

Compound Safety

Once a compound has been found to meet criteria for potential use as a drug, its safety must be extensively evaluated to ensure that the potential risk-tobenefit ratio is such that a drug will not produce significant damage under specific conditions of use. Toxicity should be clearly dissociable from efficacy.

After preclinical evaluation, a potential new drug is evaluated in acute (14 to 20 days), subchronic (28 to 90 days), and chronic (3 to 24 months) toxicity paradigms. Acute studies are performed in rodents of both sexes using oral and parenteral routes of administration. Such studies are required before Phase I studies may be conducted in humans. Dose-ranging studies are performed to identify a dose that is safe in normal subjects and that can be used as a basis for efficacy testing in the target population in Phase II trials. Subacute mutagenicity studies (Ames test) represent the first test in which a new pharmacophore is assessed before recommendation for indepth toxicological evaluation.

The duration of initial toxicity testing is very dependent on the type of drug and the plans for Phase I trials. In the case of an antibiotic that will be used for the acute treatment of opportunistic infections, the data required for human trials are significantly less than those required for a contraceptive pill for which usage is measured in years. Carcinogenicity, mutagenicity, teratogenicity, and behavioral toxicity testing occurs in more lengthy trials as a compound is moving through Phase I and Phase II trials in humans. For further information on toxicological evaluation, refer to Cavagnaro and Lewis.

DRUG DEVELOPMENT

Research/Discovery and Development may be separate units, organised along therapeutic lines reporting to separate heads of R&D. Alternatively, the R&D organisation can exist in a self-contained therapeutic organisation with a single head often known as a Strategic Business Unit. In either event, the relationship between R&D in terms of compound movement is a crucial one. Without synergy, Research may bring forward compounds for which there is no interest in Development. This can be of special concern in the present business environment where there is a continuing need for new products.

For a Development organisation charged with a well-balanced, temporally sequential product pipeline, compounds can be taken from the internal organisation or in-licensed from other companies. Resources committed to the latter usually affect Research resources and the ability to develop internal candidates. It is therefore important that communication between the two groups is optimal as well as flexible, with Discovery responding to Development needs and Development actively responding to high-risk, innovative approaches to drug therapy.

Given the nature of such innovation, the enthusiasm of the Development organisation for a totally novel compound is crucial to its introduction to the clinic and the risk taking necessary to establish a novel therapeutic target. This is exemplified in Glaxo's portfolio of serotonin receptor antagonists, which were novel compounds in search of diseases for which no known treatments existed. A popular example of perceived shortsightedness in developing new medications is that of the antiulcer medication, the histamine H2, blocker cimetidine.

When this compound was developed in the 1960s treatments for gastric ulcer encompassed antacids and surgery. The leap of faith in developing a totally new approach to ulcer therapy in light of existing effective medications was considerable. Although the retrospective viewpoint suggests that the mechanistic approach of blocking H2, receptors was obvious, there was considerable risk in bringing cimetidine into the clinic with the long lead time to the marketplace. Inevitably, development and marketing are forecasting the medical need for a new compound 8 to 10 years in the future.

For an area in which there are existing medications, there are known criteria against which new compounds can be compared. In new areas, or in areas where a totally new mechanistic approach is being targeted, the value of the innovation can be assessed only in the clinic. Yet before a compound reaches this stage, the momentum to the marketplace takes considerable faith and an element of risk taking that is not always present within large corporations. As an example, hypertension was effectively treated in the mid-1960s with diuretics and -adrenergic blockers.

The vision of Ondetti, Cushman, Horowitz, and their colleagues in the 1970s led to the discovery of the first angiotensin-converting enzyme inhibitor, captopril. This compound was considered by many to be not only superior to existing treatments for high blood pressure but also the definitive drug for this indication. Statements were made at the time that further medications for the treatment of hypertension were unnecessary, this in the face of a good percentage of "nonresponding" patients, especially in the African-American population. In the

1990s however, renin inhibitors and angiotensin-II antagonists represent newer approaches to the regulation of blood pressure that may have additional indications related to congestive heart failure and atherosclerosis, two complications of cardiovascular function that are in need of improved approaches.

The synergies between R&D have been the subject of numerous articles and have assumed the status of a research project on their own. This should not result in the trivialisation of the interaction or the impact that this relationship has on a technology-based organisation. Frequently, a productive Research organisation has less than optimal channels of communication with the Development organisation. In the pharmaceutical industry, the nature of the science is such that there is a large need for buy-in from the Development organisation to ensure that a compound with high potential receives appropriate prioritisation.

A lack of synergy between R&D can result in compounds appearing as toxicological candidates taking the Development organisation by surprise. Another facet of the R&D interface, which operates more in the management of R&D, relates to the balance in needs and resources. A highly productive Discovery group can present the Development function with more compounds than the Development organisation can handle. Management is then left with establishing priorities, either by increasing Development resources, usually at the expense of the Discovery effort, or putting compounds on the shelf and thus raising the question of the need for urgency in the Discovery process.

In the past, not a few R&D operations have disbanded Discovery efforts as compound candidates were produced, the logic being that the product pipeline was full and that further compounds from Discovery could not be accommodated. Because attrition is a major feature of the various stages of the Discovery process, the loss of compound candidates caused by unexpected findings in clinical trials with no Discovery organisation to find replacement candidates made such organisations extremely vulnerable within the global marketplace.

Clinical Evaluation

Clinical evaluation of a new compound is divided into discrete stages designated by FDA and comparable organisations in the European Economic Community (EEC). Before a drug can be tested in humans, an IND package containing information on the safety, activity, and chemical properties of a new compound is filed with FDA. In EEC, this process is known as the Clinical Trial Certificate (CTC).

FDA is obligated to respond to the IND within 30 days, at which time, if there are no objections from FDA, a company may proceed with clinical trials. Phase I studies focus on the evaluation of compound safety in normal human volunteers using dose-ranging studies to determine safety and a therapeutic window. Side effects as well as human pharmacokinetics are established at this stage. A dose in excess of that at which a therapeutic response is anticipated must also be established. Phase II studies involve open-label, single- and multiple-dose studies in the patient population. Efficacy is determined using placebo controls.

The therapeutic dose range is established as well as the route and frequency of compound administration. There is a major trend in relating compound efficacy to plasma levels rather than to dosage because there are many individual patient variables that affect the amount of drug that reaches the bloodstream. Phase III studies expand on the initial patient population, involving multicenter trials to establish uncommon (<2 percent) side effects and drug interactions.

The data derived from Phase III studies are used as the basis for the new drug application (NDA), the data required for registration of the drug with a regulatory agency for approval for sale. In EEC, the NDA is known as the Product License Application. Phase IV studies are postmarketing studies to further elucidate common side effects, to focus on patient populations not adequately covered in Phase III trials, and to gather definitive data on additional indications for the compound. The data derived from clinical trials and for which a company seeks regulatory approval relate to the uses of the drug and its side effects and safety.

The instrument to define these parameters is the package insert, the documentation accompanying a prescription drug. In seeking regulatory approval, a company should have data that will support the claims made in the package insert. Thus, the claims are the driving force in determining clinical trials and the interactions of a company with FDA. Rather than an isolated, two-stage (IND, NDA) process, frequent meetings with FDA to seek advice, opinions, and clarification can significantly accelerate the movement of a compound from the laboratory to the pharmacy.

Clinical Markers

The predictivity of animal and biochemical test procedures is unclear because, as discussed above, many models are highly empirical. The ability to diagnose disease states on the basis of blood or tissue pathology and to use such tests to determine compound efficacy is a major goal within the pharmaceutical industry. For 3-hydroxy-3-methylglutaryl CoA reductase inhibitors (lovastatin [Mevacor]) that prevent cholesterol formation, clinical endpoints were based on pharmacoepidemiological studies linking elevated cholesterol levels to atherosclerosis and other disorders of the vascular system. In the clinic, therefore, determination of efficacy is related to a decrease in plasma cholesterol levels produced by lovastatin rather than direct effects on atherosclerotic pathophysiology.

CNS Drug Discovery

The pressures and complexity of modern society have increased the use of psychotropic drugs and the incidence of anxiety and depression, creating a need for medications that are more efficacious and free of side effects than those currently available. The need for effective treatments to treat addictive disorders is a high priority in neuroscience research because of their high cost and negative impact on society.

The unmet needs in CNS disease treatment have led the U.S. Congress to declare the 1990s as the Decade of the Brain, a major initiative to facilitate the discovery and development of new medications for a variety of CNS disease states.

CNS drug discovery may be conveniently divided into three phases. The first, the age of serendipity, occurred from the early 1950s through 1975 and involved the clinical discovery of compounds originally targeted at other disease states that had unexpected CNS actions.

Iproniazid, chlorpromazine, imipramine, and L-dopa were products of this era. A second phase began in the early 1970s with the search for second-generation compounds with improved efficacy and reduced side effect liability compared with those agents discovered in the first phase.

The use of receptor binding and targeted screening led to the discovery of antagonists for the cholecystokinin. Despite the increased emphasis on molecular pharmacology, drugs discovered in this period were, to a large extent, incremental in nature or, like buspirone dependent on serendipitous evaluation in the clinic. The antipsychotic clozapine and the antidepressant fluoxetine were major therapeutic agents from this era.

Advances in molecular biology and molecular pharmacology have resulted in the identification of new drug targets: receptor subtypes and enzyme isoforms. These permit elucidation of receptor/enzyme function with the development of ligand/substrate SAR and compound selectivity. Such advances, fueling the third phase of CNS drug discovery, also have the potential to facilitate disease diagnosis and the understanding of disease etiology. The emerging computer-based structural technologies, such as CAMD and NMR, have been limited in the CNS area because many potential drug targets have yet to be crystallised and thus require approximations for structural analysis,

Limitations

Present-day understanding of brain function is limited and has become overly reductionist with minimal focus on the four principal levels of research: molecular, cellular, systems, and behaviour. Objectively integrating and interpreting data obtained at these various levels are crucial to make allowances for the complexity of function that distinguishes the brain from other organs within the body. Although considerable emphasis is placed on the density of receptors within the brain (usually 10-fold to 100-fold greater than found in other tissues), the possibility that these add to functional complexity is rarely taken into account.

Similarly, although glial cells are an important component of nervous tissue, they are frequently ignored in defining hypotheses related to drug action. It also has been noted that "neuroscience stands . . . today where atomic physics was in 1919 . . . or . . . molecular biology . . . in 1944". A lack of knowledge regarding CNS disease etiology and the descriptive nature of current psychiatric diagnosis (Baldessarini, in press) are other contributing factors that affect progress in CNS drug discovery.

Another critical issue relates to the predictive animal models. These have been highly empirical and have not always been useful in moving a compound into the clinic. In the area of depression, for instance, there are a number of biochemical and behavioral models (e.g., -receptor down-regulation, muricidal rat, swim test) in which classical antidepressants have effects, These are not especially robust test procedures, and few are on the critical path for compound characterisation.

A limitation to such tests has been that research in the area of animal behaviour as related to human CNS disease states, both in terms of determining efficacy and side effect potential, has undergone a significant deemphasis in the past decade in favor of more molecular approaches. Transgenic animals have been heralded as a more useful approach to disease pathology, but their use, to date, has been limited in the CNS. Various mouse strains have been used in anticonvulsant testing, yet these also are empirical, rather than based on definitive genetic defects related to defined CNS function.

The limitations in behaviour become self-defeating as research becomes more focused on molecular approaches. To judge the potential of behavioral paradigms based on current models, which are being improved in a very limited fashion because of funding constraints, is impractical. New knowledge regarding disease etiology cannot readily be integrated because of a paucity of researchers and the complexity of test paradigms. It is crucial that a greater focus on animal models of CNS diseases be part of the Decade of the Brain initiative.

Management

The need for innovative research to find drugs that allow the treatment or more effective treatment of human disease is a sine qua non for the pharmaceutical industry. Yet understanding of the scientific approach and what factors motivate scientists is not always a given within a research-based organisation. The R&D organisation is frequently viewed as an unpredictable, uncontrollable entity, a black hole into which vast sums of money are poured in hope that products will emerge. Communication among scientists, research management, and corporate management is not always optimal so research may often be perceived as a necessary evil rather than the lifeblood of an organisation.

To the necessarily pragmatic businessperson, the abstractly focused scientist may on one level be an icon representing the dynamics and vision of the R&D-based commercial enterprise. On another level this individual may represent a challenge to be molded and redirected into a more goaloriented, productive path. The challenges of managing and motivating scientists are formidable and are in need of attention in today's changing scientific marketplace.

The numbers of qualified scientists entering industry have been dramatically reduced in the past decade, and this is already leading to major shortages in the areas of chemistry and pharmacology. In a highly controversial public debate, some participants have focused on the inferior quality of education in the United States as a major causative factor of the shortages whereas others have directed attention to more lucrative career alternatives in investment banking and the legal profession. Whatever the reasons, there has been an exponential increase in the hiring of foreign nationals because of an absence of qualified U.S. scientists.

With such shortages and considerable in-house investments in the continued training of research staff, the effective management, motivation, and retention of scientists are as much a part of an effective strategy for drug discovery as the acquisition of enabling technologies. Many research organisations are "flat," having few managerial levels. As a result, career advancement has become limited, placing a major focus on job satisfaction. For a research organisation to provide this requires an understanding of motivational factors within the scientific arena.

Classic scientific training, especially at the graduate level, places a major premium on independent thought, on the dissemination of research results through the global scientific community, and on peer respect and acceptance. These qualities usually undergo modification within the organisational context of a corporation that places a high premium on teamwork and loyalty. However, such qualities do not disappear completely and must be factored into the research environment. This is of special concern when project priorities change and scientists have to refocus their efforts on different activities.

Ideally, scientists in industry should have the opportunity to work on interesting projects, to make their own individual contributions to research projects, to be part of the process of new project initiation, to be rewarded for their efforts in drug discovery, to publish original research findings, to attend important scientific meetings, and to have clear career goals. The assimilation of an individual into a Research organisation should be an active process, melding with the culture of the Research organisation in a synergistic manner from both a technical and a personal viewpoint.

Most large Research organisations have both managerial and scientific hierarchies to enable scientists to align their careers with science rather than having to compete for limited managerial positions for which they may not be suited. Active recognition and support from upper management for scientific excellence is a major aspect of the culture in many pharmaceutical companies. Some scientists may align their careers with a project or a therapeutic area so that when priorities change, they are more inclined to seek other opportunities than to realign with corporate needs. Such individuals are highly focused, dedicated, and often very entrepreneurial in outlook and in their ability to motivate others.

Fitzgerald has described these "drug hunters" as "having a broad knowledge of corporate science, . . . being non-compliant, disliking the status quo, risk taking, having strong convictions which they forcefully express, and being ambitious for drugs rather than themselves." Several major drugs have been discovered because of the efforts of such "swashbuckling" individuals, Although their activities were not always appreciated at the time, they have since become both corporate and industry folk heroes,

As the 21st century approaches, the urgency of scientific research has increased considerably. Capable scientists are changing companies more frequently to enhance their career prospects. This urgency has been fueled by venture capital interest in pharmaceuticals and by the global consolidation within the pharmaceutical industry and driven to a major extent by a short-term focus on research that has led to a number of mergers and takeovers with staff realignments, downsizing, and cultural dissidence.

Fifteen years ago, a scientist in the pharmaceutical industry could expect a well-paid, secure career with one company and a comfortable retirement. Today, such security is relative, even though many scientists, as evidenced by events at Genentech, Amgen, and so on, can become millionaires by (re)aligning their careers with biopharmaceutical/biotechnology startups.

The continuing high premium placed on innovative, focused biomedical science has thus provided an increasing number of career options for experienced, productive drug hunters. The high element of risk in the venture capital arena with the attendant high rewards presents a challenge to the major pharmaceutical companies to be competitive in hiring and retaining their scientific personnel. In the era of major expansion in industry research from 1976 to 1989, career needs could be met as organisations expanded. When organisations stabilise or even shrink, career opportunities become fewer. Additional dynamic factors are imposed on the Research organisation as technologies and goals change.

A major challenge to research management for the future will be to provide the leadership and the culture that effectively mesh the needs of the individual scientist with those of the Research organisation. In this context, Cuatrecasas has noted that "few, if any, large organisations have ever come close to adjusting their operational models to encourage creativity and invention. Most R&D organisations tend to be bulky, awkward, regimented, controlling, inflexible, 'conformist,' bureaucratic, formalised, overstructured, and intolerant." Against such a litany of negatives, one wonders how any technology reaches the marketplace. The imperative in upward communication is exceedingly high.

Chapter 5
Process Validation Methods

Drugs subject to terminal moist heat sterilisation may be formulated in a grade C environment, provided that the formulated bulk is immediately subjected to its subsequent processing step, e.g., filtration, sterilisation, so as to maintain low microbial and particular counts. Formulating may take place in a grade D environment if additional measures are taken to minimise contamination, such as the use of closed systems of manufacture.

Parenterals are filled in an aseptic area of at least a grade B environment or in a grade A zone with at least a grade C background before terminal moist heat sterilisation. Non-parenterals may be filled in a grade C environment before terminal moist heat sterilisation.

Validation of Moist Heat Sterilisation Processes

The validation of moist heat sterilisation processes may be performed using any of the three strategies outlined below. The approach selected should be appropriate and adequately supported. It should be stressed that the integrity of the container/closure system be established prior to validating the sterilisation process to ensure that an appropriate container/closure system has been selected.

Prospective Validation

This approach applies to new or modified processes and new equipment. The studies are conducted, evaluated, and the process and equipment system certified prior to initiating routine production.

Concurrent Validation

This approach applies to existing processes and equipment. Concurrent validation studies are conducted during regular production and should only be considered for processes which have a manufacturing and testing history indicating consistent quality production. Reworks and failures indicate potential inconsistencies in the process and should be evaluated for effect on the reproducibility of production prior to establishing validation protocol. Although suitable records may not be available for the installation of equipment, lack of this data may not compromise the balance of the studies.

Retrospective Validation

This approach can only be applied to existing products, processes and equipment and is based solely on historical information. Normal processing records generally lack sufficient detail to permit retrospective validation.

a) It must be established that the process was not modified and that the sterilising equipment is operating under the same conditions of construction and performance as documented in the records to be considered. Maintenance records and process change control documents should be available to support these claims.

b) Periods in which failures occurred should not be excluded. The incidence of failures or reworking attributed to unsatisfactory processing indicates inconsistency in the process. There should be an evaluation of these conditions for the period to be used for validation.

c) The manufacturing, maintenance and testing data should be capable of demonstrating calibration of equipment and devices, and establishing uniformity.

Validation Protocol Development

Each stage of the evaluation of the effectiveness and reproducibility of a sterilisation process should be based on a preestablished and approved detailed written protocol. A written change control procedure should be established to prevent unauthorised change to the protocol or process and restrict change during any phase of the studies until all relevant data are evaluated.

The protocol should specify the following in detail:

— the process objectives in terms of product type, batch size, container/closure system, and probability of survival desired from the process;

— preestablished specifications for the process which include the cycle time, temperature, pressures and loading pattern;

— a description of all of the equipment and support systems in terms of type, model, capacity and operating range;

— the performance characteristics of each system; performance characteristics including pressure gauge sensitivity and response, valve operation, alarm systems functions, timer response and accuracy, steam flow rates and/or pressures, cooling water flow rates, cycle controller functions, door closure gasketing, and air break systems and filters;

— for new equipment: installation requirements and installation check points for each system and subsystem;

— for existing equipment: the necessary upgrading requirements or any compensatory procedures; justification for alternate procedures should be available;

— all laboratory testing methodology;

— the personnel responsible for performing, evaluating and certifying each stage of the validation protocol and for final evaluation prior to certification of the process.

Personnel Involve

Documented evidence of the experience and training of all personnel involved in validation studies should be maintained.

— Qualified personnel should ensure that the validation protocol and testing methodology are developed in a sound engineering and scientific manner and that all studies are properly evaluated and certified.

— All personnel conducting tests should be trained and experienced in the use of the equipment and measuring devices.

— Engineering/mechanical personnel should be qualified in the operation and maintenance of sterilisers and support systems.

Laboratory Functions

— All laboratory tests, including "D" value analysis, should be performed by a competent laboratory. The laboratory should have detailed methodology and procedures covering all laboratory functions available in writing.

— In cases where outside laboratories are utilised, a suitable system for determining the competency of such laboratories should be included in the study protocol.

The range, accuracy, reproducibility and response time of all controlling and recording instruments associated with the steriliser and support equipment must be adequate to demonstrate that defined process conditions are met.

— Instruments requiring calibration include:

  — temperature recorders and sensors;

  — thermocouples;

  — pressure sensors for jacket and chamber pressure;

  — timers;

  — conductivity monitors for cooling water, if applicable;

  — flow meters for water/steam;

  — water level indicators when cooling water is used;

  — thermometers including those for thermocouple reference, chamber monitoring and all laboratory testing.

These instruments must be calibrated against traceable standards before any operational qualification can be performed. Written calibration procedures should specify the methods to be used, and records of each calibration, including actual results obtained, should be maintained.

Recalibration should be required in writing after any maintenance of instruments and, in the case of temperature sensing devices, before and after each validation run conducted as part of heat distribution or penetration studies. The instruments should be included in a written preventive maintenance programme.

INDICATOR CALIBRATION

Indicating devices used in the validation studies or used as part of post-validation monitoring or requalification must be calibrated.

— Physical and chemical indicators should be tested to demonstrate adequate predetermined response to both time and temperature.

a) Detailed written test procedures and records of test results should be available.

b) The indicators should be used before a written expiry date and stored to protect their quality.

— Biological indicators should be tested according to detailed written procedures for viability and quantitation of the challenge organism and for the time/temperature exposure response. This applies to indicators either prepared in-house or obtained commercially.

a) For commercial indicators, a certificate of testing for each lot indicating the "D" value of the lot should be available. The quantitation is acceptable if the supplier's count has been qualified and periodically confirmed.

b) If biological indicators are prepared in-house, "D" value determinations and organism characterisation are also required. In conducting "D" value studies, the choice of media (pH, electrolytes, carbohydrates, etc.) and sample carriers (suspension in ampoules, paper strips, inoculated products and inoculation on solid carriers) should be consistent with the materials used in the steriliser validation.

Records of the testing should be available.

c) The biological indicator should be used before expiry and adequately stored.

STERILISATION CYCLE DEVELOPMENT

Two basic approaches are employed to develop sterilisation cycles for moist heat processes: Overkill and Probability of Survival.

— The Overkill method is used when the product can withstand excessive heat treatment such as an F_0 \$12 without adverse effects. Bioburden and resistance data are not required to determine the required "F_0" values. Cycle parameters are adjusted to assure that the coldest point within the load receives an "F_0" that will provide at least a 12-log reduction of microorganisms having a "D_{121}" value of at least one minute.

— The Probability of Survival approach is used primarily for heat labile products. In this approach, the process for the terminal sterilisation of a sealed container is validated to achieve the destruction of pre-sterilisation bioburden to a level of 10^0, with a minimum safety factor of an additional six-log reduction ($1x10^{-6}$). The probability that any one unit is contaminated is therefore no more than one in a million; this is considered to be an acceptable level of sterility assurance.

a) The probability of survival is determined using a semi-logarithmic microbial death curve, where a plot of the log of the number of survivors versus time at a fixed temperature yields a straight line. After the line has crossed below 10^0 (less than one survivor), the y-value corresponding to a given time value is expressed as the probability of survival.

b) The determination of the minimum "F_0" value for the Probability of Survival approach is based upon the number of microorganisms (bioburden) found in a given product and their heat resistance.

c) Methods for conducting bioburden studies, estimating microbial heat resistance and determining the minimum required "F_0" value for sterilisation.

For both methods it is necessary to conduct heat distribution and heat penetration studies to determine the amount of heat delivered to the slowest heating unit in each load.

"F_0" and "D" Values

"F_0", or the Lethality Factor, is the amount of time in minutes, equivalent to time at 121°C, to which a unit has been exposed during a sterilisation process.

a) One method of calculating the "F_0" is to integrate the time the unit is exposed to heat in terms of equivalent time at 121°C.

b) A second method is based on data obtained by the use of calibrated biological indicators.

The "D" value is the time, in minutes, required to reduce a microbial population by 90%—or by one log value—under specified test conditions (i.e. fixed temperature, single species, specified medium, etc.). When heat labile products will not withstand excessive heat treatment, "D_{121}" value studies of product isolates are necessary to determine the minimum Lethality Factor (F0) that will provide an acceptable assurance of sterilisation.

The minimum "F_0" value required by a process can be related to the "D" value of the bioburden by the following equation:

$$F_0 = D_{121} \times (\log A - \log B)$$

where:

— "D_{121}" is equal to the time required at 121°C to reduce the population of the most heat resistant organism in the unit by 90%;

— "A" is the microbial count per container; and

— "B" is the maximum acceptable probability of survival ($\leq 1 \times 10^{-6}$ for pharmaceutical dosage forms).

Laboratory studies which determine the number and resistance of microorganisms associated with a product (bioburden) serve as the basis for calculating the required minimum "F0" value required for sterilisation.

A more conservative approach assumes a "D_{121}" value of 1 minute for the bioburden of the product.

Equipment Qualification

Prior to commencing heat distribution, heat penetration and/or biological challenge reduction studies, it is necessary that the equipment be checked and certified as properly installed, equipped and functioning as per its design.

Installation Requirements

a) For new equipment, qualification begins with the establishment of design, purchase and installation requirements. These requirements must be specific to the type and model of units (such as saturated steam, water immersion, water cascade, air-steam mixtures, gravity air displacement, vacuum air displacement). Included in these written requirements are all the construction materials, the sizes and tolerances of the chamber, support services and power supplies, the alarm systems, monitoring systems with response tolerance and accuracy requirements, and the operational parameter requirements as governed by the established process specifications.

   Installation qualification of new equipment should be based on written requirements and documented. The requirements should ensure that the predetermined construction and installation requirements are assessed as soon as installation permits, and that these requirements are met (correct piping materials, wiring types, alarm hookups, recorders and gauges, chamber levelling, all piping is sealed and door gasketing effects proper sealing). All installation parameters should be documented and certified prior to operational qualification of the equipment.

b) For existing equipment, subject to concurrent or retrospective validation approaches, installation qualification requires defining the existing equipment design and installation parameters from records and direct assessment. The equipment is then evaluated for its capability to satisfy the defined process specifications, and for determination of any upgrading or procedural modifications needed to meet the process requirements.

Modifications should be documented as being performed according to predetermined requirements and certified as rendering the equipment suitable for validation testing.

Operational Qualification

Operational qualification consists of testing the equipment over its pre-defined and installed operating range to verify consistent performance. Three or more test runs should be performed which demonstrate through documented evidence that:

— controls, alarms, monitoring devices and operation indicators function;

— chamber pressure integrity is maintained;

— chamber vacuum is maintained, if applicable;

— written procedures accurately reflect equipment operation;

— operation parameters are attained as preset for each test run.

Equipment should be certified as operationally qualified for any subsequent studies to be considered adequate.

HEAT DISTRIBUTION STUDIES

Heat distribution studies are performed in order to determine temperature variation throughout the steriliser chamber and should be performed prior to heat penetration studies. These studies should encompass empty chamber and loaded chamber evaluation and should be performed according to written procedures using temperature measuring sensors or probes which have been calibrated before and after use for each run.

The temperature uniformity requirements based on the type of steriliser and specific processing parameters should be specified. Heat distribution runs using an empty chamber may be performed during equipment operational qualification. These runs should be performed using the maximum and minimum cycle times and temperatures specified for the equipment.

Test runs should be repeated at each preset cycle time and temperature required in the protocol, in order to identify the heat distribution pattern of the chamber, including the slowest heating points. The studies should demonstrate that the uniformity of the sterilising medium throughout the empty chamber is within the temperature variation limits established in the protocol.

Multiple temperature sensing devices should be used in each test run. The devices should be capable of simultaneous data generation within preestablished time intervals in order to permit determination of the slowest and fastest heating zones in the chamber.

The location of each device should be documented. The placement of the devices should ensure that a uniform distribution is achieved throughout the steriliser chamber.

The data from all runs should be collated into a temperature profile of the chamber.

Heat distribution studies should also be performed on maximum and minimum chamber load configurations with consideration to the following:

a) Multiple temperature sensing devices are placed throughout the chamber but not inside the units of the load to determine the effect of any defined loading pattern on the temperature distribution within the chamber.

b) The test runs should be performed using the different container sizes to be processed using the sterilisation parameters specified for the normal production process.

c) The position of each temperature sensor in each test run must be documented.

d) The slowest heating point(s), or cold spot(s), in each run should be determined and documented.

e) Repeat runs must be performed to establish whether, for a given load configuration, the location of the cold spot(s) is fixed or variable.

f) A temperature distribution profile for each chamber load configuration should be developed and documented.

Failure to demonstrate operational consistency within the chosen criteria for acceptable temperature uniformity precludes validation to be demonstrable for the specified sterilisation cycle.

Each test run performed should be evaluated. The completed studies should be certified prior to beginning heat penetration studies.

In order to verify that the sterilising temperature has been reached in each load subjected to moist heat sterilisation, it is necessary to conduct heat penetration studies. These studies are conducted to ensure that the coolest unit within a pre-defined loading pattern (including minimum and maximum loads) will consistently be exposed to sufficient heat lethality (minimum "F_0").

Heat penetration studies should be performed according to detailed written procedures using temperature sensing devices which have been calibrated before and after each validation run which are capable of simultaneous data generation within preestablished time intervals in order to permit determination of the slowest and fastest heating units in the chamber.

The validation protocol should make provision for such variables as container size, design, material, viscosity of solution and fill volume. The container should have the maximum fill volume of a solution with heating characteristics as slow as the slowest-to-heat solution sterilised by the specified cycle. Heat penetration studies should be conducted with the maximum and minimum loading configurations for each sterilisation cycle using the sterilisation parameters specified for the normal production cycles.

Depending on the size of the container, it may be necessary to perform initial container mapping studies with temperature sensing devices placed inside the product container to identify its heat penetration characteristics and to determine the container "cold spot". During heat penetration studies, sensors should be placed in the containers at the slowest heating point in the containers, where practicable. The majority of these containers should be located at the slowest heating point in the loading pattern as determined by the heat distribution studies.

Heat delivered to the slowest heating unit of the load is monitored and this data is employed to compute the minimum lethality ("F_0" value) of the process. Once the slowest heating units of the load have been identified, at least three replicate runs should be performed to verify that the desired minimum process "F_0" value can be achieved reproducibly throughout the load. The process is considered acceptable once such consistency in lethality has been adequately established.

Biological Challenge

Introducing a known quantity of specific microorganisms with established "D" values and assessing the level of reduction with time is appropriate when the Probability of Survival approach is used. These biological challenge reduction runs may be done in conjunction with heat penetration studies.

The level of biological challenge selected for the study should consider seasonal as well as lot-to-lot variation in the product bioburden (quantity and "D" value) and should be such that a probability of survival of 1 in 106 is confirmed in all cases. A worse case bioburden using B. stearothermophilus spores is acceptable.

The placement of biological challenges should be defined in writing. The challenge should be placed in containers where practicable, so as to reflect the desired processing conditions. In addition, they must be located in direct relation to any temperature sensors when run concurrent with heat penetration studies. A minimum of three runs should be performed for each load configuration under evaluation. Positive controls should be run with each load to verify the viability of the challenge organism.

Records of the organism type, "D" value, challenge level, lot number, placement, and growth result should be available. Growth of any challenge following any of the runs indicates that sterilisation has not been achieved. The process parameters should be evaluated. If no processing error is discernable, the process is judged unacceptable.

Post-Validation Monitoring

Post-validation monitoring consists primarily of routine checking of sterilisation cycle conditions against the validated cycle, routine bioburden sampling, and ongoing equipment maintenance.

Each sterilisation cycle must be monitored to ensure that the cycle conditions were set as specified and that the time, temperature and pressure parameters were attained as per the validated cycle. These checks should be documented in the processing records.

a) The requirement to perform monitoring should be a detailed written procedure referenced in the validation protocol.

b) Biological challenges should be documented when performed in routine monitoring procedures. The location, number, type and lot number of the challenge must be included in the records along with the actual test results.

c) Deviations from defined processing conditions must be documented, investigated and assessed for compliance with the protocol. Deviations below any preestablished conditions should be judged as compromising the sterilisation process.

For sterilisation cycles based on the Probability of Survival approach, samples for bioburden testing should be obtained on each batch of drug product prior to sterilisation.

a) Samples collected at the beginning and at the end of the filling operation should be used to determine the microbial count and heat resistance of the most resistant product isolates. Routine sampling may vary according to the accumulated product testing history.

b) For any validated sterilisation process a maximum microbial count and a maximum microbial heat resistance for filled containers prior to sterilisation should be established. Microbial counts or heat resistance exceeding these levels should be judged as compromising the sterilisation.

In order to ensure that the equipment and support systems function consistently within the validation protocol specifications, there should be a written programme for the ongoing maintenance of each piece of equipment defined in the protocol. The maintenance programme should detail the items to be checked and the frequency of maintenance and calibration of monitoring devices. It should require detailed written records of all maintenance performed. The records should be reviewed by a qualified person to ensure that the process has not been compromised.

REQUALIFICATION

All changes to the steriliser system or process must be pre-authorised through the change control system or be required as part of a preestablished maintenance programme. Requalification establishes that changes to parts of the sterilising system have not invalidated the conditions outlined in the validation protocol.

Changes which require requalification include:

— replacement of sterilising medium supply components, exhaust valves or door gaskets;

— modifications to the interior chamber walls;

— modifications to the sterilising medium generating or cooling system supplies or their control systems;

— modifications to steriliser carts or unit carriers (trays).

Heat distribution should be requalified when changes to the equipment may affect the uniformity of sterilising medium in the chamber.

Heat penetration should be requalified when changes to the sterilisation process system may affect penetration of heat to the units being processed.

Requalification is performed according to detailed written procedures which require that the original validation parameters and limits be used as evaluation criteria. The requalification studies must be documented in detail and results of the studies should be compared to the original validation results and evaluated to the same extent. If the results are satisfactory, the system should be certified. If the results are not satisfactory, the modified system requires new validation studies.

Changes to loading patterns, new container/closure systems or cycle parameters do not qualify for requalification but rather require that new validation studies be performed since, the original validation parameters being different.

DOCUMENTATION

The following information should be prepared in a summary form for the purposes of inspection and evaluation by the appropriate HPFBI Bureaux.

Outline

Information required in relation to the formulation and to the filling stages of sterile drugs:

a) the type of sterile drugs; parenterals or non-parenterals;

b) the batch size;

c) description of the drug and the container/closure system to be sterilised (e.g., size(s), fill volume, or secondary packaging);

d) the air grade where the drug is formulated;

e) the air grade where the drug is filled before moist heat sterilisation.

A comprehensive outline of the protocol followed in the validation of the process should be prepared. The outline should indicate the steps performed, in proper sequence, and should encompass:

a) the approach taken;

b) justification of the approach based on the product factors;

c) summation of any modifications to the equipment required; and

d) any modifications to the protocol resulting from the study.

Process Documentation

a) If retrospective validation was conducted, the details of the lot analysis and process condition evaluation for the time period being assessed should be compiled. Evidence that process/product failures and discrepancies were included in the evaluation should be available.

b) The F0 values required to establish the validation of the process and "D" values used in the calculations should be stated giving the source of the "D" values and calculation applied.

c) The sterilisation cycle parameters used along with the load configuration(s) to which the cycle applies should be available. The details of the development of the cycle when a Probability of Survival approach was used must be included, as per Section 9 of this document and Microbiology below.

d) The heat distribution studies conducted should be summarised on a run to-run and overall basis including an evaluation. Any modifications to the studies should be detailed and study impact evaluations given. The information must encompass the level of testing undertaken, calibration requirements and chamber conditions (empty, max./min. load). Diagrams of loading patterns and sensor placement are recommended.

e) All heat penetration studies undertaken should be summarised on a run to run and overall basis. The data should demonstrate that the study parameters relate to the heat distribution study results. Any modifications to the study should be detailed and process impact assessed. The information available should be similar to that complied for the heat distribution studies.

Microbiology

a) Bioburden determinations undertaken for the product and environment in Probability of Survival approaches should be detailed. The information should include the materials or areas monitored, media and methods employed and a summary of results by number and species with "Dmin" and "Dmax" values. The laboratory conducting the "D" value determinations should be identified.

b) Biological challenge reduction studies, when performed, should be summarised and include the species used, "D" value applied, carrier method, placement, recovery methods and results obtained. Placement of the challenge should demonstrate relationship to the heat distribution and heat penetration studies.

Pharmaceutical Packaging Lines Validation

A validated process is one which enables consistent manufacturing and packaging of products in accordance with the product and market requirements in a cost effective and secure manner. Since consistency and cost effectiveness are, without doubt, key business considerations, a validation activity should be seen not as a regulatory requirement but as a business necessity. To achieve the ultimate goal of packaging product perfectly every time, equipment engineers, packaging technologists and quality teams must plan and work through a validation programme together in order to create a robust operation. As with any other multi-disciplinary project they will need to plan their work (objectives, timescales, deliverables, roles & responsibilities and key milestones) and report their findings. As you read through the notes that follow, you should view the primary objective not as regulatory compliance but as the establishment of an efficient process with minimum down time, rejects and errors. Packaging has been defined as: "the art, science and technology of preparing goods for sale in a cost effective manner."

In considering what is meant by "preparing goods for sale" in the context of pharmaceuticals we should remember that the packaging must:

— preserve the product - from degradation or contamination
— contain the product - to avoid leakage
— identify the product - providing traceability and information regarding expiry date, etc. and will also be required to provide:
— security - against tampering and counterfeiting
— information on use - an "aide memoir" for compliance.
— convenience in use - for medical staff or patient;
— a marketing tool - supporting features and/or graphics appropriate to the sales medium (OTC vs. ethical).

All this must be ensured for the life of the product and achieved within a complex regulatory environment. The latter extends beyond the pharmaceutical company packaging lines to the warehousing and distribution of packaged goods and to the manufacture of packaging components and the supply of raw materials.

There are several key areas that impact the robustness of a packaging process and should be considered in validation including:

— Packaging materials
— Packaging equipment
— Line layout
— Operator training
— Standard operating procedures.

Packaging Materials

In 2000/2001, 42% of the defects reported by MHRA in the UK related to printed packaging components; either because they were incorrectly printed or because the wrong components were used within the pack. In order to minimise the risk of defective product reaching the patient, it is therefore vital that there is strict procedural control of artwork development, review and approval and of the handling of printed components from printer to packaging line.

A good relationship with suppliers is essential, together with rigorous packaging material specifications. Pack design needs to be carried out by personnel who know how the materials are manufactured and understand what is required for production lines to operate effectively and efficiently.

It must be recognised that with most packaging materials, pharmaceuticals represent a very small market segment (for example only 4% of the LDPE (low density polyethylene) produced is destined for pharmaceutical use). With their long production runs (polymers for example are manufactured in 20 ton batches or as continuous production), packaging materials suppliers may be under significant commercial pressure from larger customers with regard to specification. In a good relationship, the supplier will have been made aware of the implications of such changes for the packaging line and technical personnel from both companies should be able to work together to address the problem.

An efficient production line needs consistent materials and the storage and handling of components is as vital in this respect as their specification. Fiber-based materials such as leaflets (inserts), cartons and labels for example, can be adversely affected by changes in temperature and relative humidity.

Packaging Materials Equipment

The design and layout of equipment has major impact on the efficiency of the packaging line. Well designed equipment will lend itself to efficient production of a consistent standard, whereas older equipment can often be inflexible and may have elements of poor design such as areas where packaging components or product may be trapped. These "traps" can result in products being incorrectly packed, e.g. a carton containing the wrong leaflet or product from a different batch. This represents a significant risk to the patient and is one of the major reasons for product recall in the industry.

The greater the number of stages there are in a packaging line, the lower its efficiency will be. With modern order patterns of short runs it may for example be better to have two slow speed fillers feeding a single cartonner rather than a single high-speed filler. Appropriate validation of the packaging lines will challenge the robustness of the packaging operation establishing the conditions under which efficiency is maximised.

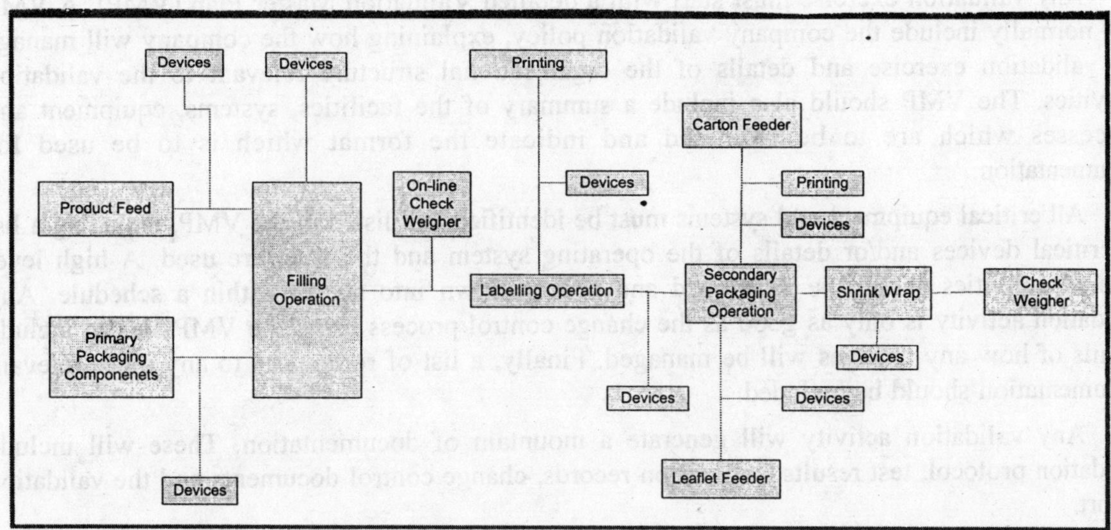

Figure 1. A typical packaging line layout

Design considerations for a line layout should include the ability to manage quick change-over, perform line clearance between batches of product and clean the line in an easy and controlled manner. The majority of problems on packaging lines are related in some way to poor line clearance; it is therefore important to design these problems out.

A typical packing line will consist of several feeders for packaging components and product. Devices will normally be located in critical positions on the line to detect presence or otherwise of the materials. For example, a device installed on the carton feeder will ensure that a carton is supplied for each product or tray of product and a barcode reader will verify that it is the correct one. A checkweigher will make certain that underfilled or overfilled bottles are identified and ensures via the reject device that they are excluded from the batch. The layout of the equipment should guarantee that easy access is provided for operators and the engineers to access this equipment when adjustments and or maintenance are required.

Operating Procedures

To manage a packaging line, adequate standard operating procedures (SOPs) will be required. It is vital that there are clear and unambiguous instructions on how to operate, adjust, and maintain each piece of equipment. In addition, there will be procedures to detail how a batch is packaged, SOP usually explains how each material is received on the line and checked for correctness, quantity, etc. by the operators. Details of In Process Control (IPC) tests will be given in these SOPs. Involving the line operators in developing the SOPs will result in documents that more accurately reflect what is actually happening on a day to day basis. Operators will also take ownership of the SOPs ensuring better compliance and hence less problems on the line.

Any validation exercise must start with a detailed Validation Master Plan (VMP). A VMP will normally include the company validation policy, explaining how the company will manage the validation exercise and details of the organisational structure relevant to the validation activities. The VMP should also include a summary of the facilities, systems, equipment and processes which are to be validated and indicate the format which is to be used for documentation.

All critical equipment and systems must be identified and listed in the VMP, including a list of critical devices and/or details of the operating system and the software used. A high level plan of activities should be developed and broken down into stages within a schedule. Any validation activity is only as good as the change control process used; the VMP should include details of how any changes will be managed. Finally, a list of references to any other relevant documentation should be included.

Any validation activity will generate a mountain of documentation. These will include validation protocol, test results, calibration records, change control documents and the validation report.

Validation protocol should be designed to test all the critical steps in the process. They provide a list of tests which are to be performed and the acceptance limits for each test. The tests must demonstrate that the system is able to do what is expected within the operating range required for the process. It is also important however, to test the system beyond the normal operating range to provide information on the system behavior, which can be used to finalise operational limits.

A classical approach to validation is to prepare test protocol for Design Qualification (DQ), Installation Qualification (IQ), Operational Qualification (OQ) and Performance Qualification (PQ). Information gathered from each of these stages must be fed into the next to ensure that the system is adequately tested. Protocol should test each piece of equipment or step in the process, however, it is important to have one overall protocol to test the interaction between different pieces of equipment and/or systems.

DQ protocol should be designed to test the conformance of the system to the original design (user requirements) and the GMP requirements. For older equipment it is worthwhile to conduct this exercise even if detailed information on the original design is not available; any potential shortfall of the system with respect to the current GMP (CGMP) requirements should be assessed. It is important to test the equipment adequately, for example it is critical to run printed components down the line, as plain components display different characteristics. It is therefore recommended that such tests are included in the factory acceptance tests.

IQ protocol should consist of checklists to ensure that the system or equipment is properly installed. At this stage engineering drawings should be checked and updated as appropriate.

OQ protocol will challenge the system to demonstrate that it can operate within the specified parameters. Tests should be developed based on the knowledge of the process and the systems, ensuring that the upper and lower operating limits are challenged. Equipment calibration should be performed at this stage and the frequency of in-process control (IPC) checks should be established. The line operating procedures (including those covering calibration, cleaning and preventative maintenance) should be finalised and operator training should be completed. The issue of procedures and assessment of operator competency with respect to the SOPs should be listed as key deliverables on the OQ protocol.

PQ protocol will be the last stage in any validation activity and should reflect the 'real' production environment, using production materials in a normal daily operation. The PQ exercise should extend over a time period sufficient to ensure that shift working patterns and normal lunch breaks etc. are included and to certify that the systems are challenged for stop/start, batch changes etc. This approach may create problems for the QA groups if they are required to release batches prior to issue of the final validation report.

The need for the PQ and its extent should therefore be evaluated when developing the VMP and the rationale for the acceptance of the validation must be documented in the VMP prior to start up of the validation activity. It is worthwhile to look for opportunities within the early production schedules to organise a matrix of PQ tests so as to speed up the collection of data while ensuring that all aspects of the system have been challenged and tested. It is important to document the rationale for a matrix approach in the VMP so that it is clear what and why it will be done.

The final validation report should include all the test results together with details of any changes made to the system. If there are test failures, these must all be reported and the resulting actions detailed. Any learning points from the activity should be logged and recommendations for future improvements documented. It is important to include a recommendation on the timescale for review of the system validation. The validation report must be reviewed and approved by QA. Some Hints and Tips Described below.

1. Spend as much time as is necessary to understand the system and its critical steps. Never underestimate the amount of time needed to develop plans, the more time you spend in design of the protocol, the less you will waste in resolving issues and investigating failures.
2. Ensure that you develop a good sound sampling plan so that your IPC tests are meaningful and provide you with useful data on the line performance (samples should reflect the normal operating conditions). The frequency of IPC tests can be reduced after review of data, so have a procedure in place to ensure that all the IPC data is routinely reviewed and assessed by knowledgeable people.
3. Device challenges will provide more information if performed before and after stoppages.
4. Finally, any validated system is as good as the associated change control process. Therefore, make sure all changes are fully assessed and documented. The impact of the

change on the validation status of the system must be fully assessed before any changes are made.

In the pharmaceutical industry we are constantly challenged to reduce costs while new markets and new packs add complexity to the operation and while an ever changing regulatory environment demands our compliance. To ensure pack integrity, manage complexity, maximise efficiency and minimise costs; appropriately designed packs, running in validated packaging lines, are a business necessity rather than a regulatory requirement. Regulators simply require that validation be documented properly to demonstrate that it has been done in accordance with the GMP expectation.

Pharmaceutical Validation and Process Control in Drug Development

Validation is an integral part of quality assurance; it involves the systematic study of systems, facilities and processes aimed at determining whether they perform their intended functions adequately and consistently as specified. A validated process is one which has been demonstrated to provide a high degree of assurance that uniform batches will be produced that meet the required specifications and has therefore been formally approved. Validation in itself does not improve processes but confirms that the processes have been properly developed and are under control. Adequate validation is beneficial to the manufacturer in many ways:

— It deepens the understanding of processes; decreases the risk of preventing problems and thus assures the smooth running of the process.
— It decreases the risk of defect costs.
— It decreases the risk of regulatory noncompliance.
— A fully validated process may require less in-process controls and end product testing.

Validation should thus be considered in the following situations:

— Totally new process;
— New equipment;
— Process and equipment which have been altered to suit changing priorities; and · Process where the end-product test is poor and an unreliable indicator of product quality.

When any new manufacturing formula or method of preparation is adopted, steps should be taken to demonstrate its suitability for routine processing. The defined process should be shown to yield a product consistent with the required quality. In this phase, the extent to which deviations from chosen parameters can influence product quality should also be evaluated.

When certain processes or products have been validated during the development stage, it is not always necessary to revalidate the whole process or product if similar equipment is used or similar products have been produced, provided that the final product conforms to the in-process controls and final product specification. There should be a clear distinction between in-process control and validation. In production, tests are performed each time on a batch to batch basis using specifications and methods devised during the development phase. The objective is to monitor the process continuously.

Major Phases in Validation

The activities relating to validation studies may be classified into three:

Phase 1: This is the Pre-validation Qualification Phase which covers all activities relating to product research and development, formulation pilot batch studies, scale-up studies, transfer of technology to commercial scale batches, establishing stability conditions and storage, and handling of in-process and finished dosage forms, equipment qualification, installation qualification, master production document, operational qualification and process capacity.

Phase 2: This is the Process Validation Phase. It is designed to verify that all established limits of the critical process parameter are valid and that satisfactory products can be produced even under the worst conditions.

Phase 3: Known as the Validation Maintenance Phase, it requires frequent review of all process related documents, including validation of audit reports, to assure that there have been no changes, deviations, failures and modifications to the production process and that all standard operating procedures (SOPs), including change control procedures, have been followed. At this stage, the validation team comprising of individuals representing all major departments also assures that there have been no changes/deviations that should have resulted in requalification and revalidation. A careful design and validation of systems and process controls can establish a high degree of confidence that all lots or batches produced will meet their intended specifications. It is assumed that throughout manufacturing and control, operations are conducted in accordance with the principle of good manufacturing practice (GMP) both in general and in specific reference to sterile product manufacture. The validation steps recommended in GMP guidelines can be summarised as follows:

— As a prerequisite, all studies should be conducted in accordance with a detailed, preestablished protocol or series of protocol, which in turn is subject to formal – change control procedures;

— Both the personnel conducting the studies and those running the process being studied should be appropriately trained and qualified and be suitable and competent to perform the task assigned to them;

— All data generated during the course of studies should be formally reviewed and certified as evaluated against predetermined criteria;

— Suitable testing facilities, equipment, instruments and methodology should be available;

— Suitable clean room facilities should be available in both the 'local' and background environment. There should be assurance that the clean room environment as specified is secured through initial commissioning (qualification) and subsequently through the implementation of a programme of re-testing – in-process equipment should be properly installed, qualified and maintained;

— When appropriate attention has been paid to the above, the process, if aseptic, may be validated by means of "process simulation" studies;

— The process should be revalidated at intervals; and · Comprehensive documentation should be available to define support and record the overall validation process.

Protocol should specify the following in detail:

— The objective and scope of study. There should already be a definition of purpose;

— A clear and precise definition of process equipment system or subsystem, which is to be the subject of study with details of performance characteristics;

— Installation and qualification requirement for new equipment;

— Any upgrading requirement for existing equipment with justification for the change(s) and statement of qualification requirement;

— Detailed stepwise statement of actions to be taken in performing the study (or studies);

— Assignment of responsibility for performing the study;

— Statement on all test methodology to be employed with a precise statement of the test equipment and/or materials to be used;

— Test equipment calibration requirements;

— References to any relevant standard operating procedures (SOP);

— Requirement for the current format of the report on the study;

— Acceptance criteria against which the success (or otherwise) of the study is to be evaluated; and

— The personnel responsible for evaluating and certifying the acceptability of each stage in the study and for the final evaluation and certification of the process as a whole, as measured against the pre-defined criteria.

All personnel involved in conducting the studies should be properly trained and qualified because they can, and often, have a crucial effect on the quality of the end product. All information or data generated as a result of the study protocol should be evaluated by qualified individuals against protocol criteria and judged as meeting or failing the requirements. Written evidence supporting the evaluation and conclusion should be available. If such an evaluation shows that protocol criteria have not been met, the study should be considered as having failed to demonstrate acceptability and the reasons should be investigated and documented. Any failure to follow the procedure as laid down in the protocol must be considered as potentially compromising the validity of the study itself and requires critical evaluation of all the impact on the study. The final certification of the validation study should specify the predetermined acceptance criteria against which success or failure was evaluated.

Analytical Assays and Test Methods

Method validation confirms that the analytical procedure employed for a specific test is suitable for its intended use. The validation of an analytical method is the process by which it is established by laboratory studies that the performance characteristics of the method meet the requirement for the intended application. This implies that validity of a method can be demonstrated only though laboratory studies. Methods should be validated or revalidated:

— before their introduction and routine use;

— whenever the conditions change for which the method has been validated, e.g., instrument with different characteristics; and

— wherever the method is changed and the change is outside the original scope of the method.

The validity of a specific method should be demonstrated in laboratory experiments using samples or standards that are similar to the unknown samples analysed in the routine. The preparation and execution should follow a validation protocol preferably written in a step-by-step instruction format as follows:

— Develop a validation protocol or operating procedure for the validation;

— Define the application purpose and scope of the method;

— Define the performance parameters and acceptance criteria;

— Define validation experiments;

— Verify relevant performance characteristics of the equipment;

— Select quality materials, e.g., standards and reagents;

— Perform pre-validation experiments;

— Adjust method parameters and/or acceptance criteria, if necessary;

— Perform full internal (and external) validation experiments;

— Develop SOPs for executing the method routinely;

— Define criteria for revalidation;

— Define type and frequency of system suitability tests and/or analytical quality control (AQC) checks for the routine; and

— Document validation experiments and results in the validation report.

Environmental Considerations

Cleaning validation is documented proof that one can consistently and effectively clean a system or equipment items. The procedure is necessary for the following reasons:

— It is a customer requirement – it ensures the safety and purity of the product;

— It is a regulatory requirement in active pharmaceutical product manufacture; and

— It also assures from an internal control and compliance point of view the quality of the process.

The FDA guide to inspections intended to cover equipment cleaning (chemical residues only) expects firms to have written procedure (SOPs) detailing the cleaning processes and also written general procedure on how cleaning processes will be validated. FDA expects a final validation report which is approved by management and which states whether or not the cleaning process is valid. The data should support a conclusion that residues have been reduced to an "acceptable level". Hardercited five crucial elements:

1. A standard operating procedure (SOP) for cleaning with a checklist;
2. A procedure for determining cleanliness (rinse or swab);
3. An assay for testing residual drug levels;
4. Preset criteria for testing chemical and microbial limit to which to equipment must be cleaned; and
5. Protocol for cleaning validation.

Harder recommended that the procedure be tested for, requiring it to be successful on three successive cleanings and there should be periodic revalidation as well as revalidation after significant changes. Jenkins and Vanderwielen presented an overview of cleaning validation covering strategy and determination of residue limits, method of sampling and analysis noting that "increased use of multipurpose equipment" has produced increased interest in cleaning validation. The cleaning protocol must be thorough and must be checked. Training is essential. A validation programme requires

— criteria for acceptance after cleaning,
— appropriate methods of sampling,
— a maximum limit set for residues, and
— test methods that must themselves be tested.

Products to be tested may be put into groups rather than testing all of them. The most important may not be the highest volume product but those capable of causing the largest possible problems if contaminated or if they contaminate the products (solubility of the drug is an important issue). Equipment may also be tested in groups.

Process Validation

Process validation is the means of ensuring and providing documentary evidence that processes (within their specified design parameters) are capable of repeatedly and reliably producing a finished product of the required quality. It would normally be expected that process validation be completed prior to the release of the finished product for sale (prospective validation). Where this is not possible, it may be necessary to validate processes during routine production (concurrent validation). Processes, which have been in use for some time without any significant changes, may also be validated according to an approved protocol (retrospective validation).

Before process validation can be started, manufacturing equipment and control instruments as well as the formulation must be qualified. The information on a pharmaceutical product should be studied in detail and qualified at the development stage, i.e., before an application for marketing authorisation is submitted. This involves studies on the compatibility of active ingredients and recipients, and of final drug product and packaging materials, stability studies, etc. Other aspects of manufacture must be validated including critical services (water, air, nitrogen, power supply, etc.) and supporting operations such as equipment cleaning and sanitation of premises. Proper training and motivation of personnel are prerequisites to successful validation.

Pharmaceutical Process Equipment

The key idea of validation is to provide a high level of documented evidence that the equipment and the process conform to a written standard. The level (or depth) is dictated by the complexity of the system or equipment. The validation package must provide the necessary information and test procedures required to provide that the system and process meet specified requirements. Validation of pharmaceutical process equipment involves the following:

— *Installation Qualification:* This ensures that all major processing and packaging equipment, and ancillary systems are in conformity with installation specification, equipment manuals schematics and engineering drawing. It verifies that the equipment has been installed in accordance with manufacturers recommendation in a proper manner and placed in an environment suitable for its intended purpose.

— *Operational Qualification:* This is done to provide a high degree of assurance that the equipment functions as intended. Operational qualification should be conducted in two stages:

  — Component Operational Qualification, of which calibration can be considered a large part.

  — System Operational Qualification to determine if the entire system operates as an integrated whole.

  — Process Performance Qualification: This verifies that the system is repeatable and is consistently producing a quality product.

These exercises assure, through appropriate performance lists and related documentation, that equipment, ancillary systems and subsystems have been commissioned correctly. The end results are that all future operations will be reliable and within prescribed operational limits.

At various stages in a validation exercise there are needs for protocol, documentation, procedures, specifications and acceptance criteria for test results. All these need to be reviewed, checked and authorised. It would be expected that representatives from the professional disciplines, e.g., engineering, research and development, manufacturing, quality control and quality assurance are actively involved in these undertakings with the final authorisation given by a validation team or the quality assurance representative.

There are two basic approaches to the validation of the process itself (apart from the qualification of equipment used in production, the calibration of control and measurement instruments, the evaluation of environmental factors, etc). These are the experimental approach and the approach based on the analysis of historical data. The experimental approach, which is applicable to both prospective and concurrent validation, may involve

— extensive product testing,
— simulation process trials,
— challenge/worst case trials, and
— control of process parameters (mostly physical).

One of the most practical forms of process validation, mainly for non-sterile products, is the final testing of the product to the extent greater than that required in routine quality control. It may involve extensive sampling, far beyond that called for in routine quality control and specifications, and often for certain parameters only. Thus, for instance, several hundred tablets per batch may be weighed to determine unit dose uniformity. The results are then treated statistically to verify the normality of the distribution and to determine the standard deviation from the average weight. Confidence limits for individual results and for batch homogeneity are also estimated. Strong assurance is provided that samples taken at random will meet regulatory requirements if the confidence limits are within compendial specifications.

In the approach based on analysis of historical data, no experiments are performed in retrospective validation, but instead all available historical data concerning a number of batches are combined and jointly analysed, if production is proceeding smoothly during the period preceding validation and the data in process inspection and final testing of the product are combined and treated statistically. The results including the outcome of process capability studies, trend analysis, etc., will indicate whether the process is under control or not.

Pharmacopoeial Testing

Past lack of rigour in testing has been responsible for some of the most controversial incidents of poisoning and drug-induced deformity. Happily, improved foresight and the thorough nature of contemporary QC culture means that such incidents are seldom encountered these days. However, this should not be seen as an excuse for allowing current standards of medicine testing to deteriorate. Control of quality in pharmaceutical and biopharmaceutical 1 formulations can be described and captured in terms of the product: purity, consistency and quality (PCQ).

The purity should be high, the consistency of product from batch to batch and outlet to outlet should be high and the general quality in terms of freedom from chemical, microbiological and physical contamination should be exemplary. Contrary to a commonly perceived flaw in thinking it is not possible to test and inspect quality into a product. This is exemplified in terms of the maintenance of a philosophy of zero-defect tolerance, product conformity to limits, specified values (specifications) and fitness for the purpose for which the product or process was intended (Figure 2). These attitudes form the basis of creating the best products via routine effective QC.

Fundamental to the best ways of working through a proper control of quality is the decision as to the main criteria in controlling the quality itself. Decision-making can be based on two general themes, either using experiential knowledge or a scientific rationale to aid judgement. There is no absolute definition as to which of these is correct, but consensus among analysts and pharmaceutical scientists is that the best quality systems (QS) incorporate the following:

- — sound scientific and most recently reviewed basis to the method;
- — effective sampling number, volume and frequency;
- — discriminatory analysis;
- — not conceding to over-reliance on one approach;
- — accountability;
- — participant willingness and personal integrity;
- — exit strategies in the event of failure; and
- — improvement culture.

Using these themes is pivotal to the effective smooth running of the total QS structure used in validation analyses (Figure 2) and manufacturing processes.

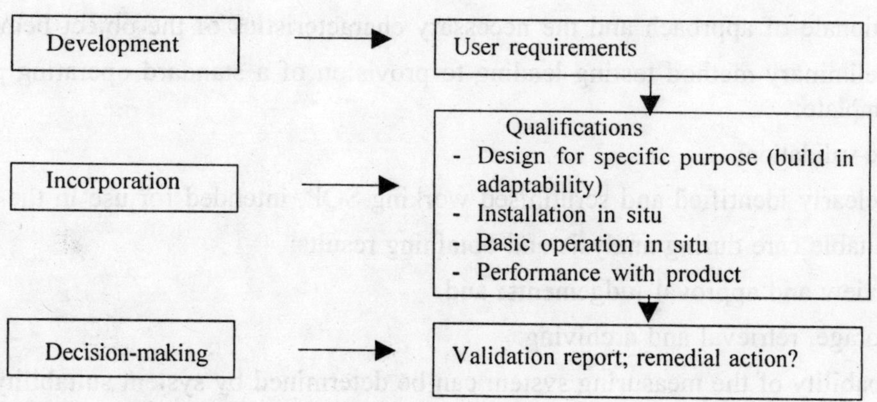

Figure 2: The Validation Life-cycle

Pharmacopoeial Testing (PT)

Pharmacopoeias and pharmacopoeial testing (PT) consist of a standardised guideline for the testing pharmaceutical ingredients and active drug substances. These are presented in the form of series of monographs (documents dealing with single substance that describe a series of parallel tests and specified limits for a substance at a range of levels from minor to major components) that perform the functions of maintaining product PCQ and fulfil the role of identifying the main constituent.

Control with a Moving Platform

It is essential to consider why control is necessary; part this derives from review of the limitations and the expectations of the method. Superimposed on demands placed by the customer and the rigour of QC, PT must focus very clearly on the latest state-of-the-art developments, such as miniaturisation technologies and understanding in the chemical, biomedical and pharmaceutical sciences. This highlights notions system suitability testing and validation parameters and puts them into the frame with incumbent notions 'keeping the analytical goalpost in sight' to ensure the analytical test docs exactly what is required of it. This means ensuring that short process steps occur between points of uncertainty and where the procedure may be most susceptible to compromise by external influences.

Pharmacopoeias should also be evolving and the International Conference on Harmonisation Technical Requirements for Registration Pharmaceuticals for Human Use (ICH) requires dutiful attention, given that products can now be processed and shipped on a fully global basis. This should also be framed against the expectations of the regulatory bodies such as the Medicines Control Agency (MCA) and the US Food and Drug Administration (FDA). Test method validation should encompass identification of the following:

— suitable expertise and those responsible;
— justification for the method selected;
— rationale of approach and the necessary characteristics of the object being investigated;
— preliminary method testing leading to provision of a standard operating procedure (SOP) template;
— pre-validation;
— a clearly identified and scrutinised working SOP, intended for use in the exercise;
— suitable care during analysis and obtaining results;
— review and approval judgements; and
— storage, retrieval and archiving.

The capability of the measuring system can be determined by system suitability testing. System suitability is fundamental to the selection of the right technology to comply with the right-first-time way of thinking and is prone to change, particularly when technology is improving in such instances as when reviewing the ability to retrieve, process and generally deal with large volumes of stored data, which can be processed in ever-decreasing times nowadays. In this case, a series of tests can be envisaged for any system and they relate to what the method measures, how data is recorded and how some degree of regularity can be obtained from the presented data and then related to physical processes that are taking place.

A typical example might include high-performance liquid chromatography or some other form of chromatography. Here, the form of graphical output in terms of the shape and position of peaks obtained on a trace or chromatogram can be likened to elution of analyte down the length of a partitioning column and past the detector in response to flow of solvent. Analytical chemists frequently talk about the number of theoretical plates, resolution or selectivity factors that describe the spatial format of measure and signals (represented as peaks) with respect to one another and a standard. In general, they can be related in a direct way to the effectiveness of the analytical tool.

Consequences of Failure

When a body gets it wrong, put very simply, in extreme cases what occurs is litigation over negligence, reputation failure events and loss of business. It then becomes clear that QC is very important in terms of the stability of the product and provision for challenge testing to support the product once beyond the jurisdiction of the manufacturer. An unchecked product, like a 'ticking time bomb' could be a catastrophic liability, as a marketed product could lead to loss of business and customer confidence and, in the worst-case scenario, the personal injury to a customer or client (Figure 3).

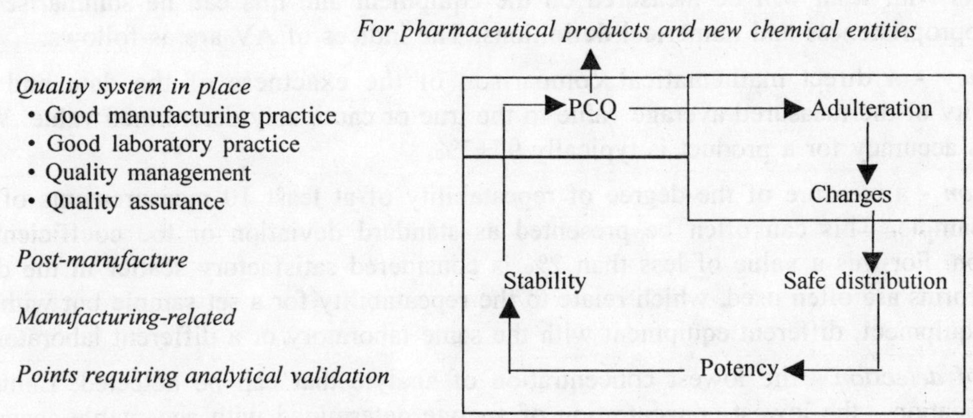

Figure 3: Risk Analysis and Damage Limitation Based on Use of a Proper Quality System

Quality-driven Need for Validation

Quality gurus in the past have stressed the need for 'fitness-for-purpose' of intercalating processes. Validation is defined as ensuring that any process or product complies with a specification, based on its intended use. In other words, a process (product) should do what it is intended to do.

Analytical validation (AV) in itself is achieved by a series of 'quality circles' and an inherent climate of continual process revision and striving for improvement, often encapsulated by kaizen—the Japanese methodology for promoting continuous improvement by reducing waste. This manifests itself as a spiral where the end of the helical process is one of obtaining an ideal product or process (Figure 3). The process itself is based on an iterative review of deficiencies in the organisation, equipment, personnel and compliance, and many other parameters that can be important to the finished product.

Process validation by analytical methods, for example, could be required as the assurance of effective cleaning prior to manufacture. There are many other examples of where a validated analytical method can support product processing. One such example would be to follow deviations in the dosage of active drug substance in a dispersed product formulation with respect to the period in a production run. In practice, AV is very commonly an integral part of the validation of other processes (Figure 3).

AV is concerned with the methodology doing what is intended and hopefully more, given that a successful QS should always allow for future developments to be taken on board and used as the quality spiral progresses. AV is primarily concerned with using a range of indices based on prior scrutiny of an analytical system via system suitability parameters, using an SOP to define what the system can reveal about a product. It is crucial, however, that the system suitability fits with what will be measured on the equipment and this can be summarised in parameter appropriateness and numerical definitions. The indices of AV are as follows:

— *Accuracy* - a direct mathematical comparison of the exactness of the data and the proximity of the measured average value to the true or cautiously determined value. With PT this accuracy for a product is typically 97±3%.

— *Precision* - a measure of the degree of repeatability of at least 10 measurements of the same sample. This can often be presented as standard deviation or the coefficient of variation. For this a value of less than 2% is considered satisfactory scatter in the data. Three forms are often used, which relate to the repeatability for a set sample but with the same equipment, different equipment with the same laboratory or a different laboratory.

— *Limit of detection* - the lowest concentration of analyte that can be detected. Limit of quantification - the lowest concentration of analyte determined with acceptable accuracy and precision.

— *Linearity* - said to be when the results obtained relate the response of the instrument being used to the concentration of the product in a linear fashion via linear regression, with a correlation coefficient of not less than 0.99.

— *Range* - the interval between the upper and lower acceptable limits. In most cases this interval should be linear.

— *Robustness* - the contingency of a method to remain unperturbed by small intentional variations in parameters that relate to the systematic variations that an analyst might introduce routinely into an analysis. Typically, in spectrophotometric analyses, this method (SOP) of robustness is challenge tested by such varying parameters as pH value, temperature and percent apolar phase.

— *Specificity* - the ability to discriminate, in an analytical chemistry context, between two or more structurally comparable analytes in a matrix or mixture.

— *Recovery* - the ability to extract all the analyte from a sample despite possible matrix intrusion.

Under foreseeable harmonisation of PT, uniformity of approach and improvements in ethics and customer focusing will be areas under intense international review over the next few years. As scientists and legislators aim for evermore effective and detailed information about products as part of this movement, the use of new developments to obtain or create a better service or product will start to become a significant part of modern-day pharmaceutical analysis and high-throughput screening.

Drug Production

Monoclonal antibodies are immunoglobulin molecules secreted from a population of identical cells (i.e., cloned cells). They are homogeneous in structure and binding specificity. In the context of this guidance, *mAb* reagents refers to monoclonal antibodies used as reagents in a drug substance manufacturing process.

The issues related to *mAb*s used as reagents are somewhat different from those of *mAb*s used as parenteral therapeutic agents. For *mAb* reagents, the primary emphasis is on assessment of the following:

— Biological safety, in particular the assessment of contamination of the *mAb* reagent with adventitious agents and/or process-related impurities from the cell substrate or cell line sources.

— Performance characteristics of the *mAb* reagent during drug substance manufacture (e.g., avidity and specificity for the target molecule).

— Potential presence of residual amounts of the *mAb* reagent in the final drug substance and/or drug product.

The recommendations in this guidance apply to the use of *mAb* reagents in the drug substance manufacturing process where the *mAb* reagent is used to purify the drug substance. The extent of characterisation required for the *mAb* reagent depends on the nature of the steps that follow use of the *mAb*, and thus will vary among submissions. While many CMC concerns regarding the use of *mAb* reagents are unique to biotechnology-produced reagents, the general concepts expressed in the FDA Guideline for Submitting Supporting Documentation in Drug Applications for the Manufacture of Drug Substances also apply. An early and continued dialogue between the applicant and the Agency is encouraged to discuss the data that should be submitted to support the use of the *mAb* reagent.

Monoclonal Antibody Reagents Production

The sponsor or applicant should submit information (e.g., production process, specification) to support the use of the *mAb* reagent or a letter of authorisation (LOA) to a drug master file (DMF) that contains this information.

A description of the *mAb* manufacturing process should be provided. The description is used to assess the potential impact on the biological safety, quality, and purity of the drug substance and/or drug product. The *mAb* reagent should be adequately characterised and its identity, purity, and structural integrity should be assessed, as these factors are vital to its efficient and uninterrupted performance during production of drug substances. Reagents that have not been fully characterised for viral safety should not be introduced into facilities where biologics and drugs from mammalian cell culture are produced because of the potential for cross-contamination. Additional recommendations relating to *mAb* reagents are:

— For *mAb* reagents prepared using hybridoma propagation, serum additives in culture media should be free of contaminants and adventitious agents.

— Manufacturers should use bovine-derived materials only from cattle that were born, raised, and slaughtered in countries that are free of BSE (bovine spongiform encephalopathy).

The predominant concern with the use of *mAb* reagents in drug substance manufacture is the introduction of adventitious agents (e.g., viruses, bacteria, fungi, mycoplasma) and/or process-related impurities (e.g., protein and DNA contaminants, column leachables, media components) into the drug substance. Of particular concern are those that are not removed during drug substance manufacture steps after the introduction of the *mAb* reagent. In many instances, the extent of the cell bank safety characterisation and the clearance studies for adventitious agents and/or process-related impurities should follow the established standards for *mAb*s intended for human use.

A reduced level of testing of cell banks and/or validation of the procedures used to remove or inactivate adventitious agents and/or process-related impurities during purification of the *mAb* may be appropriate under certain circumstances, with justification. Early dialogue with the Agency is encouraged when a reduced level of testing and/or validation is planned. A reduced level can be justified when, for example:

— The drug product is terminally sterilised.

— The use of the reagent is followed by adequate steps for the removal and/or inactivation of the adventitious agents and/or process-related impurities. In this instance, the overall assessment of the removal and/or inactivation process can take into account validation data from steps in the manufacture of the reagent and manufacture of the drug substance.

— Processing steps downstream of the reagent include extremes of pH or organic solvents, and there are reliable data in the scientific literature that the extremes remove and/or inactivate adventitious agents and/or process-related impurities.

— The *mAb* reagent is produced in an expression system in which human infectious agents do not propagate (e.g., plants, bacteria, fungi, insect cultures).

Drug Manufacturing

A major use of *mAb* reagents is in the purification of drug substance by *mAb*s attached to a solid support (e.g., immunoaffinity chromatography). Issues relating to and recommendations on the information to submit in support of the use of *mAb* reagents in the purification process are discussed below. The information that should be submitted to support other uses of *mAb* reagents in drug manufacture will depend on the use and are not discussed in this guidance. Sponsors or applicants with questions on documentation to support other uses of *mAb* reagents are encouraged to contact the Agency.

Drug substance purification process

The drug substance purification processes should be described in the application. The drug substance manufacturer should establish a specification for the incoming *mAb* reagent, and perform testing before using the reagents in the manufacturing process. In addition to identity testing for the incoming *mAb* reagent, drug substance manufacturers should carry out additional testing (e.g., binding activity, adventitious agents) to ensure that the reagent will perform as intended. Affinity and specificity studies are recommended to assess whether the characteristics of a *mAb* reagent are optimal for targeted binding to the appropriate substrate during the manufacture of the drug substance.

Leaching of *mAb* or impurities from the solid support into the final product should be considered when specifications are established for the drug substance. The amount of column leachables is not uniform over the column lifespan and depends on several factors (e.g., length of storage, solutions used in the regeneration and/or sanitisation steps, column operating parameters). A variety of methods can be used to test for leachables such as sampling the buffer flow-through prior to the load of the drug substance intermediate, in-process testing of the intermediate bulk, or testing the final drug substance. Alternatively, if documentation is available that the production steps that follow the use of the reagent *mAb* reduce the maximum amount of column leachables to appropriate levels, this documentation can be provided in lieu of routine testing for leachables.

Data on the ability of the affinity column to achieve the intended purity under specified working conditions should be submitted. The stability of the *mAb* reagent during use, the column performance, and the microbial contaminants should be monitored during production of drug substance and documented by the drug substance manufacturer. Tests and acceptance criteria for residual *mAb* should be included in the specifications for drug substances processed with *mAb* reagents. Residual *mAb* should be monitored by sensitive and specific assay (e.g., enzyme-linked immunosorbent assay (ELISA)).

Changes in the *mAb* supplier or changes in the manufacturing process of *mAb* or solid support are considered to be drug substance manufacturing process changes that can have an effect on the biological safety and effectiveness of the drug substance and, consequently, the final product. In cases where significant changes have been implemented in the *mAb* manufacturing process that may change the purity or the performance of the reagent (e.g., specificity, avidity, microbiological safety), appropriate product comparability testing should be performed.

The guidance document entitled FDA Guidance Concerning Demonstration of Comparability of Human Biological Products, Including Therapeutic Biotechnology-Derived Products contains a discussion of comparability testing for *mAb*s used parenterally. Comparability testing for *mAb* reagents should focus mainly on the performance characteristics of the reagent and its purity and stability. This is particularly important when changes in the reagent manufacture are likely to have an impact on the biological safety, purity, quality, or stability of the drug substance and/or drug product.

Monoclonal Antibody Reagents Specifications

Specifications for the *mAb* reagents should be provided. A certificate of analysis (COA) should be available for each individual reagent lot. For monoclonal antibodies linked to a solid support, COAs should be provided for both forms, unconjugated and linked. A copy of a representative COA should be provided. The COA should provide the test results, including those for adventitious agents, expiration date, and a disclaimer statement in large bold lettering: Reagent use only; not intended for Human use.

Unconjugated monoclonal antibody reagents

Tests to adequately characterise the unconjugated *mAb* reagent typically include:

— Identity (e.g., reducing and nonreducing sodium dodecyl sulfate polyacrylamide gel electrophoresis (SDS-PAGE) pattern, isoelectric focusing (IEF) profile) C Purity (e.g., high performance liquid chromatography (HPLC), SDS-PAGE, capillary electrophoresis)
— Protein concentration
— Binding to the target molecule
— pH
— Microbial and/or bacterial endotoxin limits, as appropriate
— Preservatives, as appropriate

Monoclonal antibody reagents linked to solid support

Tests for *mAb* reagents linked to solid support should include, at minimum, the following:

— Physical characteristics (e.g., mean particle size, matrix structure)
— Concentration of *mAb* (e.g., milligrams of *mAb* per gram of resin)
— Specific binding capacity at recommended temperature and buffer ranges
— Amount of leaching of *mAb*
— Microbial and/or bacterial endotoxin limits, as appropriate
— Preservatives, as appropriate

Highly Variable Drugs

In traditional bioequivalence study designs based on 2-periods, the factors in the ANVOVA model are: Formulation, Period, Sequence and Subjects nested within Sequence. These factors account for all the identifiable sources of between subject variability. Within-subject variability is contained in the Residual Variance. The residual variance is made up of several components:

(i) WSV in absorption, distribution, metabolism and excretion (ADME) combined with a component of analytical variability,

(ii) within-formulation variability (WFV),

(iii) the subject by formulation interaction (S*F) and

(iv) unexplained, random variability.

The components of the residual variance cannot be subdivided further in a 2-period design. The hope is that the two products in a bioequivalence study are of good pharmaceutical quality so there is little within formulation variability and there is negligible subject by formulation interaction. An advantage of replicate designs, in which the test and reference formulations are each administered twice is that the subject by formulation interaction can be 'teased out' of the residual variance and it is possible to estimate within subject variabilities associated with the test (Swt) and reference (Swr) formulations.

Concept of Bioequivalence

The modern concept of bioequivalence is based on a survey of physicians carried out by Westlake in the 1970s which concluded that a 20% difference in dose between two formulations would have no clinical significance for most drugs. Hence bioequivalence limits were set at 80 - 120%. Plasma concentration dependent measures such as Cmax or AUC are not normally distributed; they are log normal, and hence bioequivalence limits became 80 - 125%. In traditional average bioequivalence based on the Two One-Sided Test, the 90% confidence interval around the geometric mean ratio of the test and reference formulations is therefore required to fall within bioequivalence limits of 80 - 125%. The width of the 90% confidence interval depends on the number of subjects in the study and the magnitude of the residual variance. The ANOVA-CV is simply the square root of the residual variance multiplied by 100.

Problem with highly variable drugs

The results of two bioequivalence studies on formulations of drugs A and B. There are the same number of subjects in each study and the GMR is the same in both. As far as the Two One-Sided Test is concerned, the only difference between the two studies is the magnitude of the ANOVA-CV. Drug A has a low within-subject variability (ANOVACV 15%) and the 90% confidence interval falls comfortably within the bioequivalence limits of 80 - 125%. Drug B is highly variable, however, with an ANOVA-CV of 35%.

The study fails because the lower bound of the 90% confidence interval falls below the lower bioequivalence limit (80%). In other words, the study on drug B was underpowered, the simple remedy for which would be to repeat the study with a greater number of subjects. Highly variable drugs are usually safe drugs with flat dose response curves and application of the present preset bioequivalence limits of 80-125% amounts to imposition of unwarranted tougher bioequivalence requirements than for lower variability drugs.

A highly variable drug product (HVDP) is a formulation of poor pharmaceutical quality in which the drug itself is not highly variable, but there is a big component of within formulation (tablet to tablet, capsule to capsule, patch to patch) variability (WFV). HVDPs pose a problem because they are cannot be detected in traditional 2-treatment, 2-period, 2-sequence cross-over design studies. Replicate designs, however, facilitate their detection because the within-subject variabilities of the test and reference formulations can be estimated separately. When they are very different, the probable explanation is that one of the formulations is a HVDP. Now if the brand is a HVDP, then a better quality test product should not be penalised by forcing it to meet the variability of the poor quality reference product.

Chlorpromazine

The ANOVA-CVs from three different types of studies on chlorpromazine conducted at different times by three different analysts by three completely different analytical methods. Solution data gives the best estimate of true pharmacokinetic within-subject variability since, in the absence of a formulation, there is no subject by formulation interaction, and there is no component of within formulation variability included in the estimate.

The results of the bioequivalence study on two formulations of chlorpromazine (unpublished data) which is a good illustration of the kind of problems that beset bioequivalence studies on highly variable drugs. Despite the large number of subjects (n=37), all comparisons of Cmax failed US-FDA conditions which require a 90% confidence interval around this measure to be within 80-125%. The most interesting point here is that a reference to reference comparison also failed decisively.

An example of a HVDP

After a traditional 2-treatment, 2-period, 2-sequence cross-over bioequivalence study on two formulations of the beta-blocker nadolol failed, it was decided to investigate the sources of variability by conducting a 4-period replicate study. Thus a 2-treatment, 4-period, 4-sequence cross-over study was conducted in 22 healthy volunteers.

The results indicated a failure of both AUClast and Cmax in terms of the 90% confidence intervals failing to fall within preset bioequivalence limits of 80 - 125%, although Cmax passed the Health Canada requirement for the GMR to fall within these bioequivalence limits. Examination of the two administrations of the test formulation demonstrated that the drug itself was not highly variable in terms of either measure and the GMR for both was 97%, close to the ideal. In contrast, however, the reference to reference comparison showed both Cmax and AUClast very highly variable, the GMRs of both measures was 87%, and the reference formulation failed when tested against itself.

After the earlier 2-period bioequivalence study in which within formulation variation and subject by formulation interaction term were inseparable components of the residual variance, it was tempting to attribute failure to subject by formulation interaction. The four period design, however, showed clearly failure was attributable to a very different problem. One could say that the 'right' answer was that the test formulation was not bioequivalent with the reference formulation simply because their variances were so different.

Example of a subject by formulation interaction

A bioequivalence study on two percutaneous patch formulations of nitroglycerin was carried out in 37 subjects in a 2-treatment, 4-period, 4-sequence cross over design. Serial blood samples were collected over 12 hours after which the patch was removed to facilitate measurement of the elimination phase.

The test formulation met bioequivalent requirements in Cmax and AUClast, despite high variability in both measures. This was a consequence of the study being adequately powered with a total of 148 observations in the data set. The test to test and the reference to reference comparison also met bioequivalence requirements. Examination of the variabilities associated with the test and reference formulations showed them to be roughly comparable, but there were large subject by formulation interactions associated with both Cmax (28%) and AUClast (21%).

Two important points arise from this study. One is the lack of sensitivity of average bioequivalence to a substantial subject by formulation interaction. Individual bioequivalence is very sensitive to the interaction and failed the study. The second point concerns the clinical significance of a subject by formulation interaction with any given drug, which is a difficult question to study prospectively. Problems in judging the clinical significance of subject by formulation interaction in general may have contributed to the demise of individual bioequivalence at US-FDA.

Non-linear highly variable drug

Two bioequivalence studies were carried out on two formulations of propafenone which is a non-linear, highly variable drug. Both studies were traditional 2-treatment, 2-period, two sequence cross-over studies. In the first study, 74 healthy subjects were dosed after an overnight fast, and in the second, 25 healthy subjects were dosed after a standardised high fat breakfast. The first study was successful in that both measures met bioequivalence requirements despite high within-subject variability The Fed study was not powered sufficiently for the 90% confidence interval around ln Cmax to fall within bioequivalence limits of 80-125%.

Possible methods of dealing with drug products

Cmax is often the most variable of the two measures, partly because it is a single point determinant which is dependent upon an adequate blood sampling schedule around tmax. A simple method of dealing with highly variable drugs would be to treat them as 'uncomplicated drugs' and not require a 90% confidence interval around Cmax. Each of the four examples discussed in this paper were also highly variable in terms of AUClast but its variability was less than Cmax which means a smaller number of subjects would have been required to achieve adequate statistical power.

Since highly variable drugs are generally safe drugs with shallow dose response curves, it is reasonable to tolerate greater than 20% differences between test and reference formulations. The EU-CPMP guidelines, for example, permit a sponsor prospectively to justify broadening the bioequivalence limits from 80 - 125% to, say, 75 - 133%.

The bioequivalence limits can be scaled to the within-subject variability of the reference formulation by the use of the residual variance in a two-period design or the within-subject variance associated with the reference formulation in a replicate design. The fundamental concept is shown in Equation 1. which implies the 90% confidence interval around the difference between the log transformed means of the test and reference formulation must fit between bioequivalence limits of qABE which is set by the drug regulatory body. The commonly accepted bioequivalence limits are set at 80 - 125% (0.8 - 1.25) which is ±0.225 on the natural log scale. In scaling, the bioequivalence

$$-0.223 \leq (\mu_t - \mu_r) = 0.223 \qquad \therefore\ (\mu_t - \mu_r)^2 \leq 0.223^2 \tag{1}$$

limits are divided by the within-subject standard deviation at which the limits are to be permitted to be broadened (σ_{W0}). The latter is to be set by a drug regulatory agency. The left hand side of Equation 1 is divided by the within subject standard deviation of the reference formulation (σ_{WR}) Equation 2. Rearrangement of Equation 2 gives Equation 3 which broadens the bioequivalence limits for highly variable drugs in a systematic way.

$$\frac{(\mu_t - \mu_r)}{\sigma_{WR}} \leq \frac{0.223}{\sigma_{W0}} \tag{2}$$

$$(\mu_t - \mu_r) \leq \frac{0.223}{\sigma_{W0}} \times \sigma_{WT} \tag{3}$$

The method of Boddy and Co-workers for widening the bioequivalence limits for highly variable drugs/products is a slightly different approach to the same concept. Here the bioequivalence limits are set as a fixed multiple (k) of the standard deviation (σ_{WR} or σ_{RES}). In other words, ($\theta_{ABE} = k\sigma_{WR}$), such that k represents the number of standard deviations by which the means are allowed to vary. Thus, when *k* is set at ($0.223/\sigma_{W0}$) the relationship becomes exactly the same as Equation 3.

Scaling the ABE metric amounts to the same thing as scaling the bioequivalence limits, since the relationships shown in Equations 1-3 are used for both methods. For the purposes of illustration, the point at which the bioequivalence limits are permitted to be broadened by scaling (σ_{W0}) was set at 0.20 or 0.25. The value σ_{W0} = 0.20 was selected by US-FDA during the decade long debate on individual bioequivalence, although for scaled ABE, we prefer the more conservative σ_{W0} = 0.25.

Validation of Analytical Methods

Scientists have various analytical methods requirements at different stages of the development lifecycle, method validation needs also adjust throughout the lifecycle. The objective during the late-development stages is to provide substantial information about whether a method can be run accurately and consistently under less-controlled circumstances. The methods used in early development, however, generally do not face these challenges. Requirements for method validation are clear for new drug applications (NDA) and many other worldwide marketing applications. These requirements are specified in documents from the International Conference on Harmonisation (ICH), regulatory agencies, and pharmacopeias.

The validation guidelines applicable to early drug development phases, however, are not as specific. This lack of guidance, coupled with a generally conservative, risk-averse environment within the pharmaceutical industry can result in the application of more-stringent late-phase method validation requirements to products in early development.

Recognising the dilemma many pharmaceutical companies face, the PhRMA Analytical Technical Group selected "method validation by phase of development" as a topic in need of an "acceptable analytical practice" or an industry-led guidance. The scope was limited to small-molecule drug substances and drug products in the clinical phase of development. Biopharmaceuticals, raw materials, intermediates, in-process controls, excipients, and bioanalytical and preclinical methods were excluded. A committee presented starting-point views on the topic at the September 2003 PhRMA workshop and the subject was debated by attendees.

The group preferred a phased approach to method validation. Consensus could not be reached, however, regarding the specific details of what should be included, delayed, or eliminated when validating methods in early development.

Analytical Methods by Phase of Development

According to ICH and Food and Drug Administration guidances, the objective of method validation is to demonstrate that analytical procedures "are suitable for their intended purpose". Therefore, to understand how a method should be validated at various phases of development, it is important to understand the analytical method's purpose at various developmental stages. The method's purpose should be linked to the clinical studies' purpose and the pharmaceutical purpose of the product being studied.

The purposes of initial clinical trials is to determine a safe dosing range and key pharmacological data, typically in healthy human volunteers. As development continues, clinical studies are conducted on increasing numbers of patients to prove efficacy while continuing to study the drug's safety profile.

The purposes of pharmaceutical products in early phases is to deliver a known dose that is bioavailable. As product development continues, increasing emphasis is placed on identifying a stable, robust formulation from which multiple, bioequivalent lots can be manufactured and ultimately scaled-up, transferred, and controlled for commercial manufacture.

The purposes of initial analytical methods are to ensure potency, which can relate directly to the requirement of a known dose; to identify impurities in the drug substance and product, which can relate to the drug's safety profile; and to help evaluate key drug characteristics such as crystal form, drug release, and drug uniformity because these properties can compromise bioavailability. As development continues, the purposes of the analytical methods mirror those of the pharmaceutical product. The methods should be stabilityindicating and capable of measuring the effect of key manufacturing parameters to help ensure that the drug substance and product are consistent. Ultimately, in the subsequent development stages, the methods must be robust, cost effective, transferable, and of sufficient accuracy and precision for specification setting and stability assessment of marketed products. Method validation plays a key role in ensuring analytical methods are suitable for these intended purposes. Validation studies conducted during early development should ensure that analytical methods are appropriately assessing the product's potency and safety.

Benefits and Risks

Although performing validation in phases has clear benefits, it also must be noted that potential risk is associated with this approach. The risk can be reduced significantly if the analytical scientist has a good understanding of the analytical methodology's limitations and a basic understanding of the chemistry or process used to produce the drug substance or product. With a strong technical base and the use of good method development practices, analytical scientists are much more likely to develop a suitable method for its intended purpose and limit the risk of delaying some method validation experiments.

Ultimately, analytical scientists are responsible for the scientific defence of their methods; and thus, it is useful to review potential benefits and risks associated with performing method validation in phases.

Reasons for implementing a phased approach to method validation in early development include ongoing method development and optimization, a changing synthetic route for the drug substance, a changing formulation, and a high product-attrition rate. Given the desire to rapidly implement change in early development and the business driver to do more with less, a phased method validation approach can lead to benefits such as:

— fewer resources devoted to method validation;
— lower costs;
— more flexibility in early development;
— more time to focus on analytical science.

These benefits help analytical scientists focus more on the items that truly affect product quality and on the advancement of pharmaceutical medicines in general. It also is important that a phased approach to method validation not compromise product safety or increase other risks associated with the development of new drugs.

To help assess those risks, a two-step approach was taken at the September 2003 workshop. First, attendees were asked to share problems encountered later in development that could have been detected and avoided by more method validation in early development. Second, attendees were asked to numerically assess (on a 1 to 6 scale) the likelihood and the impact of the following predefined risks, using their experiences and their company practices for methods, method validation, specification setting, and/or product quality in general:

— clinical hold (regulatory risk);
— unknown impurity (including degradation product) in a drug substance batch not used in toxicological studies;

- incorrect potency administered;
- key drug substance or product property not discovered;
- inconsistent product not discovered;
- increased out-of-specification (OOS) results;
- invalid/inadequate method not discovered until later in development;
- method not rugged and cannot be run by other laboratories;
- imprecise or inaccurate method leading to poor specification setting or stability assessment.

In response to the first question, the problems shared by workshop attendees were able to be resolved and had little longterm effect on the products in question. The issues mostly related to inadequate method ruggedness (e.g., changing instruments leading to different HPLC gradients and linear ranges, and discovering problems not seen when the method was run by fewer analysts).

In response to the second question, survey results indicated that the likelihood of the predefined risks occurring is low. If they did occur, however, their effect could be relatively high (Figure 4). Consistent with the feedback from the first question in which method ruggedness issues were raised but were resolved, the response with the highest likelihood (method ruggedness) was rated with one of the lowest impact scores.

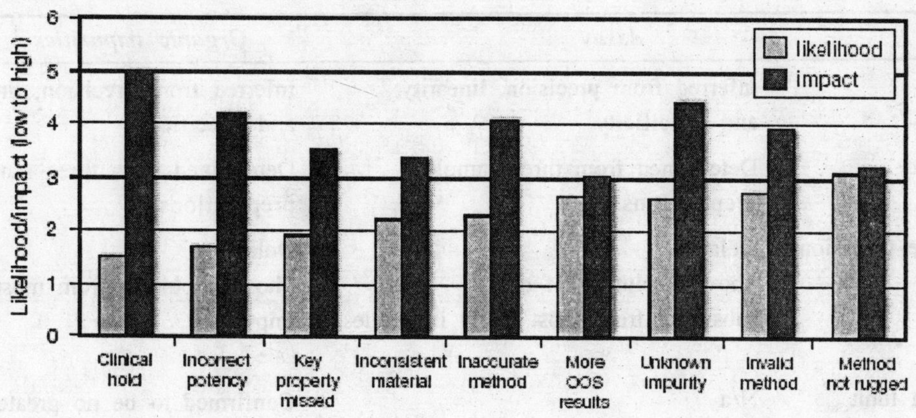

Figure 4: Method validation risk assessment.

At the end of the workshop, after discussing potential reductions in method validation, attendees were asked to take a second look at the survey and determine whether their rating on the likelihood of any predefined risks would change as a consequence of reducing method validation. The consensus was that the likelihood of the risks would not change and remained low.

Recommended Approaches

At the September 2003 workshop, method validation characteristics for several drug-substance and drug-product methods were discussed. These methods are listed in Table I for drug substance. Time constraints prevented discussions about other methods such as those that detect various crystalline forms.

Consensus was not reached on which the specific details of which aspects of method validation studies should be eliminated or delayed during early development. Participants agreed, however, that method validation should be phased.

Experiments that should be considered in a phased method validation programme are described. In some cases, the suggested number of tests may not be sufficient to perform formal statistical analyses (e.g., least-squares analysis of linearity data, relative standard deviation of precision data), but the number of tests should be sufficient to determine whether the method validation characteristic is likely to cause a problem.

In addition, the suggested experiments assume that one analysis (e.g., one injection for HPLC) will be conducted for each sample preparation leading to one reportable result from the method. If the method requires different replication (e.g., multiple injections from each preparation), then this should be taken into account during method validation.

Table I: Recommended drug substance method validation during early development.

	Assay	*Organic impurities*
Accuracy	Inferred from precision, linearity, and specificity	Inferred from precision, linearity, and specificity
Repeatability	Determined from three sample preparations	Determined from three sample preparations
Intermediate precision	Delay	Delay
Specificity	Show resolution of drug substance from most likely impurities	Show resolution from most likely impurities
Quantitation limit	N/a	Confirmed to be no greater than the reporting limit
Detection limit	N/a	Delay
Linearity	Determine from impurity linearity if appropriate or three levels 80–120% of the concentration specified in the method	Determine from three concentrations (e.g., for area % methods, test at sample concentration, at 1% of that level, and at the quantitation limit)
Range	Defined by the linearity work	Defined by the linearity and quantitation limit work
Robustness	Solution stability and information gathering	Solution stability and information gathering

Phased validation of drug substance methods: Two key drug substance methods required to help ensure the safety and potency of pharmaceutical products are methods for assay and organic impurities. Specificity and quantitation limit are the primary validation characteristics to ensure that these methods meet their intended purposes of potency and safety. Experiments that demonstrate specificity, quantitation limit, and other ICH method validation characteristics (including ones that can be delayed) are summarised in Table 1. To simplify terms, organic impurity methods will be referred to as impurity methods.

Accuracy: Because it is rare to have more than one assay and impurity method available early in development, it is often difficult to determine the accuracy of an assay or impurity method by comparison with a secondary method. Rather, accuracy can be inferred from the precision, linearity, and specificity studies. In addition, it may be useful to assess the overall mass balance of the main component and known impurities to verify the accuracy of these methods.

Repeatability: The repeatability of the assay and impurity methods should be assessed by testing three sample preparations. The results from these studies should give the analytical scientist a sufficient estimate of the assay's and impurity methods' precision.

Intermediate precision: During early stages of development, when methods are operated typically in one laboratory by a few analysts, it is not necessary to determine the intermediate precision of an assay or impurity method.

Specificity: Assay and impurity methods specificity should be evaluated during the early development stages and then regularly reviewed and re-evaluated as changes are made to the drug substance synthetic process. During early development, the assay and impurity methods should separate the most likely impurities (e.g., synthetic impurities, degradation products). In addition, it is important to show separation of the main component and impurities from the raw materials and intermediates, particularly those used in subsequent parts of the synthetic process. Furthermore, it is useful to demonstrate the separation of known and likely sideproducts in the final synthetic steps.

As the synthetic process continues to change, the analytical scientist should evaluate the potential for generating new impurities or side-products and demonstrate the capability of the assay and the impurity methods to separate new intermediates, side-products, and raw materials as appropriate. Once a method is used to monitor the drug substance's stability attributes, the stability-indicating capabilities of the method must be demonstrated. In general, this task is accomplished by showing that the method can separate major degradation products generated from forced degradation studies.

Quantitation limit: Regardless of the phase of development, the quantitation limit for an impurities method should be no greater than its reporting limit. As specified in ICH Q2A, it is not necessary for the quantitation limit to be determined for the assay method.

Detection limit: During early development, it is not critical to have a defined detection limit for an impurities method because verifying that the reporting limit can be quantified is sufficient. Rather, determination of the detection limit can be delayed until later development when the ICH Q3A reporting limits are required.

Linearity: When performing full method validation according to ICH guidelines, a minimum of five concentrations normally is used to establish the linear range. With good method development practices (e.g., operating in the linear range of the detector, proper column loading), however, the number of concentrations evaluated can be limited during early development while adding little risk that the methods will later be significantly nonlinear.

For early-phase impurity methods, the linear range can be evaluated by ensuring proper quantification at three concentrations. Which concentrations to test will depend on the sample preparation and the type of standardisation. For area percentage methods, three concentrations are suggested: at the sample concentration, at 1% of that level, and at the quantitation limit. Data from these three samples ensure that the method's linear range and information on the quantitation limit are acceptable.

If the assay method is the same or similar to the impurity method and the assay concentration is within the limits tested for the impurity method, no additional linearity data are needed. If the assay method is different, then linearity should be assessed using three concentrations that are 80-120% of the concentration specified by the method.

Range: The working ranges for the two methods are supported by the linearity and quantitation limit experiments described.

Robustness: During early development, robustness testing can be limited to demonstrating that solutions are adequately stable for their duration of use in the laboratory. During method development and early stages of the project, an analyst should begin to develop an experience base and gather information about which method parameters have the greatest effect on the analytical results and method performance. This experience base can be used in later stages to develop specific robustness experiments and to help establish appropriate system suitability requirements.

Phased validation of drug product methods: During the 2003 workshop, four types of drug product methods were discussed: assay, impurities, dissolution, and content uniformity (CU). The key characteristics for helping ensure product potency and safety are accuracy and specificity. Table II summarises minimally acceptable method validation studies is provided. The discussions used traditional (immediate release) tablets as a model, and though the principles apply to other dosage forms, the specifics must be interpreted and adapted by an analytical scientist.

Accuracy: ICH requirements state that accuracy may be inferred once precision, linearity, and specificity have been established. With an emphasis on expediting method validation in early development, a minimum number of recovery studies are suggested. These condensed recovery studies are performed in lieu of more extensive linearity and precision studies to demonstrate adequate accuracy and linearity of the methods.

For assay, it is recommended that recovery of the drug substance be determined in the presence of excipients at 100% of the dosage form strength. For dissolution, recovery of the drug substance in the presence of excipients is recommended at 50, 75, and 100% of the dosage form strength. For content uniformity, recovery of the drug substance in the presence of excipients is recommended at 70, 100, and 130% of the dosage form strength. In the case of multiple strengths of similar formulations, further efficiencies may be gained by conducting recovery experiments that bracket the full concentration or strength range.

Early in development, samples of degradation products may be in very short supply, if available at all. Hence, a minimum requirement for demonstrating the accuracy of the impurities method is that recovery is determined using drug substance (in the presence of excipients) at two or three levels.

Repeatability: Performing the 100% recovery experiments using three sample preparations for assay, dissolution, and content uniformity should generate a sufficient estimate of the repeatability of the methods. Similarly, conducting the recovery experiment using three sample preparations at the standard concentration or, if applicable, the highest individual specification limit should provide a sufficient estimate of the repeatability of the impurity method. For multiple strengths of similar formulations, bracketing the full concentration or strength range should be sufficient.

Intermediate precision: Similar to the drug-substance recommendations, intermediate precision can be delayed until the methods are used in multiple laboratories and/or by several different analysts and instruments.

Specificity: Early phase methods must be reliable for determining the potency and safety of the drug product. Therefore, assurance of the assay and impurities method(s) specificity is important even early in development. Demonstrating that the assay result is unaffected by the presence of impurities and formulation excipients is suggested as the minimum for the assay method. For the impurities method at this early stage, the drug product should be appropriately degraded to demonstrate that the degradation products have nearbaseline resolution from the main component and synthetic impurities. The analyses for content uniformity and dissolution also should be unaffected by the extracting solvent or media and excipients.

Quantitation and detection limits: Identical to the drug substance recommendations, the quantitation limit for the drug product impurities method should be no greater than its reporting limit. Determination of the detection limit can be delayed until later development when the ICH Q3B reporting limits are required. It is not necessary for the quantitation and detection limits for the assay, CU, and dissolution methods to be determined, as per ICH Q2A.

Linearity: When standard concentrations are matched or roughly matched to the expected analyte concentration(s) and good method development practices are used, it is not unreasonable to delay ICH-type linearity studies. Rather, adequate linearity for dissolution, CU, and impurities methods can be inferred from the accuracy studies that demonstrate good recovery at various concentrations of key analyte. For the assay method, determining the accuracy at various dosage strengths may help define the linearity. In the absence of a range of strengths, it is reasonable to expect that the results will cover a relatively narrow range, and thus ICH linearity experiments can be delayed.

Range: The working ranges for the dissolution, CU, and impurity methods are supported by the experiments described for accuracy. For assay, determination of range can be delayed for the same reasons described for linearity.

Robustness: Early development is a good time to gather information about the robustness of the methods, but probably too early to begin to conduct designed experiments. Experimentally determined solution stabilities should be established to cover their duration of use in the laboratory.

Other Aspects of Method

In addition to optimising the experiments performed to validate methods during early development, other aspects of method validation can and should be scaled back or delayed to achieve all the benefits of phased method validation. The phasing of documentation, acceptance criteria, and the role of the quality assurance unit were discussed during the workshop. The role of the quality assurance unit is outside the scope of this topic, but recommendations were made for the other aspects.

Regardless of the phase of development, the laboratory raw data used to demonstrate the validity of analytical methods must be properly documented in a notebook or using another good manufacturing practices-compliant data storage format. A detailed method validation report was not felt to be required by workshop attendees until submission of the final marketing application.

Concerning acceptance criteria and method validation protocol, attendees felt that internal guidelines or best practice documents are useful for early development. Preapproved protocol and/or rigid acceptance criteria could unnecessarily restrict the scientific evaluation of methods and lead to extensive, unnecessary investigations, however, when the focus in early development should be on the larger issues of potency and safety.

During later development when the drug substance and product and corresponding methods/specifications are more established and better understood; when multiple laboratories and stakeholders are involved; and when the method purposes are expanded, acceptance criteria and more defined method validation standard operating procedures or protocol may be useful.

Chapter 6

Design of Biopharmaceuticals

Terms such as 'biologic', 'biopharmaceutical' and 'products of pharmaceutical biotechnology' or 'biotechnology medicines' have now become an accepted part of the pharmaceutical literature. However, these terms are sometimes used interchangeably and can mean different things to different people. Although it might be assumed that 'biologic' refers to any pharmaceutical product produced by biotechnological endeavour, its definition is more limited. In pharmaceutical circles, 'biologic' generally refers to medicinal products derived from blood, as well as vaccines, toxins and allergen products. 'Biotechnology' has a much broader and long-established meaning. Essentially, it refers to the use of biological systems or biological molecules for/in the manufacture of commercial products.

The term 'biopharmaceutical' was first used in the 1980s and came to describe a class of therapeutic proteins produced by modern biotechnological techniques, specifically via genetic engineering or, in the case of monoclonal antibodies, by hybridoma technology. Although the majority of biopharmaceuticals or biotechnology products now approved or in development are proteins produced via genetic engineering, these terms now also encompass nucleic-acid-based, i.e. deoxyribonucleic acid (DNA)- or ribonucleic acid (RNA)-based products, and whole-cell-based products.

The pharmaceutical industry, is barely 60 years old. From very modest beginnings, it has grown rapidly, reaching an estimated value of US$100 billion by the mid 1980s. There are well in excess of 10 000 pharmaceutical companies in existence, although only about 100 of these can claim to be of true international significance. These companies manufacture in excess of 5000 individual pharmaceutical substances used routinely in medicine. (Table 1) Some pharmaceuticals that were traditionally obtained by direct extraction from biological source material. Many of the protein-based pharmaceuticals mentioned are now also produced by genetic engineering

The first stages of development of the modern pharmaceutical industry can be traced back to the turn of the twentieth century. At that time (apart from folk cures), the medical community had at their disposal only four drugs that were effective in treating specific diseases:

— Digitalis (extracted from foxglove) was known to stimulate heart muscle and, hence, was used to treat various heart conditions.

— Quinine, obtained from the barks/roots of a plant (Cinchona genus), was used to treat malaria.

— Pecacuanha (active ingredient is a mixture of alkaloids), used for treating dysentery, was obtained from the bark/roots of the plant genus Cephaelis.

— Mercury, for the treatment of syphilis.

This lack of appropriate, safe and effective medicines contributed in no small way to the low life expectancy characteristic of those times.

Table 1. Some pharmaceuticals that were traditionally obtained by direct extraction from biological source material. Many of the protein-based pharmaceuticals mentioned are now also produced by genetic engineering

Substance	*Medical application*
Blood products (e.g. coagulation factors)	Treatment of blood disorders such as haemophilia A or B
Vaccines	Vaccination against various diseases
Antibodies	Passive immunisation against various diseases
Insulin	Treatment of diabetes mellitus
Enzymes	Thrombolytic agents, digestive aids, debriding agents (i.e. cleansing of wounds)
Antibiotics	Treatment against various infections agents
Plant extracts (e.g. alkaloids)	Various, including pain relief

Developments in biology (particularly the growing realisation of the microbiological basis of many diseases), as well as a developing appreciation of the principles of organic chemistry, helped underpin future innovation in the fl edgling pharmaceutical industry. The successful synthesis of various artificial dyes, which proved to be therapeutically useful, led to the formation of pharmaceutical/ chemical companies such as Bayer and Hoechst in the late 1800s. Scientists at Bayer, for example, succeeded in synthesizing aspirin in 1895.

Despite these early advances, it was not until the 1930s that the pharmaceutical industry began to develop in earnest. The initial landmark discovery of this era was probably the discovery, and chemical synthesis, of the sulfa drugs. These are a group of related molecules derived from the red dye prontosil rubrum. These drugs proved effective in the treatment of a wide variety of bacterial infections (Figure 1.). Although it was first used therapeutically in the early 1920s, large-scale industrial production of insulin also commenced in the 1930s.

The medical success of these drugs gave new emphasis to the pharmaceutical industry, which was boosted further by the commencement of industrial-scale penicillin manufacture in the early 1940s. Around this time, many of the current leading pharmaceutical companies (or their forerunners) were founded. Examples include Ciba Geigy, Eli Lilly, Wellcome, Glaxo and Roche. Over the next two to three decades, these companies developed drugs such as tetracyclines, corticosteroids, oral contraceptives, antidepressants and many more. Most of these pharmaceutical substances are manufactured by direct chemical synthesis.

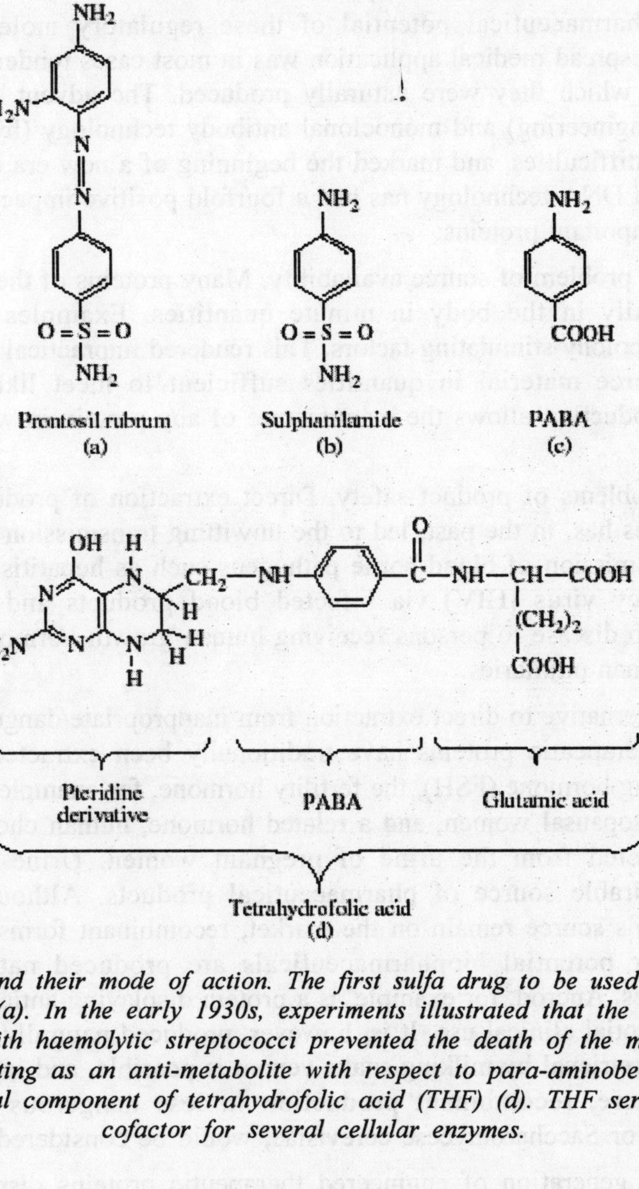

Prontosil rubrum (a) | Sulphanilamide (b) | PABA (c)

Pteridine derivative | PABA | Glutamic acid

Tetrahydrofolic acid (d)

Figure 1. Sulfa drugs and their mode of action. The first sulfa drug to be used medically was the red dye prontosil rubrum (a). In the early 1930s, experiments illustrated that the administration of this dye to mice infected with haemolytic streptococci prevented the death of the mice. (b). Sulfanilamide induces its effect by acting as an anti-metabolite with respect to para-aminobenzoic acid (PABA) (c). PABA is an essential component of tetrahydrofolic acid (THF) (d). THF serves as an essential cofactor for several cellular enzymes.

AGE OF BIOPHARMACEUTICALS

Biomedical research continues to broaden our understanding of the molecular mechanisms underlining both health and disease. Research undertaken since the 1950s has pinpointed a host of proteins produced naturally in the body that have obvious therapeutic applications. Examples include the interferons and interleukins (which regulate the immune response), growth factors, such as erythropoietin (EPO; which stimulates red blood cell production), and neurotrophic factors (which regulate the development and maintenance of neural tissue).

Although the pharmaceutical potential of these regulatory molecules was generally appreciated, their widespread medical application was in most cases rendered impractical due to the tiny quantities in which they were naturally produced. The advent of recombinant DNA technology (genetic engineering) and monoclonal antibody technology (hybridoma technology) overcame many such difficulties, and marked the beginning of a new era of the pharmaceutical sciences. Recombinant DNA technology has had a fourfold positive impact upon the production of pharmaceutically important proteins:

— It overcomes the problem of source availability. Many proteins of therapeutic potential are produced naturally in the body in minute quantities. Examples include interferons, interleukins and colony-stimulating factors. This rendered impractical their direct extraction from native source material in quantities sufficient to meet likely clinical demand. Recombinant production allows the manufacture of any protein in whatever quantity it is required.

— It overcomes problems of product safety. Direct extraction of product from some native biological sources has, in the past, led to the unwitting transmission of disease. Examples include the transmission of blood-borne pathogens such as hepatitis B and C and human immunodeficiency virus (HIV) via infected blood products and the transmission of Creutzfeldt-Jakob disease to persons receiving human growth hormone (GH) preparations derived from human pituitaries.

— It provides an alternative to direct extraction from inappropriate/dangerous source material. A number of therapeutic proteins have traditionally been extracted from human urine. Folliclestimulating hormone (FSH), the fertility hormone, for example, is obtained from the urine of postmenopausal women, and a related hormone, human chorionic gonadotrophin (hCG), is extracted from the urine of pregnant women. Urine is not considered a particularly desirable source of pharmaceutical products. Although several products obtained from this source remain on the market, recombinant forms have now also been approved. Other potential biopharmaceuticals are produced naturally in downright dangerous sources. Ancrod, for example, is a protein displaying anticoagulant activity and, hence, is of potential clinical use. It is, however, produced naturally by the Malaysian pit viper. Although retrieval by milking snake venom is possible, and indeed may be quite an exciting procedure, recombinant production in less dangerous organisms, such as Escherichia coli or Saccharomycese cerevisiae, would be considered preferable by most.

— It facilitates the generation of engineered therapeutic proteins displaying some clinical advantage over the native protein product. Techniques such as site-directed mutagenesis facilitate the logical introduction of predefined changes in a protein's amino acid sequence. Such changes can be as minimal as the insertion, deletion or alteration of a single amino acid residue, or can be more substantial. Such changes can be made for a number of reasons, and several engineered products have now gained marketing approval. An overview summary of some engineered product types now on the market is provided in Table 2.

Table 2. Selected engineered biopharmaceutical types/products that have now gained marketing approval.

Product description/type	Alteration introduced	Rationale
Faster acting insulins	Modified amino acid sequence	Generation of faster acting insulin
Slow acting insulins	Modified amino acid sequence	Generation of slow acting insulin
Modified tissue plasminogen activator	Removal of three of the five native domains of tPA	Generation of a faster acting thrombolytic (clot degrading) agent
Modified blood factor VIII	Deletion of 1 domain of native factor VIII	Production of a lower molecular mass product
Chimaeric/humanised antibodies	Replacement of most/virtually all of the murine amino acid sequences with sequences found in human antibodies	Greatly reduced/eliminated immunogenicity. Ability to activate human effector functions
'Ontak', a fusion protein	Fusion protein consisting of the diphtheria toxin linked to interleukin-2 (IL-2)	Targets toxin selectively to cells expressing an IL-2 receptor

Despite the undoubted advantages of recombinant production, it remains the case that many protein-based products extracted directly from native source material remain on the market. In certain circumstances, direct extraction of native source material can prove equally/more attractive than recombinant production. This may be for an economic reason if, for example, the protein is produced in very large quantities by the native source and is easy to extract/purify, e.g. human serum albumin. Also, some blood factor preparations purified from donor blood actually contain several different blood factors and, hence, can be used to treat several haemophilia patient types. Recombinant blood factor preparations, on the other hand, contain but a single blood factor and, hence, can be used to treat only one haemophilia type.

The advent of genetic engineering and monoclonal antibody technology underpinned the establishment of literally hundreds of start-up biopharmaceutical (biotechnology) companies in the late 1970s and early 1980s. The bulk of these companies were founded in the USA, with smaller numbers of start-ups emanating from Europe and other world regions. Many of these fledgling companies were founded by academics/technical experts who sought to take commercial advantage of developments in the biotechnological arena. These companies were largely financed by speculative monies attracted by the hype associated with the establishment of the modern biotech era. Although most of these early companies displayed significant technical expertise, the vast majority lacked experience in the practicalities of the drug development process. Most of the well-established large pharmaceutical companies, on the other hand, were slow to invest heavily in biotech research and development. However, as the actual and potential therapeutic signifi- cance of biopharmaceuticals became evident, many of these companies did diversify into this area.

Table 3. Pharmaceutical companies who manufacture and/or market biopharmaceutical products approved for general medical use in the USA and EU

Sanofi-Aventis	Hoechst AG
Bayer	Wyeth
Novo	Nordisk Genzyme
Isis	Pharmaceuticals Abbott
Genentech	Roche
Centocor	Novartis
Boehringer	Manheim Serono
Galenus	Manheim Organon
Eli Lilly	Amgen
Ortho Biotech	GlaxoSmithKline
Schering Plough	Cytogen
Hoffman-la-Roche	Immunomedics
Chiron	Biogen

Most either purchased small, established biopharmaceutical concerns or formed strategic alliances with them. An example was the long-term alliance formed by Genentech and the well-established pharmaceutical company Eli Lilly. Genentech developed recombinant human insulin, which was then marketed by Eli Lilly under the trade name Humulin. The merger of biotech capability with pharmaceutical experience helped accelerate development of the biopharmaceutical sector.

Many of the earlier biopharmaceutical companies no longer exist. The overall level of speculative finance available was not sufficient to sustain them all long term. Furthermore, the promise and hype of biotechnology sometimes exceeded its ability actually to deliver a final product. Some biopharmaceutical substances showed little efficacy in treating their target condition, and/or exhibited unacceptable side effects. Mergers and acquisitions also led to the disappearance of several biopharmaceutical concerns. Table 3. lists many of the major pharmaceutical concerns which now manufacture/market biopharmaceuticals approved for general medical use.

Status and Future of Biopharmaceuticals

Approximately one in every four new drugs now coming on the market is a biopharmaceutical.

By mid 2006, some 160 biopharmaceutical products had gained marketing approval in the USA and/or EU. Collectively, these represent a global biopharmaceutical market in the region of US$35 billion (Table 4.), and the market value is estimated to surpass US$50 billion by 2010. The products include a range of hormones, blood factors and thrombolytic agents, as well as vaccines and monoclonal antibodies (Table 5.). All but two are protein-based therapeutic agents. The exceptions are two nucleic-acid-based products: 'Vitravene', an antisense oligonucleotide, and 'Macugen', an aptamer. Many additional nucleic-acid-based products for use in gene therapy or antisense technology are in clinical trials, although the range of technical difficulties that still beset this class of therapeutics will ensure that protein-based products will overwhelmingly predominate for the foreseeable future.

Many of the initial biopharmaceuticals approved were simple replacement proteins. The ability to alter the amino acid sequence of a protein logically coupled to an increased understanding of the relationship between protein structure and function has facilitated the more recent introduction of several engineered therapeutic proteins (Table 2.). Thus far, the vast majority of approved recombinant proteins have been produced in the bacterium E. coli, the yeast S. cerevisiae or in animal cell lines (most notably Chinese hamster ovary (CHO) cells or baby hamster kidney (BHK) cells.

Although most biopharmaceuticals approved to date are intended for human use, a number of products destined for veterinary application have also come on the market. One early such example is that of recombinant bovine GH (Somatotrophin), which was approved in the USA in the early 1990s and used to increase milk yields from dairy cattle. Additional examples of approved veterinary biopharmaceuticals include a range of recombinant vaccines and an interferon-based product (Table 6.).

At least 1000 potential biopharmaceuticals are currently being evaluated in clinical trials, although the majority of these are in early stage trials. Vaccines and monoclonal antibody-based products represent the two biggest product categories. Regulatory factors (e.g. hormones and cytokines) and gene therapy and antisense-based products also represent significant groupings. Although most protein-based products likely to gain marketing approval over the next 2-3 years will be produced in engineered E. coli, S. cerevisiae or animal cell lines, some products now in clinical trials are being produced in the milk of transgenic animals. Additionally, plant-based transgenic expression systems may potentially come to the fore, particularly for the production of oral vaccines.

Interestingly, the first generic biopharmaceuticals are already entering the market. Patent protection for many first-generation biopharmaceuticals (including recombinant human GH (rhGH), insulin, EPO, interferon-a (IFN-a) and granulocyte-CSF (G-CSF)) has now/is now coming to an end. Most of these drugs command an overall annual market value in excess of US$1 billion, rendering them attractive potential products for many biotechnology/pharmaceutical companies. Companies already/soon producing generic biopharmaceuticals include Biopartners (Switzerland), Genemedix (UK), Sicor and Ivax (USA), Congene and Microbix (Canada) and BioGenerix (Germany). Genemedix, for example, secured approval for sale of a recombinant CSF in China in 2001 and is also commencing the manufacture of recombinant EPO. Sicor currently markets hGH and IFN-a in eastern Europe and various developing nations. A generic hGH also gained approval in both Europe and the USA in 2006.

Table 4. Approximate annual market values of some leading approved biopharmaceutical products. Data gathered from various sources, including company home pages, annual reports and industry reports

Product (Company)	Product description (use)	Annual sales value (US$, billions)
Procrit (Amgen/Johnson & Johnson)	EPO (treatment of anaemia)	4.0
Epogen & Aranesp combined (Amgen)	EPO (treatment of anaemia)	4.0
Intron A (Schering Plough)	IFN-α (treatment of leukaemia)	0.3
Remicade (Johnson & Johnson)	Monoclonal antibody based (treatment of Crohn's disease)	1.7
Avonex (Biogen)	Interferon-α (IFN-α; treatment of multiple sclerosis)	1.2
Embrel (Wyeth)	Monoclonal antibody based (treatment of rheumatoid arthritis)	1.3
Rituxan (Genentech)	Monoclonal antibody based (non-Hodgkin's lymphoma)	1.5
Humulin (Eli Lilly)	Insulin (diabetes)	1.0

To date, no gene-therapy-based product has thus far been approved for general medical use in the EU or USA, although one such product has been approved in China. Although gene therapy trials were initiated as far back as 1989, the results have been disappointing. Many technical difficulties remain in relation to, for example, gene delivery and regulation of expression. Product effectiveness was not apparent in the majority of trials undertaken and safety concerns have been raised in several trials.

Only one antisense-based product has been approved to date (in 1998) and, although several such antisense agents continue to be clinically evaluated, it is unlikely that a large number of such products will be approved over the next 3-4 years. Aptamers represent an additional emerging class of nucleic-acid-based therapeutic. These are short DNA- or RNA-based sequences that adopt a specific three-dimensional structure, enabling them to bind (and thereby inhibit) specific target molecules. One such product (Macugen) has been approved to date. RNA interference (RNAi) represents a yet additional mechanism of achieving downregulation of gene expression. It shares many characteristics with antisense technology and, like antisense, provides a potential means of treating medical conditions triggered or exacerbated by the inappropriate overexpression of specific gene products. Despite the disappointing results thus far generated by nucleic-acid-based products, future technical advances will almost certainly ensure the approval of gene therapy and antisense-based products in the intermediate to longer term future.

Table 5. Summary categorisation of biopharmaceuticals approved for general medical use in the EU and/or USA by 2006

Product type	*Examples*	*No. approved*
Blood factors	Factors VIII and IX	8
Thrombolytic agents	tPA	12
Hormones	Insulin, GH, gonadotrophins	33
Haematopoietic growth factors	EPO, CSFs	8
Interferons	IFN-α, -β, -γ	16
Interleukin-based products	IL-2	3
Vaccines	Hepatitis B-surface antigen	20
Monoclonal antibodies	Various	30
Nucleic acid based	Antisense and aptamer	2
Additional products	Tumour necrosis factor (TNF), therapeutic enzymes	18

Technological developments in areas such as genomics, proteomics and high-throughput screening are also beginning to impact significantly upon the early stages of drug development. By linking changes in gene/protein expression to various disease states, for example, these technologies will identify new drug targets for such diseases. Many/most such targets will themselves be proteins, and drugs will be designed/developed specifically to interact with. They may be protein based or (more often) low molecular mass ligands.

Additional future innovations likely to impact upon pharmaceutical biotechnology include the development of alternative product production systems, alternative methods of delivery and the development of engineered cell-based therapies, particularly stem cell therapy. As mentioned previously, protein-based biotechnology products produced to date are produced in either microbial or in animal cell lines. Work continues on the production of such products in transgenic-based production systems, specifically either transgenic plants or animals.

Virtually all therapeutic proteins must enter the blood in order to promote a therapeutic effect. Such products must usually be administered parenterally. However, research continues on the development of non-parenteral routes which may prove more convenient, less costly and obtain improved patient compliance. Alternative potential delivery routes include transdermal, nasal, oral and bucal approaches, although most progress to date has been recorded with pulmonary-based delivery systems. An inhaled insulin product was approved in 2006 for the treatment of type I and II diabetes.

Table 6. Some recombinant (r) biopharmaceuticals recently approved for veterinary application in the EU

Product	Company	Indication
Vibragen Omega (r-feline interferon omega; IFN-ω)	Virbac	Reduction of mortality/clinical symptoms associated with canine parvovirus
Fevaxyl Pentafel (combination vaccine containing r-feline leukaemia viral antigen as one component)	Fort Dodge Laboratories	Immunisation of cats against various feline pathogens
Porcilis porcoli (combination vaccine containing r-E. coli adhesins)	Intervet	Active immunisation of sows
Porcilis AR-T DF (combination vaccine containing a recombinant modified toxin from Pasteurella multocida)	Intervet	Reduction in clinical signs of progressive atrophic rhinitis in piglets
Porcilis pesti (combination vaccine containing r-classical swine fever virus E_2 subunit antigen)	Intervet	Immunisation of pigs against classical swine fever
Bayovac CSF E_2 (combination vaccine containing r-classical swine fever virus E2 subunit antigen)	Intervet	Immunisation of pigs against classical swine fever

A small number of whole-cell-based therapeutic products have also been approved to date. All contain mature, fully differentiated cells extracted from a native biological source. Improved techniques now allow the harvest of embryonic and, indeed, adult stem cells, bringing the development of stem-cell-based drugs one step closer. However, the use of stem cells to replace human cells or even entire tissues/organs remains a long term goal. Overall, therefore, products of pharmaceutical biotechnology play an important role in the clinic and are likely to assume an even greater relative importance in the future.

Biotechnology in Drug Production

Biotechnology and bio-industry are becoming an integral part of the knowledge-based economy, because they are closely associated with progress in the life sciences and in the applied sciences and technologies linked to them. A new model of economic activity is being ushered in -the bio-economy—in which new types of enterprise are created and old industries are revitalised. The bio-economy is defined as including all industries, economic activities and interests organised around living systems.

The bio-economy can be divided into two primary industry segments: the bio-resource industries, which directly exploit biotic resources crop production, horticulture, forestry, livestock and poultry, aquaculture and fisheries; and related industries that have large stakes as either suppliers to or customers of the bio-resource sector—agrochemicals and seeds, biotechnologies and bio-industry, energy, food and fibre processing and retailing, pharmaceuticals and health care, banking and insurance. All these industries are closely associated with the economic impact of human-induced change to biological systems.

The potential of this bio-economy to spur economic growth and create wealth by enhancing industrial productivity is unprecedented. It is therefore no surprise that high-income and technologically advanced countries have made huge investments in research and development (R&D) in the life sciences, biotechnology and bio-industry. In 2001, bio-industries were estimated to have generated US$34.8 billion in revenues worldwide and to employ about 190,000 people in publicly traded firms. These are impressive results given that, in 1992, bio-industries were estimated to have generated US$8.1 billion and employed fewer than 100,000 persons.

The main beneficiaries of the current "biotechnology revolution" and the resulting bio-industries are largely the industrialised and technologically advanced countries, i.e. those that enjoy a large investment of their domestic product in R&D and technological innovation. Thus, the United States, Canada and Europe account for about 97 per cent of the global biotechnology revenues, 96 per cent of persons employed in biotechnology ventures and 88 per cent of all biotechnology firms. Ensuring that those who need biotechnology have access to it therefore remains a major challenge. Similarly, creating an environment conducive to the acquisition, adaptation and diffusion of biotechnology in developing countries is another great challenge. However, a number of developing countries are increasingly using biotechnology and have created a successful bio-industry, at the same time increasing their investments in R&D in the life sciences.

Over the past decade, a clutch of companies has amassed significant profits from a relatively limited portfolio of drugs. There is, today, heightened recognition that lucrative opportunities await companies that can develop even a single life-saving biotechnology drug. For instance, Amgen's revenues increased by over 40 per cent between 2001 and 2002 owing to the US$2 billion it made in 2002 from sales of Epogen and the US$1.5 billion earned from sales of Neupogen. Over US$1 billion in sales of Rituxan—a monoclonal antibody against cancer—in 2002 helped Genentech record a 25 per cent growth over its 2001 performance.

In California, there are two biotechnology "clusters" of global importance: one in San Diego-La Jolla, south of Los Angeles, and the other in the Bay Area, near San Francisco. A cluster is defined as a group of enterprises and institutions in a particular sector of knowledge that are geographically close to each other and networked through all kinds of links, starting with those concerning clients and suppliers. In neither biotechnology cluster does it take more than 10 minutes to travel from one company to another.

The San Diego cluster is supported in all aspects of its functioning, including lobbying politicians and the various actors in the bio-economy, by Biocom—a powerful association of 450 enterprises, including about 400 in biotechnology, in the San Diego region. The cluster relies on the density and frequency of exchanges between industry managers and university research centres. For instance, one of its objectives is to shorten the average time needed to set up a licensing contract between a university and a biotechnology company; it generally takes 10 months to establish such a contract, which is considered too long, so the cluster association is bringing together all the stakeholders to discuss this matter and come to a rapid conclusion.

The clusters have developed the proof of concept, to show that from an idea, a theory or a concept there could emerge a business model and eventually a blockbuster drug. Such an endeavour between the researchers and bio-industry would lead to licensing agreements that rewarded the discovery work. A strategic alliance between politics, basic research and the pharmaceutical industry (whether biotechnological or not) within the cluster would be meaningless without capital.

In fact, bio-industries' success is above all associated with an efficient capital market, according to David Pyott, chief executive officer of Allergan, the world leader in ophthalmic products and the unique owner of Botox -a product used in cosmetic surgery and the main source of the company's wealth. No cluster can exist without a dense network of investors, business angels, venture capitalists and bankers, ready to get involved in the setting up of companies.

The European bio-industry is less mature than its US counterpart. Actelion of Switzerland qualified as the world's fastest-growing drugs group in sales terms following the launch of its first drug, Tracleer, but it did not achieve profitability until 2003. Similarly, hardly any European biotechnology companies are earning money. Only Serono SA—the Swiss powerhouse of European biotechnology—has a market capitalisation to rival US leaders. Serono SA grew out of a hormone extraction business with a 50-year record of profitability and is the world leader in the treatment of infertility; it is also well known in endocrinology and the treatment of multiple sclerosis.

In 2002, Serono SA made US$333 million net profit from US$1,546 million of sales; 23 per cent of the revenue from these sales was devoted to its R&D division, which employs 1,200 people. The Spanish subsidiary of Serono SA in Madrid is now producing recombinant human growth hormone for the whole world, whereas factories in the United States and Switzerland have ceased to produce it.

The Spanish subsidiary had to invest @36 million in order to increase its production, as well as another @5 million to upgrade its installations for the production of other recombinant pharmaceuticals to be exported worldwide. In spite of a wealth of world-class science, the picture in much of Europe is of an industry that lacks the scale to compete and is facing the financial crunch, which may force many companies to seek mergers with stronger rivals.

Germany has overtaken the United Kingdom and France, and is currently home to more biotechnology companies than any country except the United States. But, far from pushing the boundaries of biomedical science, many companies are putting cutting-edge research on hold and are selling valuable technology just to stay solvent. Until the mid-1990s, legislation on genetic engineering in effect ruled out the building of a German bio-industry.

According to Ernst & Young, the more than 400 companies set up in Germany since then needed to raise at least US$496 million from venture capitalists over 2004 to refinance their hunt for new medicines. Most were far from having profitable products and, with stock markets in effect closed to biotechnology companies following the bursting of the bubble in 2000, they were left to seek fourth or even fifth rounds of private financing.

The biggest German biotechnology companies, such as GPC Biotech and Medigene, were able to raise significant sums in initial public offerings at the peak of the Neuer Markt, Germany's market for growth stocks. But when the technology bubble burst in 2000, it became clear to GPC Biotech that investors put very little value on "blue-sky" research. "They wanted to see proven drug candidates in clinical trials", said Mirko Scherer, chief financial officer. The only option for companies such as GPC Biotech and Medigene was to buy drugs that could be brought to market more quickly.

GPC Biotech has used the cash it earned from setting up a research centre for Altana, the German chemicals and pharmaceutical group, to acquire the rights to satraplatin, a cancer treatment that was in the late stages of development. In October 2003, regulators authorised the initiation of the final round of clinical trials. After a series of clinical setbacks, Medigene has mothballed its early-stage research to cut costs and has licensed in late-stage products to make up for two of its own drugs that failed. The strategy will help the company eke out its cash; but cutting back on research will leave little in its pipeline.

Many of Germany's biotechnology companies have abandoned ambitious plans to develop their own products and chosen instead to license their drug leads to big pharmaceutical companies in exchange for funding that will allow them to continue their research. This approach is supported by the acute shortage of potential new medicines in development by the world's biggest pharmaceutical companies. But Germany's bioindustry has few experimental drugs to sell—about 15 compared with the more than 150 in the United Kingdom's more established industry. Moreover, most of Germany's experimental drugs are in the early stages of development, when the probability of failure is as high as 90 per cent. That reduces the price that pharmaceutical companies are willing to pay for them.

Companies also have to struggle with less flexible corporate rules than their rivals in the United Kingdom and the United States. Listed companies complain that the Frankfurt stock exchange does not allow injections of private equity, which are common in US biotechnology. As a result, few of Germany's private companies state that they expect to float in Frankfurt. Most are looking to the United States, the United Kingdom or Switzerland, where investors are more comfortable with high-risk stocks. However, many German companies may not survive long enough to make the choice.

A number of investors in Germany's bio-industry are already pushing in this direction. TVM, the leading German venture capital group, had stakes in 14 German biotechnology companies and was trying to merge most of them. TVM sold off all Cardion's drug leads after failing to find a merger partner for the arthritis and transplant medicine specialists. After raising US$14.1 million in 2002, Cardion has become a shell company that may one day earn royalties if its discoveries make it to market.

UK-based Apax Partners was said to have put almost its entire German portfolio up for sale. The fate of MetaGene Pharmaceuticals, one of Apax's companies, may await many others. In October 2003, the company was bought by the British Astex, which planned to close the German operation after stripping out its best science and its US$15 million bank balance.

GPS Biotech's chief financial officer was critical of the investors who turned their backs on Germany and put 90 per cent of their funds in the United States, when a lot of European companies were very cheap. And although Stephan Weselau, chief financial officer of Xantos, was frustrated that venture capitalists saw little value in his young company's anti-cancer technology, he was adamant about the need for Germany's emerging biotechnology to consolidate if it was to compete against established companies in Boston and San Diego.

The market for initial public offerings in the United Kingdom was all but closed to biotechnology for the three-year period 2000-2002; it reopened in the United States in 2003. City of London institutions, many of which took huge losses on biotechnology, were reluctant to back new issues and have become more fussy about which quoted companies they are prepared to finance.

The United Kingdom is home to one-third of Europe's 1,500 biotechnology companies and more than 40 per cent of its products in development. Although the United Kingdom had 38 marketed biotechnology products and 7 more medicines awaiting approval by the end of 2003, analysts stated that there were too few genuine blockbusters with the sort of sales potential needed to attract investors' attention away from the United States.

A dramatic case is that of PPL (Pharmaceutical Proteins Ltd) Therapeutics—the company set up to produce drugs in the milk of a genetically engineered sheep (Polly). By mid-December 2003, the company had raised a paltry US$295,000 when auctioneers put a mixed catalogue of redundant farm machinery and laboratory equipment under the hammer. This proved that exciting research (Dolly and Polly sheep) does not always lead to commercial success. The profitable British companies reported pre-tax profits of £145 million in 2003, less than 15 per cent of the US$1.9 billion pre-tax profits reported by Amgen. By mid-2003, the British biotechnology sector seemed to be coming of age.

Investors could choose between three companies that had successfully launched several products and boasted market capitalisations in excess of US$884 million. Since then they have seen PowderJect Pharmaceuticals plc acquired by Chiron Corp., the US vaccines group, for a deal value of £542 million in May 2003; and General Electric swooped in with a £5.7 billion bid for Amersham, the diagnostics and biotechnology company, in October 2003. Earlier, in July 2000, Oxford Asymmetry had been purchased by the German company Evotec Biosystems for £343 million, and, in September 2002, Rosemont Pharma was acquired by the US firm Bio-Technology General for £64 million.

In May 2004, Union Chimique Belge (UCB) agreed to buy Celltech, the United Kingdom's biggest biotechnology company, for £1.53 billion (@2.26 billion). UCB decided Celltech could be its stepping stone into biotechnology after entering an auction for the marketing rights to Celltech's new treatment for rheumatoid arthritis (CPD 870), touted as a blockbuster drug with forecast annual sales of more than US$1 billion. After seeing trial data not revealed to the wider market, UCB decided to buy the whole company. The surprise acquisition was accompanied by a licensing deal that gives UCB the rights to CPD 870, which accounted for about half the company's valuation. Goran Ando, the Celltech chief executive who will become deputy chief executive of UCB, stated: "we will immediately have the financial wherewithal, the global commercial reach and the R&D strength to take all our drugs to market." News of the deal, which will be funded with debt, sent Celltech shares 26 per cent higher to £5.42, whereas UCB shares fell 4 per cent to @33.68.

Celltech had been the grandfather of the British biotechnology sector since it was founded in 1980. With a mixture of seed funding from the Thatcher government and the private sector, the company was set up to commercialise the discovery of monoclonal antibodies that can become powerful medicines. Listed in 1993, the company made steady progress in its own research operations, but gained products and financial stability only with the acquisitions of Chiroscience in 1999 and Medeva in 2000. It also acquired Oxford GlycoSciences in May 2003 in a deal worth £140 million. The great hopes Celltech has generated were based largely on CPD 870, the arthritis drug it planned to bring to market in 2007 that could be by far the best-selling product to come out of a British biotechnology company.

After the UCB-Celltech deal, the group ranked fifth among the top five biopharmaceutical companies, behind Amgen, @6.6 billion in revenue in 2003; Novo Nordisk, @3.6 billion; Schering, @3.5 billion; and Genentech, @2.6 billion. Based on 2003 results, the combined market capitalisation of UCB Pharma and Celltech will be @7.14 billion; revenues, @2,121 million; earnings before interest, tax and amortisation, @472 million; pharmaceutical R&D budget, @397 million; number of employees, approximately 1,450.

Celltech is the biggest acquisition by UCB, which branched out from heavy chemicals only in the 1980s. Georges Jacob, its chief executive since 1987, stated that when he joined UCB he found a company "devoted to chemicals, dominated by engineers, pretty old-fashioned and very much part of heavy industry". UCB had been built entirely on internal growth, and its only other sizeable acquisition was the speciality chemicals business of US-based Solutia in December 2002 for US$500 million, a move that split the Belgian group's @3 billion revenues evenly between pharmaceuticals and chemicals.

One constant was the continued presence of a powerful family shareholder, owning 40 per cent of UCB's equity via a complicated holding structure. UCB made its first foray into pharmaceuticals in the 1950s with the development of a molecule it sold to Pfizer, Inc. This became Atarax, an anti-histamine used to relieve anxiety. The relationship with Pfizer was revived in a more lucrative fashion for UCB following the 1987 launch of Zyrtec, a blockbuster allergy treatment that Pfizer helped to distribute in the United States. Although UCB has a follow-up drug to Zyrtec, it faces the loss of the US patent in 2007.

UCB also had to fight patent challenges to its other main drug, Keppra, an epilepsy treatment. With the takeover of Celltech, UCB will gain a pipeline of antibody treatments for cancer and inflammatory diseases to add to its allergy and epilepsy medicines. According to most analysts, the expansion in health-care activities will lead the group to divest itself of its remaining chemical business.

After this takeover and following the earlier acquisition of PowderJect Pharmaceuticals and Amersham by US companies, there is not much left in the United Kingdom's biotechnology sector except Acambis, another vaccine-maker, valued at about £325 million, and a string of companies below the £200 million mark where liquidity can be a problem for investors. The industry was therefore afraid it would be swamped by its much larger rivals. Martyn Postle, director of Cambridge Healthcare and Biotech, a consultancy, stated that "we could end up with the UK performing the role of the research division of US multinationals".

According to the head of the Bioindustry Association (BIA), "it is clearly the fact that US companies are able to raise much, much more money than in the United Kingdom, which puts them in a much stronger position". The BIA called for changes in the rules on "pre-emption rights", which give existing shareholders priority in secondary equity offerings. Because Celltech was by far the most liquid stock in the sector, there could be a broader impact on the way the financial sector treats biotechnology, including a reduction in the number of specialist investors and analysts covering the sector.

It is important for the United Kingdom to create an environment in which biotechnology can flourish. The industry has called for institutional reform, including measures to make it easier for companies to raise new capital. The British government must also ensure that its higher education system continues to produce world-class scientists. That reinforces the need for reforms to boost the funding of universities. The Celltech takeover need not be seen as a national defeat for the United Kingdom.

The combined company may end up being listed in London. Even if it does not, Celltech's research base in the United Kingdom will expand. Its investors have been rewarded for their faith and, if its CPD 870 drug is approved, UCB's shareholders will also benefit. But, for Celltech's executives, the acquisition is a victory for Europe. The takeover creates an innovative European biotechnology company that is big enough, and has sufficient financial resources, to compete globally. "The key was to have viable European businesses that have a sustainable long-term presence," stated Goran Ando, who confirmed that UCB's research will be run from Celltech's old base in Slough.

In France in 2003, according to the France Biotech association, there were 270 biotechnology companies focused on the life sciences and less than 25 years old. They employed 4,500 people—a number that could be multiplied four or five times if about @3 billion were to be invested in public research over three years. In 2003, France invested only @300 million of private funds and @100 million of public funds in biotechnology, far behind Germany and the United Kingdom, which each invested about @900 million per year. In 2003, France launched a five-year Biotech Plan aimed at restoring the visibility and attractiveness of France in 2008-2010. Three areas—human health, agrifood and the environment—were expected to attract the funds as well as the efforts of universities, public and private laboratories, hospitals, enterprises and investors.

SangStat, a biotechnology company created in 1989 in the Silicon Valley by Philippe Pouletty, is working on organ transplants. It was established in California because, at the time of its creation, venture capital in France was only just starting to support such endeavours in biotechnology. Between FFr 600 million and FFr 2 billion were needed to set up a biotechnology corporation to develop one or perhaps two new drugs, and bankruptcy was very likely in France. SangStat is now a world leader in the treatment of the rejection of organ transplants and intends to extend its expertise and know-how to the whole area of transplantation. It is already marketing two drugs in the United States and three in Europe. A second corporation, DrugAbuse Sciences (DAS), was established by Pouletty in 1994, by which time venture capital was becoming a more common practice in Europe.

Two companies were created at the same time: DAS France and DAS US in San Francisco, both belonging to the same group and having the same shareholders. Being established in Europe and the United States, greater flexibility could be achieved from the financial viewpoint and better resilience to stock exchange fluctuations. DAS was able to increase its capital by FFr 140 million (@21.3 million) in 1999 with the help of European investors. DAS specialises in drug abuse and alcoholism. Its original approach was to study neurological disorders in the patient so as to promote abstinence, treat overdoses and prevent dependence through new therapies.

Pouletty had surveyed 1,300 existing biotechnology companies in 1994 and found that hundreds were working on cancer and dozens on gene therapy, diabetes, etc., but not one was working on drug and alcohol addiction. Even the big pharmaceutical groups had no significant activity in this area, although drug and alcohol addiction is considered the greatest problem for public health in industrialised countries. For instance, 2.5 per cent of the annual gross domestic product in France is spent on these illnesses, and some US$250 billion in the United States.

A first product, Naltrel, improves on the current treatment of alcoholism by naltrexone. The latter, to be efficient, must be taken as pills every day. But few alcoholics can strictly follow this kind of treatment. In order to free patients from this daily constraint, a monthly intramuscular injection of a delayed-action micro-encapsulated product has been developed, which helps alcoholics and drug addicts to abstain from their drug. The molecule developed inhibits the receptors in the brain that are stimulated by opium-related substances.

Another successful product, COC-AB, has been developed for the emergency treatment of cocaine overdoses. This molecule recognises cocaine in the bloodstream and traps it before it reaches the brain; it is then excreted through the kidneys in urine. Commercialisation of the medicine was expected to help the 250,000 cocaine addicts who are admitted annually to the medical emergency services.

In the long term, DAS intends to develop preventive compounds that can inhibit the penetration of the drug into the brain. DAS was expected to become a world-leading pharmaceutical company by 2005-2007 in the treatment of alcoholism and drug addiction or abuse. This forecast was based on the current figures of 30 million chronic patients in the United States and Europe, comprising 22 million alcoholics, 6 million cocaine addicts and 2 million heroin addicts.

Another success story is the French biotechnology company Eurofins, founded in Nantes in 1998 to exploit a patent .led by two researchers from the local faculty of sciences. Eurofins currently employs 2,000 people worldwide and in four years increased its annual turnover 10-

fold (to @162 million). Its portfolio contains more than 5,000 methods of analysing biological substances. The company is located in Nantes, where 130 people carry out research on the purity and origin of foodstuffs.

Despite the closure of some of Eurofins' 50 laboratories in order to improve the company's financial position in the face of the slowdown in the economy, Eurofins wants to continue to grow. This success story has led the city of Nantes to think about creating a biotechnology city. It has also given a strong impetus to medical biotechnology at Nantes' hospital, where the number of biotechnology researchers soared from 70 to 675.

In October 2003, the Institute of Genetics Nantes Atlantique initiated the analysis of human DNA for forensic purposes. This institute, which received venture capital from two main sources, was expected to employ 50 people within two years in order to meet the demand generated by the extension of the national automated database of genetic fingerprinting.

Oryzon Genomics is a genomics company based in Madrid, Spain. It applies genomics to new cereal crops, grapevines and vegetables, as well as to the production of new drugs (especially for Parkinson's and Alzheimer's diseases). It is a young enterprise, an offshoot of the University of Barcelona and the Spanish Council for Scientific Research (CSIC), located in Barcelona's Science Park. With a staff of 22 scientists, the company is experiencing rapid growth and is developing an ambitious programme of functional genomics.

It was the first genomics enterprise to have access to special funding from the NEOTEC Programme, in addition to financial support from the Ministry of Science and the Generalitat of Catalonia. Moreover, the National Innovation Enterprise (ENISA), which is part of the General Policy Directorate for Medium and Small Sized Enterprises of the Ministry of the Economy, has invested @400,000 in Oryzon Genomics—this was ENISA's first investment in the biotechnology sector. At the end of 2002, Najeti Capital, a venture capital firm specialising in investments in technology, acquired 28 per cent of Oryzon Genomics in order to support the young corporation. In 2003, Oryzon Genomics' turnover was estimated at @500,000, and its clients comprised several agrifood and pharmaceutical companies as well as public research centres.

Japan is well advanced in plant genetics and has made breakthroughs in rice genomics, but it is lagging behind the United States in human genetics. Its contribution to the sequencing of the human genome (by teams of researchers from the Physics and Chemistry Research Institute of the Science and Technology Agency, as well as from Keio University Medical Department) was about 7 per cent. In order to reduce the gap with the United States, the Japanese government has invested significant funds in the Millennium Project, launched in April 2000.

The project covers three areas: the rice genome, the human genome and regenerative medicine. The 2000 budget included ¥347 billion for the life sciences. The genomics budget, amounting to ¥64 billion, was twice that of the neurosciences. Within the framework of the Millennium Project, the Ministry of Health aimed to promote the study of genes linked with such diseases as cancer, dementia, diabetes and hypertension; results for each of these diseases were expected by 2004.

The Ministry of International Trade and Industry (MITI) set up a Centre for Analysis of Information Relating to Biological Resources. This had a very strong DNA-sequencing capacity—equivalent to that of Washington University in the United States (sequencing of over 30 million nucleotide pairs per annum)—and will analyse the genome of micro-organisms used in fermentation and provide this information to the industrial sector. In addition, following the project launched in 1999 by Hitachi Ltd, Takeda Chemical Industries and Jutendo Medical Faculty aimed at identifying the genetic polymorphisms associated with allergic diseases, a similar project devoted to single-nucleotide polymorphisms (SNPs) was initiated in April 2000 under the aegis of Tokyo University and the Japanese Foundation for Science. The research work is being carried out in a DNA-sequencing centre to which 16 private companies send researchers with a view to contributing to the development of medicines tailored to individuals' genetic make-up.

On 30 October 2000, the pharmaceutical group Daiichi Pharmaceutical and the giant electronics company Fujitsu announced an alliance in genomics. Daiichi and Celestar Lexico Science (Fujitsu's biotechnology division) were pooling their research efforts over the five-year period 2000-2005 to study the genes involved in cancer, ageing, infectious diseases and hypertension. Daiichi devoted about US$100 million to this research in 2001-2002, and about 60 scientists were involved in this work of functional genomics.

On 31 January 2003, the Japan Bioindustry Association (JBA) announced that, as of December 2002, the number of "bioventures" in Japan totalled 334 firms. This announcement was based on a survey -the first of its kind—conducted by the JBA in 2002 to have a better understanding of the nation's bio-industry. A "bioventure" was defined as a firm that employs, or develops for, biotechnology applications; that complies with the definition of a small or medium-sized business as prescribed by Japanese law; that was created 20 years ago; and that does not deal primarily in sales or imports/exports. The 334 bioventures had a total of 6,757 employees, sales amounting to ¥105 billion and R&D costs estimated at ¥51 billion. The average figures per bioventure were: 20 employees, sales worth ¥314 million and R&D costs of ¥153 million.

The three regions with the highest concentrations of bioventures were Kanto (191, or 57 per cent of the national total), Kinki/Kansai (55, or 16 per cent) and Hokkaido (32, or 10 per cent). One-third of all ventures (112) were located in Tokyo (within the Kanto region). The most common field of bioventure operations was pharmaceuticals and diagnostic product development (94 bioventures), followed by customized production of DNA, proteins, etc. (78 bioventures), bioinformatics (41 ventures), and reagents and consumables development (38 bioventures).

In its 2003 global biotechnology census, the consultancy firm Ernst & Young ranked Australia's A$12 billion biotechnology and, bio-industry as number one in the Asia-Pacific region and sixth worldwide. Australia accounts for 67 per cent of public biotechnology revenues for the Asia-Pacific region. The Australian government gave a boost to the bio-industry by providing nearly A$1 billion in public biotechnology expenditure in 2002-2003. There were around 370 companies in Australia in 2002 whose core business was biotechnology—an increase from 190 in 2001.

Human therapeutics made up 43 per cent, agricultural biotechnology 16 per cent and diagnostics companies 15 per cent. Over 40 biotechnology companies were listed on the Australian stock exchange (ASX) and a study released by the Australian Graduate School of Management reported that an investment of A$1,000 in each of the 24 biotech companies listed on the ASX between 1998 and 2002 would have been worth more than A$61,000 in 2003—an impressive 150 per cent return. During the same period, shares in listed Australian biotechs significantly outperformed those of US biotechs, and the overall performance of listed Australian biotech companies was higher than that of the Australian stock market as a whole.

Over A$500 million was raised by listed Australian life science companies in 2003, and the ASX health-care and biotechnology sector had a market capitalisation of A$23.4 billion in 2003, up 18 per cent on 2002. There has been a maturing of the Australian biotechnology sector, with greater attention paid to sustainable business models and the identification of unique opportunities that appeal to investors and partners. The industry is supported by skilled personnel—Australia is considered to have a greater availability of scientists and engineers than the United Kingdom, Singapore or Germany.

Australia is ranked in the top five countries (with a population of 20 million or more) for the number of R&D personnel. In terms of public expenditure on R&D as a percentage of GDP, it outranks major OECD countries, including the United States, Japan, Germany and the United Kingdom. For biomedical R&D, Australia is ranked the second most effective country—ahead of the United States, the United Kingdom and Germany—particularly with respect to labour, salaries, utilities and income tax. Australia is ranked third after the Netherlands and Canada for the cost competitiveness of conducting clinical trials.

Australian researchers indeed have a strong record of discovery and development in therapeutics. Recent world firsts include the discovery that Helicobacter pylori causes gastric ulcers, and the purification and cloning of three of the major regulators of blood cell transformation -granulocyte colony-stimulating factor (GCSF), granulocyte macrophage colony-stimulating factor (GMCSF) and leukaemia inhibiting factor (LIF). Australia is cementing its place at the forefront of stem cell research with a transparent regulatory system and the establishment of the visionary National Stem Cell Centre (NSCC). An initiative of the Australian government, this centre draws together expertise and infrastructure; in 2003 it entered into a licensing agreement with the US company LifeCell.

Strong opportunities exist in areas such as immunology, reproductive medicine, neurosciences, infectious diseases and cancer. There are also opportunities for bioprospecting given that Australia is home to almost 10 per cent of global plant diversity, with around 80 per cent of plants and microbes in Australia found nowhere else in the world. Although 25 per cent of modern medicines come from natural products, it is estimated that only 1 per cent of plants in Australia have been screened for natural compounds.

Australia is the most resilient economy in the world, has the lowest risk of political instability in the world and possesses the most multicultural and multilingual workforce in the Asia-Pacific region. Its geographical location has not been a deterrent to the establishment of partnerships. According to Ernst & Young's 2003 "Beyond Borders" global biotechnology report, Australia had 21 cross-border alliances in 2002—more than France and Switzerland, and 18 more than its nearest Asia-Pacific competitor.

All the major pharmaceutical companies have a presence in Australia and pharmaceuticals are the third-highest manufactures export for Australia, generating over US$1.5 billion. The largest drugexploration partnership in Australian history, between Merck & Co., Inc. and Melbourne-based Amrad to develop drugs against asthma, other respiratory diseases and cancer, was valued at up to US$112 million (plus royalties) in 2003. It is therefore no wonder that the pharmaceutical industry in Australia, which has annual revenues of US$9.2 billion, is increasingly viewed by the main global players as a valuable source of innovative R&D and technology.

Linear Model of Medical Innovation

Several OECD governments have established biotechnology science parks as a means to strengthen industry-university links and create new employment. This reflects an assumption that innovation is the product of a linear pattern of events in which, briefly, innovation is initiated by basic scientific research, which is followed by applied and more product-oriented research activities, clinical development and testing, commercial manufacturing, and finally marketing and diffusion. The assumption is that, if technological innovation is strongly linked to basic scientific research, science parks or the "clustering" of young firms around a basic research centre would provide an "incubator" conducive to more rapid and effective technology transfer.

In support of this linear concept, Jaffe has shown for the United States that university research causes industry R&D and not vice versa. In addition, university research, particularly in biotechnology, seems to increase local innovation by attracting clusters of similar firms to one geographical area. Moreover, the history of the biotechnology industry confirms these assumptions. The biotechnology industry originated in California, near San Francisco, in an area where several research centres were located, and firms were founded in co-operation with academic scientists at those centres.

There are obvious benefits to being part of a cluster. On the supply side, they include availability of specialised labour, specialised intermediate inputs, and knowledge spillovers. On the demand side, the strength of some high-technology sectors may come from clustering with important users in other industries or domestic users. Some of the drawbacks of clustering include congestion costs and increased competition. By 1991, in the United States, 50 per cent of the biotechnology industry was still significantly clustered. Science parks were created in the hope that clusters of young firms around a science base could foster innovation. However, several recent studies seem to indicate that science park firms are not more innovative than other firms.

A recent analysis of the dynamics of industrial clustering in biotechnology points to some of the reasons. The science base attracts new biotechnology firms in sectors where entries are already flourishing. However, the effects on firm growth are negative in some other biotechnology sectors and much weaker in others. This means that new firms can absorb "spillovers" from within their own and closely related sectors but are not good at absorbing spillovers from the science base of other sectors. In the biotechnology industry, intersectoral feedback or links do not seem to encourage entry. This is due in part to the fact that the various biotechnology sectors do not all share technological links. For example, developments in the health care sector do not necessarily lead to entries in sectors such as chemicals and food. Furthermore, strength of employment in a specific sector in a cluster seems to discourage similar firms from entering, perhaps for reasons of competition.

Product and Process Development

A main reason for government intervention is to protect citizens from the uncertainties and risks of new technologies. In addition, all governments have developed mechanisms to steer research into priority areas, to ban controversial or undesirable research, and to balance innovation against the need to contain health-care costs. What are the effects of government policies on product and process development and how does uncertainty about these policies affect output in the health care sector?

Regulatory policies

Over the past decade, both the individual states and the federal government have adopted measures designed to ease the financial and regulatory burden on the biotechnology sector, to take account of the circumstances unique to early stages of product development in this industry; and to respond to public health concerns that innovative products be made available to patients as quickly as possible. Many of the intended effects of these policies and proposals relate to reducing out-of-pocket costs, making the process more predictable, and moving effective and safe products to market faster. If realised, any of these effects will increase incentives for firms to engage in and for investors to invest in biopharmaceutical R&D.

Cost of clinical trials

As highlighted by Gosse et al., developing new biopharmaceuticals and getting them approved for marketing is a lengthy, uncertain, and costly process. The times from the initiation of clinical testing in the United States to submission of a product license application (PLA) with the Food and Drug Administration (FDA), and to approval of the PLA by the FDA, averaged 3.9 and 5.7 years, respectively, for new biopharmaceuticals approved in the United States between 1990 and 1994. Policies to reduce these times would lower the cost of bringing new biopharmaceuticals to market and increase the returns that may be expected from successful product introductions.

Although new drug development costs can change significantly over time, the relative contributions of various components of the development and regulatory review processes are likely to be much more stable and can be assessed. DiMasi et al. estimated R&D costs for a sample of new drugs that first entered clinical testing anywhere in the world from 1970 to 1982. When the costs of research failures and preclinical expenditures are included in cost estimations, they found that time costs represent more than half of total costs.

Time costs are measured as the amount that could have been earned if the funds spent on R&D expenditures up to the date of marketing approval had instead been invested in a financial instrument of similar risk. Thus, reductions in the amount of time spent in development or regulatory review can significantly reduce costs. Shows the percentage declines in cost per approved new drug (failures included) that can be achieved from a reduction of one year in the clinical trial and regulatory review phases.

Since the late 1980s, several aspects of the drug development and review process have been modified to reduce the time to market for new therapies. Initially, the changes were introduced to improve access to new therapies to treat serious or life-threatening conditions. Investigational new drug (IND) regulations allowed for patient access to new therapies outside standard clinical trials. Fast-track initiatives (Subpart E regulations and accelerated approval regulations) were implemented to expedite time to market of drugs for life-threatening illnesses. This was accomplished by allowing more lenient risk-benefit ratios and clinical endpoints

Since 1993, under the authority of the *Prescription Drug User Fee Act of* 1992 (PDUFA-Public Law No. 102-571), the FDA has collected user fees from applicants seeking FDA approval for certain new drug applications (NDAs), PLAs, and supplemental applications. The Act established a five-year programme for the payment of user fees, which generated almost $80 million in fiscal year 1996.

The pharmaceutical and biotechnology industries' expectations for speedier FDA review of applications for new drugs and biologics have figured prominently in the implementation of the user fee programme. A crucial component of the programme is a series of performance goals designed to achieve specific incremental improvements in the speed and efficiency of the drug review process, the ultimate goal being review and ruling on an application within 12 months. In 1996, the agency took action on 269 original applications, with 131 approvals. Of these, 53 were new molecular entities (NMEs), i.e. a drug based on active ingredients never marketed before.

NMEs approved in a given year are an important industry marker and an indicator of the rate of innovation. By charting the number of NMEs and median approval times since 1986, it is apparent that even if not designed specifically to expedite regulatory review, early access, together with fast track mechanisms and PDUFA, have been successful regulatory reforms. On the other hand, treatment IND regulations are also associated with longer clinical development times. The longer development time may reflect difficulties in expanding distribution and monitoring to physicians and patients who would not ordinarily be included in the compressed clinical trial protocols.

It is widely recognised that R&D is influenced by public policy. What is less understood is the reverse, i.e. the extent to which new technological developments can influence policy making and regulatory bodies. It is apparent that the relation between regulatory frameworks and new science and technology is increasingly complex. There is no doubt that the application of molecular biological techniques has spurred a revolution in drug development. Since many of these biopharmaceutical products have altered traditional drug development by targeting innovative therapeutic methods or treatments of the genetic basis of disease, the policies and regulations mandated by regulatory agencies in all OECD countries have required modification. Regulations, some dating from 1902, had not kept pace with technological change. Thus, proposals for regulatory reform were advocated by government, industrial, and academic groups.

In developing regulatory guidelines for new technologies, policy makers are challenged to strike a balance between public concern over unknown technological risks, and guidelines that foster, rather than impede, research on promising new treatments. Biotechnology provides a useful example of the difficulties and complexities that regulatory authorities face.

The Recombinant Advisory Committee (RAC) was founded in 1974 to advise the Secretary of Health and Human Services, the Assistant Secretary of Health, and the Director of the NIH on "the current state of knowledge and technology regarding DNA recombinants and to recommend guidelines to be followed by investigators with recombinant DNA". *The RAC's role was to assure the public that genetic research was being done in the open and in the right way.*

Over the years, the RAC has proved useful in addressing sensitive issues of safety and medical ethics in a public forum; proposing (and progressively adapting) guidelines for recombinant DNA experiments, generation of transgenic animals, and, more recently, human gene therapy protocols. The RAC met quarterly to review these protocols and to ensure that proposals fell within the guidelines of an NIH points-to-consider document. Prior to mid-1995, all gene therapy protocols arising from federally funded research had to be submitted for RAC review. The RAC proceeded to make specific recommendations, ensured that safety precautions were addressed, and reviewed the scientific and ethical basis of the proposal. The time needed to obtain RAC approval of a protocol was affected by the limited meeting schedule. The Director of the NIH awarded final NIH approval.

The second federal government mechanism to approve a human gene therapy trial is the standard IND submitted to the FDA. As gene research moved into the mainstream, the apparent redundancy of the two review mechanisms seemed cumbersome. The dual review process increased the time to commencement of human clinical trials. Thus, the seemingly redundant process of protocol review by the NIH and the FDA drew criticism from industry, academia, and AIDS activists. This prompted the director of the NIH to reconsider the role and function of the RAC.

As a result, RAC is no longer responsible for approvals, but is responsible for identifying novel human gene transfer experiments deserving public discussion and transmitting comments/recommendations to the NIH, for identifying novel ethical issues relevant to specific human applications of gene transfer, for identifying novel scientific and safety issues relevant to specific human applications of gene transfer, and for publicly reviewing human gene transfer clinical trial data.

The RAC set a precedent for the review of human gene therapy trials. In 1989, the government of the United Kingdom established the Committee on the Ethics of Gene Therapy, under the chairmanship of Sir Cecil Clothier. Based upon the recommendations of the Clothier Committee, the UK Gene Therapy Advisory Committee (GTAC) was established in 1992 to review proposals for genetic therapy for human disease. The GTAC has prepared a manual, the GTAC Guidance on Making Proposals to Conduct Gene Therapy Research on Human Subjects, for preparing human gene therapy proposals in the United Kingdom.

GTAC serves to complement local research ethics committees (LREC) and at the present time, will not consider proposals for germ cell gene therapy. Outside of the United States, GTAC is the closest equivalent to the RAC. The GTAC review of a human gene therapy protocol is similar to the initial US RAC/FDA separate and parallel review; the GTAC and the Medicines Control Agency (MCA, the UK counterpart of the FDA) receive the proposal simultaneously. GTAC evaluations and recommendations are then submitted to the MCA, LREC, and the principal applicant. Although the GTAC is similar to the RAC, GTAC does not have a history of public debate and access. It is a smaller group, is more likely to seek external *ad hoc* reviewers and thus is ultimately more able to streamline review.

Industrial Property Rights

"Industrial property" systems have been developed by states as a means for recognising and promoting innovation. Patents, for example, protect the innovator for a limited period against use by third parties of the protected subject matter without his consent. Patent systems promote innovation by encouraging the early and effective public disclosure of inventions. They universally involve publication of a full description of the invention upon grant or, in many systems, 18 months after patent protection is originally sought.

A patent cannot hamper the free use of whatever is already in the public domain; it can only control the use by others of the inventor's novel addition to the previously existing technology. The principle of providing a temporary period of legal protection encourages the climate for innovation, to the ultimate benefit of the public as a whole. This period of protection is not yet uniform in all countries, but the period is most commonly set at 20 years from the patent application date, subject to the payment of annual renewal fees. Patents also encourage investment in R&D and in the production and marketing of new products and processes.

Statutory intellectual property rights provide a basic framework for voluntary technology transfer through intellectual property right licensing, supplemented and reinforced by provisions based on the supply of know-how and other factors which may be less easy to define. Patent law demands clear definition of the protected technology and thereby establishes the scope of the rights of the innovator, identifies what is transferred to a licensee, and allows for the corresponding freedoms of third parties to be assessed.

Subject to international agreements designed to improve and unify patent protection throughout the world, a country is free to develop its own policy towards legal protection systems and legal enforceability procedures. Thus, a country is free to develop and implement measures to encourage technological innovation, technology transfer and other technology-related objectives, provided these measures conform to the minimum standards of protection mandated by the TRIPS Agreement and other multilateral treaties in the field of intellectual property law.

Important factors affecting national patent policy are:

— the current level of national technology transfer from the research base and expectations as to its future development;

— the need to encourage technology transfer from other countries;

— the desire to attract foreign investment to the country or region (a strong patent system is more likely to do so).

The freedom to carry out research is safeguarded under patent laws. Under patent law "experimental use" for research purposes is not considered to be an infringement of the rights of the patent owner. But what is purely experimental (rather than experimental for commercial purposes) is a matter of interpretation, mainly through case law, and can therefore vary according to national jurisprudence. The freedom to commercialise the products of research depends on whether or not patents are infringed, or for plants, whether they are essentially derived or dependent varieties under plant variety rights.

Pharmaceutical innovation

To develop a new drug requires an average of 12 years and \$300-500 million. Regulations governing clinical research are also one of the primary reasons for rising R&D costs. Most of the industry's innovative efforts, as mentioned previously proceed in a fairly linear manner, with clearly defined stages, many of them determined and regulated by law. Pharmaceutical companies must follow a lengthy R&D process.

Pre-clinical tests study the potential risks that a compound poses to humans and the environment by using animals, tissue cultures, and other test systems to examine the relationship between factors such as dose level, frequency of administration, and duration of exposure to both the short-and long-term survival of living organisms. This is followed by three phases of clinical testing to assess both safety and efficacy in humans.

Since companies typically patent early during pre-clinical testing, the development and approval process, discussed above, can consume a significant portion of a new chemical entity's patent life. Today, when a drug reaches the market, it typically has 8-11 years of patent protection remaining, a number that has been declining steadily for the past three decades. When the patent on a pharmaceutical product expires, other companies can make generic copies without spending hundreds of millions of dollars on discovery, development and testing.

The second or third product in a class, the so-called "me-too's", will often be marketed at a discount. As part of the efforts to contain costs, purchasers will shift prescriptions to generic products as early as possible, and this will include extensive use of the first generic available in a class of products. The price of generics may be as low as 20-30 per cent of that of the branded product, and it has been shown that, in the United States for example, sales of a branded product will drop as much as 50-70 per cent within one year after its patent expires; in addition, there will be a substantial effect on the second and third product in the class.

Thus, the pharmaceutical industry is more dependent on strong intellectual property protection than any other industry. If pharmaceutical companies could not patent their drugs they would be unlikely to invest in new research. Furthermore, it is frequently argued that relatively weak intellectual property rights protection in a country may lower the probability that firms will invest there, and that, if they do, they may restrict investment to their own subsidiaries and will also restrict the transfer of "know-how".

In Canada, for example, for almost two decades, patent protection of prescription drugs was weakened by allowing compulsory licensing of drug imports. Compulsory licensing facilitated the proliferation of cheaper generic substitutes for brand-name prescription drugs and contributed in a major way to the development of a strong, mostly Canadian-owned generic drug industry.

The multinational drug companies objected to the weakening of their intellectual property rights and publicised their reluctance to invest and conduct R&D in Canada. Pressure to repeal the legislation gained additional impetus when compulsory licensing became an obstacle to successful completion of the free trade agreement between Canada and the United States.

In 1987, the government enacted Bill C-22, which provided for protection from compulsory licensing for a period of seven years in the case of licence to manufacture, and ten years in the case of licence to import. Bill C-91, which was enacted in 1992, abolished compulsory licensing completely, in accordance with the provisions of the General Agreement on Tariffs and Trade (GATT) and the North American Free Trade Agreement (NAFTA).

A survey of institutions belonging to the "Canadian biotechnology community" reported average annual growth of R&D expenditures of 41 per cent during the period 1989-93, with the agri-food sector growing at 112 per cent a year, followed by the health care sector at 77 per cent. The slowest growth (5 per cent a year) was recorded in the research sector, where federal government biotechnology expenditures were affected by government spending restrictions.

Measured in terms of total revenue, the Canadian biotechnology industry is today about 5.6 per cent that of the United States, up from 2.9 per cent in 1994. Furthermore, the total number of core biotechnology companies increased from 121 in 1994 to 224 in 1997 with the small and very small companies accounting for 42 per cent and 30 per cent, respectively. Industry revenues have increased from $353 million to $1.1 billion, and total financing activity during 1996 exceeded $1 billion, approximately the same amount of financing as was raised in total over the preceding five years.

It would be difficult to explain the dramatic increase in R&D activity in the Canadian pharmaceutical industry exclusively in terms of the economics of patent protection and it is unlikely that the economic A number of indicators of pharmaceutical R&D spending in Canada show an increase in R&D activity starting around the year 1987. A survey of institutions belonging to the "Canadian biotechnology community" reported average annual growth of R&D expenditures of 41 per cent during the period 1989-93, with the agri-food sector growing at 112 per cent a year, followed by the health care sector at 77 per cent. The slowest growth (5 per cent a year) was recorded in the research sector, where federal government biotechnology expenditures were affected by government spending restrictions.

Measured in terms of total revenue, the Canadian biotechnology industry is today about 5.6 per cent that of the United States, up from 2.9 per cent in 1994. Furthermore, the total number of core biotechnology companies increased from 121 in 1994 to 224 in 1997 with the small and very small companies accounting for 42 per cent and 30 per cent, respectively. Industry revenues have increased from $353 million to $1.1 billion, and total financing activity during

1996 exceeded $1 billion, approximately the same amount of financing as was raised in total over the preceding five years.

It would be difficult to explain the dramatic increase in R&D activity in the Canadian pharmaceutical industry exclusively in terms of the economics of patent protection and it is unlikely that the economic benefits of increased patent protection alone would cause such an increase. Indeed other contributing factors should be noted. For example, the Canadian pharmaceutical companies made a commitment during the debate on the merits of Bill C-22 to double the ratio of R&D to sales from less than 5 per cent in 1984 to 10 per cent in 1996. In addition between 1985 and 1987 legislation on tax incentives for R&D was amended to include experimental development, and to extend the carry forward period for R&D tax credit from seven to ten years.

Benefits of Biotechnology

We can now detect many diseases and medical conditions more quickly and with greater accuracy because of the sensitivity of new, biotechnology-based diagnostic tools. A familiar example of biotechnology's benefits is the new generation of home pregnancy tests that provide more accurate results much earlier than previous tests. Tests for strep throat and many other infectious diseases provide results in minutes, enabling treatment to begin immediately in contrast to the two- or three-day delay of previous tests.

Biotechnology has also decreased the costs of diagnostics. A new blood test, developed through biotechnology, measures the amount of low-density lipoprotein (LDL), or "bad" cholesterol, in blood. Conventional methods require separate and expensive tests for total cholesterol, triglycerides and high-density lipoprotein cholesterol. Also, a patient must fast 12 hours before the test. The new biotech test measures LDL in one test, and fasting is not necessary. We now use biotechnology-based tests to diagnose certain cancers, such as prostate and ovarian cancer, by taking a blood sample, eliminating the need for invasive and costly surgery.

In addition to diagnostics that are cheaper, more accurate and quicker than previous tests, biotechnology is allowing us to diagnose diseases earlier in the disease process, which greatly improves a patient's prognosis. Most tests detect diseases once the disease process is far enough along to provide measurable indicators. Proteomics researchers are discovering molecular markers that indicate incipient diseases before visible cell changes or disease symptoms appear. Soon physicians will have access to tests for detecting these biomarkers before the disease begins.

The wealth of Genomics information made available by the Human Genome Project will greatly assist doctors in early diagnosis of hereditary diseases, such as type I diabetes, cystic fibrosis, early-onset Alzheimer's Disease, and Parkinson's Disease ailments that previously were detectable only after clinical symptoms appeared. Genetic tests will also identify patients with a propensity to diseases, such as various cancers, osteoporosis, emphysema, type II diabetes and asthma, giving patients an opportunity to prevent the disease by avoiding triggers such as diet, smoking and other environmental factors.

Biotechnology-based diagnostic tests are not only altering disease diagnosis but also improving the way health care is provided. Many tests are portable, so physicians conduct the tests, interpret results and decide on treatment literally at the patient's bedside. In addition, because many of these diagnostic tests are based on colour changes similar to a home pregnancy test, the results can be interpreted without technically trained personnel, expensive lab equipment or costly facilities, making them more available to poorer communities and people in developing countries.

The human health benefits of biotechnology detection methodologies go beyond disease diagnosis. For example, biotechnology detection tests screen donated blood for the pathogens that cause AIDS and hepatitis. Physicians will someday be able to immediately profile the infection being treated and, based on the results, choose the most effective antibiotics.

Therapeutics Regimes

Biotechnology will make possible improved versions of today's therapeutic regimes as well as treatments that would not be possible without these new techniques. Biotechnology therapeutics approved by the U.S. Food and Drug Administration (FDA) to date are used to treat many diseases, including anemia, cystic fibrosis, growth deficiency, rheumatoid arthritis, hemophilia, hepatitis, genital warts, transplant rejection, and leukemia and other cancers. All are derived from biological substances and processes designed by nature. Some use the human body's own tools for fighting infections and correcting problems. Others are natural products of plants and animals. The large-scale manufacturing processes for producing therapeutic biological substances also rely on nature's molecular production mechanisms.

Many living organisms produce compounds that have therapeutic value for us. For example, many antibiotics are produced by naturally occurring microbes, and a number of medicines on the market, such as digitalis, are also made by plants. Plant cell culture, recombinant DNA technology and cellular cloning now provide us with new ways to tap into natural diversity.

A fungus produces a novel, antioxidant enzyme that is a particularly efficient at mopping up free radicals known to encourage tumour growth. Byetta™ (exenatide), an incretin mimetic, was chemically copied from the venom of the gila monster and approved in early 2005 for the treatment of diabetes. PRIALT ® (ziconotide), a recently approved drug for pain relief, is a synthetic version of the toxin from a South Pacific marine snail.

The ocean presents a particularly rich habitat for potential new medicines. Marine biotechnologists have discovered organisms containing compounds that could heal wounds, destroy tumours, prevent inflammation, relieve pain and kill microorganisms. Shells from marine crustaceans, such as shrimp and crabs, are made of chitin, a carbohydrate that is proving to be an effective drug-delivery vehicle.

Proteins

Some diseases are caused when defective genes don't produce the proteins (or enough of the proteins) the body requires. Today we are using recombinant DNA and cell culture to produce the missing proteins. Replacement protein therapies include

— factor VIII-a protein involved in the blood-clotting process, lacked by some hemophiliacs.
— insulin-a protein hormone that regulates blood glucose levels. Diabetes results from an inadequate supply of insulin.

Gene Therapy

Gene therapy is a promising technology that uses genes, or related molecules such as RNA, to treat diseases. For example, rather than giving daily injections of missing proteins, physicians could supply the patient's body with an accurate instruction manual-a nondefective gene-correcting the genetic defect so the body itself makes the proteins. Other genetic diseases could be treated by using small pieces of RNA to block mutated genes.

Only certain genetic diseases are amenable to correction via replacement gene therapy. These are diseases caused by the lack of a protein, such as hemophilia and severe combined immunode deficiency disease (SCID), commonly known as the "bubble boy disease." Some children with SCID are being treated with gene therapy and enjoying relatively normal lives. Hereditary disorders that can be traced to the production of a defective protein, such as Huntington's disease, are best treated with RNA that interferes with protein production.

Medical researchers have also discovered that gene therapy can treat diseases other than hereditary genetic disorders. They have used briefly introduced genes, or transient gene therapy, as therapeutics for a variety of cancers, autoimmune disease, chronic heart failure, disorders of the nervous system and AIDS. In late 2003, China licensed for marketing the first commercial gene therapy product, Gendicine, which delivers the P53 tumour suppressor gene. The product treats squamous cell carcinoma of the head and neck, a particularly lethal form of cancer.

Cell Transplants

Approximately 10 people die each day waiting for organs to become available for transplantation. To circumvent this problem, scientists are investigating ways to use cell culture to increase the number of patients who might benefit from one organ donor. Liver cells grown in culture and implanted into patients kept them alive until a liver became available.

In one study of patients with type 1 diabetes, researchers implanted insulin-producing cells from organ donors into the subjects' livers. Eighty percent of the patients required no insulin injections one year after receiving pancreatic cells; after two years, 71 percent had no need for insulin injections. In another study, skeletal muscle cells from the subject repaired damage to cardiac muscle caused by a heart attack.

Expensive drugs for suppressing the immune response must be given if the transplanted cells are from someone other than the patient. Researchers are devising new ways to keep the immune system from attacking the transplanted cells. One method being used is cell encapsulation, which allows cells to secrete hormones or provide a specific metabolic function without being recognised by the immune system. As such, they can be implanted without rejection. Other researchers are genetically engineering cells to express a naturally occurring protein that disables immune system cells that bind to it. Other conditions that could potentially be treated with cell transplants are cirrhosis, epilepsy and Parkinson's Disease.

Immune System

Like the armed forces that defend countries, the immune system is made up of different branches, each containing different types of "soldiers" that interact with each in complex, multifaceted ways. For example, the cytokine branch, which stimulates other immune system branches, includes the interleukins, interferons and colony-stimulating factors all of which are proteins. Because of biotechnology, these proteins can now be produced in sufficient quantities to be marketed as therapeutics.

Small doses of interleukin-2 have been effective in treating various cancers and AIDS, while interleukin-12 has shown promise in treating infectious diseases such as malaria and tuberculosis. Researchers can also increase the number of a specific type of cell, with a highly specific function, from the cellular branch of the immune system. Under certain conditions, the immune system may not produce enough of the cell type a patient needs. Cell culture and natural growth factors that stimulate cell division allow researchers to provide or help the body create the needed cell type.

Cancer vaccines that help the immune system find and kill tumours have also shown therapeutic potential. Unlike other vaccines, cancer vaccines are given after the patient has contracted the disease, so they are not preventative. They work by intensifying the reactions between the immune system and tumour. Despite many years of research, cancer vaccines have not yet emerged as a viable strategy to fight cancer. Nonetheless, researchers are optimistic that this kind of approach to battling cancer would be a major improvement over the therapies used today.

Suppressing the Immune System

In organ-transplant rejections and autoimmune diseases, suppressing our immune system is in our best interest. Currently we are using monoclonal antibodies to suppress, very selectively, the type of cell in the immune system responsible for organ-transplant rejection and autoimmune diseases, such as rheumatoid arthritis and multiple sclerosis.

Patients given a biotechnology-based therapeutic often show significantly less transplant rejection than those given cyclosporin, a medicine that suppresses all immune function and leaves organ-transplant patients vulnerable to infection. Inflammation, another potentially destructive immune system response, can cause diseases characterised by chronic inflammation, such as ulcerative colitis. Two cytokines, interleukin-1 and tumour necrosis factor, stimulate the inflammatory response, so a number of biotechnology companies are investigating therapeutic compounds that block the actions or decrease production of these cytokines.

Xenotransplantation

Organ transplantation provides an especially effective, cost-efficient treatment for severe, lifethreatening diseases of the heart, kidney and other organs. According to the United Network of Organ Sharing (UNOS), in the United States more than 87,000 people are on organ waiting lists. Organs and cells from other species-pigs and other animals-may be promising sources of donor organs and therapeutic cells. This concept is called xenotransplantation. The most significant obstacle to xenotransplantation is the immune system's self-protective response. When nonhuman tissue is introduced into the body, the body cuts off blood flow to the donated organ. The most promising method for overcoming this rejection may be various types of genetic modification. One approach deletes the pig gene for the enzyme that is the main cause of rejection; another adds human genetic material to disguise the pig cells as human cells.

The potential spread of infectious disease from other species to humans through xenotransplantation needs close attention. However, a 1999 study of 160 people who had received pig cells as part of treatments showed no signs of ill health related to this exposure. In addition, scientists have succeeded at deleting the gene that triggers immune activity from a type of pig that cannot be infected with the virus that causes the most concern.

Biopolymers

Nature has also provided us with biological molecules that can serve as useful medical devices or provide novel methods for drug delivery. Because they are more compatible with our tissues and our bodies absorb them when their job is done, they are superior to most man-made medical devices or delivery mechanisms. For example, hyaluronate, a carbohydrate produced by a number of organisms, is an elastic, water-soluble biomolecule that is being used to prevent postsurgical scarring in cataract surgery, alleviate pain and improve joint mobility in patients with osteoarthritis and inhibit adherence of platelets and cells to medical devices, such as stents and catheters.

A gel made of a polymer found in the matrix connecting our cells promotes healing in burn victims. Gauze-like mats made of long threads of fibrinogen, the protein that triggers blood clotting, can be used to stop bleeding in emergency situations. Adhesive proteins from living organisms are replacing sutures and staples for closing wounds. They set quickly, produce strong bonds and are absorbed.

Regenerative Medicine

Biotechnology permits the use of the human body's natural capacity to repair and maintain itself. The body's toolbox for self-repair and maintenance includes many different proteins and various populations of stem cells that have the capacity to cure diseases, repair injuries and reverse age-related wear and tear.

Tissue Engineering

Tissue engineering combines advances in cell biology and materials science, allowing us to create semi-synthetic tissues and organs in the lab. These tissues consist of biocompatible scaffolding material, which eventually degrades and is absorbed, plus living cells grown using cell culture techniques. Ultimately the goal is to create whole organs consisting of different tissue types to replace diseased or injured organs.

The most basic forms of tissue engineering use natural biological materials, such as collagen, for scaffolding. For example, two-layer skin is made by infiltrating a collagen gel with connective tissue cells, then creating the outer skin with a layer of tougher protective cells. In other methods, rigid scaffolding, made of a synthetic polymer, is shaped and then placed in the body where new tissue is needed. Other synthetic polymers, made from natural compounds, create flexible scaffolding more appropriate for soft-tissue structures, like blood vessels and bladders.

When the scaffolding is placed in the body, adjacent cells invade it. At other times, the biodegradable implant is spiked with cells grown in the laboratory prior to implantation. Simple tissues, such as skin and cartilage, were the first to be engineered successfully. Recently, however, physicians have achieved remarkable results with a biohybrid kidney that maintains patients with acute renal failure until the injured kidney repairs itself.

A group of patients with only a 10 to 20 percent probability of survival regained normal kidney function and left the hospital in good health because the hybrid kidney prevented the events that typically follow kidney failure: infection, sepsis and multi-organ failure. The hybrid kidney is made of hollow tubes seeded with kidney stem cells that proliferate until they line the tube's inner wall. These cells develop into the type of kidney cell that releases hormones and is involved with filtration and transportation. In addition to carrying out these expected metabolic functions, the cells in the hybrid kidney also responded to signals produced by the patient's other organs and tissues.

The human body produces an array of small proteins known as growth factors that promote cell growth, stimulate cell division and, in some cases, guide cell differentiation. These natural regenerative proteins can be used to help wounds heal, regenerate injured tissue and advance the development of tissue engineering described in earlier sections.

As proteins, they are prime candidates for large-scale production by transgenic organisms, which would enable their use as therapeutic agents. Some of the most common growth factors are epidermal growth factor, which stimulates skin cell division and could be used to encourage wound healing; erythropoietin, which stimulates the formation of red blood cells and was one of the first biotechnology products; fibroblast growth factor, which stimulates cell growth and has been effective in healing burns, ulcers and bone and growing new blood vessels in patients with blocked coronary arteries; transforming growth factor-beta, which helps fetal cells differentiate into different tissue types and triggers the formation of new tissue in adults; and nerve growth factors, which encourage nerve cells to grow, repair damage and could be used in patients with head and spinal cord injuries or degenerative diseases such as Alzheimer's Disease.

Conventional Vaccines

Vaccines help the body recognise and fight infectious diseases. Conventional vaccines use weakened or killed forms of a virus or bacteria to stimulate the immune system to create the antibodies that will provide resistance to the disease. Usually only one or a few proteins on the surface of the bacteria or virus, called antigens, trigger the production of antibodies. Biotechnology is helping us improve existing vaccines and create new vaccines against infectious agents, such as the viruses that cause cervical cancer and genital herpes.

Most of the new vaccines consist only of the antigen, not the actual microbe. The vaccine is made by inserting the gene that produces the antigen into a manufacturing cell, such as yeast. During the manufacturing process, which is similar to brewing beer, each yeast cell makes a perfect copy of itself and the antigen gene. The antigen is later purified. By isolating antigens and producing them in the laboratory, it is possible to make vaccines that cannot transmit the virus or bacterium itself.

This method also increases the amount of vaccine that can be manufactured because biotechnology vaccines can be made without using live animals. Using these techniques of biotechnology, scientists have developed antigen-only vaccines against life-threatening diseases such as hepatitis B and meningitis. Recently researchers have discovered that injecting small pieces of DNA from microbes is sufficient for triggering antibody production. Such DNA vaccines could provide immunisation against microbes for which we currently have no vaccines. DNA vaccines against HIV, malaria and the influenza virus are currently in clinical trials.

Biotechnology is also broadening the vaccine concept beyond protection against infectious organisms. Various researchers are developing vaccines against diseases such as diabetes, chronic inflammatory disease, Alzheimer's Disease and cancer.

Vaccine Delivery Systems

Whether the vaccine is a live virus, coat protein or a piece of DNA, vaccine production requires elaborate and costly facilities and procedures. And then there's the issue of injections, which can sometimes be painful and which many patients dislike. Industrial and academic researchers are using biotechnology to circumvent both of these problems with edible vaccines manufactured by plants and animals.

Genetically modified goats have produced a possible malaria vaccine in their milk. Academic researchers have obtained positive results using human volunteers who consumed hepatitis vaccines in bananas, and E. coli and cholera vaccines in potatoes. In addition, because these vaccines are genetically incorporated into food plants and need no refrigeration, sterilisation equipment or needles, they may prove particularly useful in developing countries. Researchers are also developing skin patch vaccines for tetanus, anthrax, influenza and E. coli.

Preparation of Peptide Libraries

Optimisation of the peptide sequences over the past 17 years has involved the synthesis and screening of thousands of analogs of the original biologically active sequences. Although thousands of analogs have been prepared and tested, they represent only a small fraction of the possible pentapeptides (205 for the L-amino acids alone). Existing methods for the synthesis and screening of many peptides are severely limited in their ability to generate and screen such numbers (i.e., millions) and/or in their ability to generate unmodified free peptides in quantities capable of interacting in solution at concentrations appropriate for relevant in vitro assays and Pinilla and colleagues have developed synthetic peptide combinatorial libraries (SPCLs) composed of mixtures of free peptides that in total exceed 50 million hexapeptides and in quantities that can be used directly in virtually all existing assay systems. Thus, in the example presented here, a library composed of 52,128,400 hexapeptides along with an iterative selection process was used to confirm the utility of the SPCL approach for the identification of active sequences in existing radio-receptor assays.

Methods of Preparation

Preparation of Synthetic Peptide Combinatorial Libraries

An SPCL consisting of six-residue peptide sequences having free N-terminals and amidated C-terminals was synthesised in which the first two amino acids in each peptide were individually and specifically defined, whereas the last fouramino acids consisted of equimolar mixtures of 19 of the 20 natural L-amino acids. (Cysteine was omitted from this library.) This synthesis generated 400 different peptide mixtures, each represented by the formula O1O2XXXX-NH2 [O1O2=AA, AC, AD, AE, etc., through YV, YW, YY at positions O1 and O2; each X represents an equimolar mixture of the 19 amino acids] and containing 130,321 combinations, This library contains 400x130,321=52,128,400 hexapeptides.

The SPCL was assembled using the solid-phase approach on methylbenzhydrylamine (MBHA) polystyrene resin in combination with simultaneous multiple peptide synthesis using t-Boc protected amino acids. The XXXX-resin was prepared using a process of division, coupling, and recombination (DCR) of individual resins, which ensures the equimolarity of each peptide within the XXXX-resin. For this procedure, 19 equally weighed portions of resin (and, therefore, equal numbers of milliequivalents) were placed into porous polypropylene packets and then coupled to each of the protected N-a-t-Boc amino acids. Completion of coupling was determined by Kaiser's ninhydrin test. The resins were combined and thoroughly mixed. The resulting mixture (X-resin) was then divided into 19 equal portions, the N-a-t-Boc protecting groups were removed, and trifluoroacetic acid salts were neutralised.

Each individual portion was then coupled to completion using one of the 19 different activated amino acids to generate 361 dipeptide resin combinations (XX-resin). The DCR process was repeated twice more to yield a XXXX-resin, representing an equimolar mixture of 130,321 tetramers. This XXXX-resin was then divided into 400 equal portions, and the two defined positions, O1, and O2 were coupled using the solid-phase multiple synthesis method.

Amino acid analysis confirmed the expected equimolarity (±10 percent). Following deprotection and cleavage from the resins, each of the 400 peptide mixtures was extracted with water to yield a final peptide concentration of 1 to 3 mg/mL, which ensures that there is a sufficient concentration of each individual peptide within a mixture for use in standard in vitro assays. At 1.0 mg/mL, each of the 130,321 peptides within each peptide mixture is present at a concentration of approximately 10.3 nM. Mixture concentrations as high as 5.0 mg/mL can be utilised readily.

Radioreceptor Assay

Particulate membranes were prepared using a modification of the method described by Pasternak and colleagues. Rat brains frozen in liquid nitrogen were obtained from Rockland,

Inc. The brains were defrosted, the cerebella were removed, and the remaining tissue was weighed. Each brain was individually homogenized in 40 mL Tris-HCI buffer (50 mM, pH 7.4, 4 °C) and centrifuged (16,000 rpm) for 10 minutes.

The pellets were resuspended in fresh Tris-HCI buffer and incubated at 37 °C for 40 minutes. Following incubation, the suspensions were centrifuged as before, the resulting pellets were resuspended in 100 volumes of Tris-HCI buffer, and the suspensions were combined. Membrane suspensions were prepared and used in the same day. Protein content of the crude homogenates ranged from 0.15 to 0.2 mg/mL as determined using the method described by Bradford.

Binding assays were carried out in polypropylene tubes. Each tube contained 0.5 mL of membrane suspension, 8 nM [3H]-DAGO (specific activity 36 Ci/mmol 160,000 cpm), 0.08 mg/mL peptide mixture, and Tris-HCI buffer in a total volume of 0.65 mL. Assay tubes were incubated for 60 minutes at 25 °C. The reaction was terminated by filtration through GF-B filters. The filters were subsequently washed with 6 mL Tris-HCI buffer, 4 °C. Bound radioactivity was counted on an LKB Beta-plate Liquid Scintillation Counter and expressed in counts per minute (cpm).

To determine interassay and intra-assay variation, standard curves in which [3H]-DAGO was incubated with a range of concentrations of unlabelled DAGO (0.13 to 3,900 nM) were included on each plate of each assay (using a 96-well format). Competitive inhibition assays were performed as above using serial dilutions of the peptide mixtures. IC50 (the concentration necessary to inhibit 50 percent of [3H]-DAGO binding) values were then calculated using the software GRAPHPAD (ISI, San Diego) and were found to be consistent in three determinations.

Preparation of Large Peptide Libraries

Most biological processes are controlled and modulated by intermolecular interactions. These interactions can occur with a change in the covalent structure of one or more of the participants (e.g., an enzyme substrate interaction) or with no change in covalent structure (e.g., an antibody antigen interaction). In the latter case, in general, the three-dimensional structures of both the ligand and the acceptor molecule(s) change as a consequence of the interaction, which in turn can lead to a change in the physical and chemical properties of the acceptor molecule(s) in a way that modulates cellular structure and function. Thus, these interactions are critical requirements for the conformational, dynamic, and stereoelectronic changes that are central to the "chemistry of life" in biological systems.

In this regard, peptides and proteins and their post translationally modified derivatives constitute the most widely used "molecules of life" and can serve many functional roles (e.g., as antibodies, enzymes, growth factors, immunomodulators, hormones, neurotransmitters, and receptors) and the many other functions that are critical to cellular function and to intercellular communication in complex living systems. It is no accident that nature uses proteins as the major functional molecules in living systems, which undoubtedly is related to the enormous physical and chemical diversity that is possible for these compounds.

For example, if one utilises only the 20 standard amino acid residues found in proteins and examines the number of distinct chemical species available, millions of molecules already are possible at the pentapeptide stage (3.2x106); that number becomes 1.28x109 at the heptapeptide stage. Thus, for even a small protein of 100 amino acid residues, there are an astronomical number of possibilities. It is not clear how many of these possibilities nature has explored, but it is clear that only a small fraction of those possible are used.

There is a great opportunity in the possibility for utilising enormous chemical diversity to obtain a better understanding of how nature works and for the discovery of novel lead molecules that can serve as starting points for the development of agonist or antagonist drugs with specific biological effects. It also is a challenge to develop a simple method to prepare such large and diverse chemical libraries in a cost-effective manner that will allow examination of the binding properties of a particular species in the library and at the same time have each chemical species present in sufficient quantities for structure determination.

The authors recently proposed and developed a methodology for preparing large, statistically diverse peptide libraries (104 to 108 individual species) in a short time and for examining their ligand-binding activities with acceptor macromolecules such as antibodies and enzymes.

Results and Discussion

The creation of a large peptide library creates several problems. The most important is that of scale. The basic question posed was how much of each peptide is needed so that, on the one hand, sufficient concentrations are available to screen for binding and, on the other hand, sufficient amounts are available for structure determination. After examining several approaches, the authors devised a method that maximises chances for success with the minimum amount of peptide. This method exploits the idea of one peptide for one bead.

The synthetic methodology used is the Merrifield method in which the peptide of interest is synthesised on a solid support. This method has revolutionised peptide chemistry (and synthetic chemistry in general) in that it greatly simplifies the multistep synthetic processes of preparing a peptide. The growing peptide chain is assembled on a resin bead, and as a consequence, the solvents and reagents required for the synthesis can be removed by the simple expedient of washing. This methodology provides two other previously unexploited advantages. First, depending on the substitution level and size of the bead (in standard Merrifield syntheses, the substitution level is generally 0.2 to 1.0 mmol/g resin, and the bead size is generally from 50 to 200 microns), a high local concentration of peptide can be present on each bead.

Calculations suggest that the local concentration of peptide on a single bead is in the millimolar to micromolar range and that the amount of peptide present would be from 50 to 300 pmol, more than sufficient to determine the sequence, because modern sequencers can sequence in the 2 to 5 pmol range. Second, a bead provides a unique surface (like a cell) for interaction of the ligand present on the surface of the bead with a macromolecule in the surrounding medium. Such a surface should be excellent for large-scale screening in a minimum volume but with a large surface area.

The next question posed was, given the above considerations, how to prepare a large, chemically diverse peptide mixture in which each peptide in the mixture would be localised to a single resin bead and each bead would possess a single peptide and in which each peptide in the library would be present in approximately the same concentration. The answer to the latter part of the question is to have each bead in the mixture approximately the same size and substituted to the same extent. To ensure that each bead has a unique peptide and only that peptide, it is necessary that each bead be exposed to only a single coupling reaction at a time and that the reaction be driven to completion.

The approach is similar to that presented by Furka and colleagues, who, however, did not recognise the potential of having a unique peptide sequence on every bead. Finally, for diversity, one must turn to statistics. For example, if the 20 standard amino acids are used for the construction of a library, by dividing the resin into 20 equal parts, adding each amino acid to only one of these parts, then thoroughly mixing all the parts, by dividing into 20 equal parts again, adding each amino acid to only one of these parts, and so forth, one can rapidly develop a library of millions of peptides on millions of beads. Because a gram of standard-size solidphase resin contains about 1 million 100-micron beads, very large libraries are feasible using Merrifield solid-phase methodology.

It is important to recognise two important synthetic issues in the construction of such a large, diverse peptide library. First, different amino acid residues have very different chemical reactivities. For example, activate -Fmocalanine is much more reactive than -Fmoc-isoleucine. Second, and even more important, when a large peptide library is constructed, the peptide products become very diverse chemically and hence differ greatly in their reactivity (nucleophilicity). Therefore, every reaction must be driven to completion. As a practical matter, we found that using a threefold to fourfold excess of the amino acid, a 1- to 2-hour reaction time in a minimum volume, and optimised Merrifield synthetic procedures generally leads to completion of the reaction even for difficult sequences such as Val to Val-peptide coupling.

To check on the fidelity of the methodology for producing single peptide moieties on a bead, we examined a large number of single resin beads chosen both randomly and from our binding assay for their structure and for the synthetic fidelity of the synthetic peptide on the bead using a Pulsed Liquid Automatic Peptide Sequencer to determine the sequence and quantitate the amount of peptide on a single bead and then used modern preview analysis to determine the fidelity of the peptide on a single bead. These studies showed that each bead contains between 50 and 300 pmols of peptide as predicted, and preview analysis demonstrated that the peptides on each bead were homogeneous, with the percentage of a single peptide species being between97 to 99.9 percent in a pentapeptide library of more than 2 million peptides.

Next, these libraries were utilised to screen for binding to acceptor macromolecules. For this purpose, the authors prepared the libraries to leave the peptide attached to the bead, but with all the protecting groups (amino terminal and side-chain moieties) removed. Thus, it was necessary to develop a synthetic strategy so that all side-chain protecting groups could be removed following construction of the peptide library while the peptide remained on the resin and, in addition, to ensure that the peptide on the surface of the bead was accessible for binding to the macromolecular acceptor by construction of a spacer of suitable length that is "biocompatible." One approach is to use polyamide resins that have been modified with a spacer arm that consisted of a -alanine, an -amino caproic acid moiety, and an ethylenediamine moiety attached to the polyamide polymer.

In this strategy, Fmoc protection is used for -amino groups, and tert- butyloxycarbonyl, tert-butyl esters, and tert-butyl ether type side-chain protections are used (-Boc protection in conjunction with Fmoc-based side-chain protecting groups also can be used). The -Fmoc groups were removed with piperidine, and following construction of the peptide library, the side-chain protecting groups were removed by 90 percent trifluoroacetic acid in N,N-dimethylformamide (v/v) containing 1 percent anisole and 0.9 percent ethanedithiol.

The peptide-resin beads were then neutralised with 10 percent diisopropylethylamine in N,N-dimethylformamide and thoroughly washed with several solvents (including water) before use in screening. Utilising this methodology, we obtained a number of peptide libraries suitable for rapid screening of the type described below. To screen a library composed of millions of different chemical species requires careful consideration. Among the most common problems for consideration are the signal-to-noise (background signal) ratio, nonspecific chemical reactions, unexpected chemical reactions, and the usual problems of sensitivity and specificity.

To overcome these problems, the authors developed a rapid screening method that utilises an enzyme-linked immunoassay method in which the acceptor molecule (e.g., a monoclonal antibody) is coupled to the enzyme alkaline phosphatase, which can then catalyse a reaction in which those beads that interact with the monoclonal antibody become coloured as a result of the enzyme-catalysed reaction. These beads can be easily distinguished from those that do not react because they are colourless. The reacting beads (those that are coloured) can be removed easily from the incubation medium by a micromanipulator under a low-power dissecting microscope as previously discussed.

The coloured beads are then washed, the bound monoclonal antibodyenzyme complex removed by treatment with denaturing reagents that can solubilise proteins (e.g., 6M guanidine hydrochloride), and the single bead subjected to sequence analysis. In this way, unique new structures can be discovered that bind with high affinity (micromolar to nanomolar) to acceptor molecules. Ordinarily, we separately synthesise the binding peptides discovered by these procedures and examine their binding to the acceptor molecules by standard radioreceptor binding assays. Generally, there is a good correspondence between the binding seen on the bead and that obtained in the solution binding experiments.

Computer Design of Bioactive Compounds

The computer design of bioactive molecules is now a reality. The design is based on the observed or postulated threedimensional (3-D) properties of the ligand as bound to the target macromolecule. Single crystal x-ray crystallography of the ligand macromolecule complex can supply the necessary information. However, an x-ray structure may not be available, at least at the beginning stages of a medicinal chemistry investigation.

As an alternative, ligand structure-activity relationships are a sensitive probe of the shape and chemical properties of the binding site on a macromolecule of unknown 3-D structure. This structure-activity relationship can be used to map the binding site from the inside out instead of from the outside in as one would do with protein crystallography.The resulting pharmacophore maps are 3-D summaries of the structure-activity relationships on which they are based. Beyond this, they provide the necessary information for computer techniques that design new compounds to meet the 3-D criteria and for those that forecast the potency of compounds suggested by people or computer. Thus, there are three aspects of the structure-activity-based molecular design strategy: pharmacophore mapping, 3-D searching and molecular design, and 3-D quantitative structure-activity relationships. Each of these pieces forms a part of the strategy to convert two-dimensional (2-D) structure-activity information into a novel bioactive molecule by consideration of the 3-D properties of the molecules.

Pharmacophore Mapping

The goal of pharmacophore mapping is to establish the bioactive conformations of the ligands and how to superimpose these conformations. For pharmacophoremapping, one needs structure-activity relationships of structurally diverse and conformationally informative molecules. From this information, one first proposes a pharmacophore, that is, the chemical nature of the groups required for bioactivity and the geometric relationships between them. The structureactivity relationships of the ligands establish the required groups, answering the question, Activity is destroyed by removal of what group? Conformationally constrained compounds that are also active may help establish the bioactive conformation of all the compounds. The molecules are superimposed, in their proposed bioactive conformations, over the atoms of the pharmacophore or their projected binding points on the macromolecule. The union of the volumes occupied by the active compounds as superimposed suggests the regions in space that can be occupied by any newly designed active ligand. In addition, new regions in space occupied by compounds that meet the pharmacophore requirements but are inactive define "forbidden regions" that, if occupied, destroy activity.

Application to D1 Agonists

Martin and colleagues' work started with the observation that the phenyl group of SKF 38393 increases the affinity for the D1 dopaminergic receptor by 100X compared with II. The goal was to find potent D1 agonists that have little D2 activity. Distance geometry generation of conformations and energy minimisation revealed that the axial and equatorial conformations are approximately equal in energy and are the lowest found. To establish which is the bioactive conformation, we synthesised several compounds that placed an added phenyl in an axial or equatorial position. Only those with the phenyl in the equatorial position show the phenyl boost. Thus, the bioactive conformation of I is equatorial.

3-D Databases in Molecular Modelling

To organise the pharmacophore modelling of many compounds by the small molecule group at Abbott Laboratories, Martin and colleagues developed a 3-D database system based on the

Daylight Chemical Information System. The coordinates and charges as well as literature and project biological properties are stored. In addition, the compounds can be searched in the database by substructure. An advantage to using a chemical information database is that all sets of coordinates of a compound are together regardless of their original source.

Abbott Laboratories' small-molecule molecular graphics program reads and writes directly to these 3-D databases. This permits the graphics program to be used to display the bioactive conformation without the user's knowing its dataset name, to display all stored conformations of a molecule, or to display all members of a group used to derive a pharmacophore or 3DQSAR model. Because the bioactivity associated with each bioactive conformation is identified, the database also can be asked whether the same conformation is responsible for different bioactivities.

3-D Substructure Searching

Gund and colleagues had suggested 3-D searching much earlier but had created no 3-D database. Esaki followed this work with another prototype system. Simultaneously with the author and colleagues' work, Jakes and Willett, Jakes and coworkers, Brint and Willett, DesJarlais and colleagues, Sheridan and Venkataraghavan, Lewis and Dean, Bartlett and coworkers, and Sheridan and colleagues were addressing the same problem from different viewpoints. The field has grown so much that there are now six 3-D database-searching systems available to researchers other than that of the original developer. Dozens of laboratories around the world are doing research on the topic. The impetus for this work is the increasing availability both of computer hardware for 3-D molecular modelling and of 3-D protein structures.

Description

The aim of 3-D substructure searching is to find or design molecules that meet 3-D criteria by examining the 3-D structures of hundreds or thousands of molecules. In contrast to pharmacophore mapping, a 3-D search needs no existing structure-activity relationships. However, the more information used, the more likely the correct search question will be posed.

There are three main types of searches. Geometric search questions deal with the intramolecular relationships between geometric objects (points, lines, and planes) calculated from a structure. They are independent of the enantiomer of the compound and its orientation in space. Similarity searching asks how similar a database molecule is in 3-D properties to the reference molecule. In contrast, steric searches ask whether a candidate structure can fit into a particular volume. The result of a steric search is different for enantiomers of a molecule. The allowed orientations of the molecule in the target space are determined by some steric searching programs or specified by the user in others.

Uses of 3-D Searching

3-D searching has three distinct applications in medicinal chemistry. First, 3-D searches may recognise known compounds that meet 3-D criteria (new bioactivities in old molecules). Second,

3-D searches may test a proposed pharmacophore. Only if the search identifies all active molecules is the pharmacophore correct. Third, 3-D searching may help design new compounds that mimic one or another of the low-energy conformations of an active molecule. The synthesis and testing of such a set of compounds may identify which is the bioactive conformation. Note that 3-D searching may help design new compounds that mimic the bioactive conformation of a molecule. These may show improved features such as improved bioavailability, selectivity, ease of synthesis, or patentability.

Sources of 3-D Structures

Of course, one needs 3-D structures to search. In our original work, the only coordinates available were in databases of modelled compounds, Somewhat later the CONnectivity to COoRDinates (CONCORD) program, which generates a 3-D structure of a molecule in a few seconds, became available.' We used CONCORD to build 3-D databases of our corporate and commercially available compounds. Sometimes it would serve no use for coordinates to be in a database; thus, files of 3-D structures also can be searched with ALADDIN. Recently, we added the option to generate the structure with CONCORD as part of the 3-D searching process.

Design of Novel D1 Agonists

ALADDIN was used to search Abbott's small-molecule modelling group's database of compounds modelled for various projects to find existing compounds that might have dopaminergic activity. This search identified V as well as several other compounds that were later shown to be active. Molecular graphics of V showed where to add the phenyl group to impart D1 selectivity, compound VI.

Traditional medicinal chemistry of this new lead led to a more potent analog, VII. This compound is the most potent and selective D1 dopaminergic agonist known. Notice that the pharmacophore N and meta OH groups are in roughly the same geometric relationship in these active dopaminergic compounds. The pendant phenyl group occupies slightly different regions in space in the different compounds. This suggested that the phenyl might be replaced with other bulky groups. Accordingly, the adamantyl analog VIII was synthesised. It is also a potent agonist. Thus, we successfully applied the strategy of finding weakly active compounds with a 3-D search and using molecular graphics and traditional medicinal chemistry to suggest more potent and selective analogs.

Design Novel Compounds With 3-D Searching

3-D searching also can design novel compounds that match a pharmacophore. Table 2 shows the strategy. The core of this strategy is to identify molecules that match the pharmacophore in geometric relationships but not atom types, The appropriate atoms are then mutated into those required for the pharmacophore. Thus, the search covers a database of molecules included for their geometric properties only. Notice that we use CONCORD to generate the 3-D structures of the designed molecules.

To implement the strategy, we invented a language (MODify SMIles [MODSMI]) that is used to tell the computer how to change the structure of the database molecule into that expected to be active. This MODSMI language transforms the SMILES description of the 2-D structures of the database molecules into the target 2-D structures. The four verbs of MODSMI are "nibble," to remove an atom: "replace," to change one atom into another; "axe," to break a bond or change its bond order; and "join," to make a bond between two atoms. Because the atoms to be transformed into the pharmacophore atoms are identified in the SMILES of the database molecules, the transformations can be applied only to certain atoms. The MODSMI language was used for two purposes in the design of potential dopamine agonists. First, the pharmacophore atoms were added to the appropriate places in the structure. Second, geometrically irrelevant substituents were removed from the structures, and nonpharmacophore heteroatoms were changed into carbons, Thisprevents the computer suggestion of a series of close analogs.

Application of Novel Dopaminergic Agonists

To evaluate this procedure, I tested its ability to design dopaminergic agonists. Compounds IX through XVII are the essential substructures of known dopaminergic agonists in which ail bonds between the N and O are in a ring.

There are three databases:

(1) the Fine Chemicals Directory of 80,000 commercially available compounds, (2) the Pomona College Medicinal Chemistry Project database of 27,000 compounds with measured solvent-water partition coefficients (the 3-D structures in these databases were generated with CONCORD), and (3) the Abbott small-molecule modelling group's database of carefully modelled compounds, 9,000 3-D structures from 3,000 compounds, Compounds XVIII through XXI in figure 9 are examples of the types of compounds suggested.

There is a strong resemblance between the 3-D structures of the two compounds. Does this strategy design the known molecules? Yes, it suggested eight of nine known classes of fused-ring dopaminergics. Does it design new molecules? Yes, it designed 75 novel series compounds in which all atoms between the O and N of the pharmacophore are in a ring (a total of >300 molecules). It also designed more than 100 other compounds with one rotatable bond in the path for a total of 508 molecules.

Evaluation of the Strategy by the Design of Morphine Mimics

Similar strategies can be used to design mimics of peptides in their bioactive conformations. If one does not know the bioactive conformation, one can use these methods to design mimics of the various low-energy conformations. Similarly, one can use 3-D searching to design compounds that probe the direction of binding of heteroatoms to a macromolecule.

I decided to test the strategy by using the bioactive conformation of enkephalin for the search criteria and asked whether morphine is designed. To not bias the results with structures we had modelled or tested at Abbott, we searched the Fine Chemicals Directory for 3-D templates and transformed them as had been done in the dopaminergic example. The search criteria included an unsubstituted aromatic atom to which the required OH would be added. Thus, morphine would not meet the search criteria.

Quantitative Forecast of Potency of Suggested Molecules

It is not sufficient to design novel compounds. These compounds also must be potent. Thus, the third aspect of the computer design of bioactive molecules involves the understanding of the 3-D quantitative structure-activity relationships, We have successfully used a special implementation of comparative molecular field analysis (CoMFA) for this purpose.

Description of CoMFA

For CoMFA one needs to have a biological potency measured for at least 15 molecules, In addition, one needs the superposition rule and bioactive conformations derived from pharmacophore mapping. A CoMFA starts with calculating fields around each molecule at intersections of a 2Å lattice. The fields are calculated using traditional potential energy equations. Typically, energies are calculated for at least 1,000 points. In the analysis, high positive steric energies are truncated to a more modest value (4 to 25 kcal/mol, for example). Lattice locations with low standard deviations are discarded from the calculations. The relationship between the remaining fields and potency is evaluated using partial least squares, a variant of principal components. Because there are more energy values per compound than compounds, crossvalidation is an essential aspect of the method. In cross-validation, the potency of each compound is forecast from a model from which it had been deleted.

The result of a CoMFA analysis is an equation that describes the contribution of each lattice energy value to potency. Such equations are used for forecasting the potency of additional compounds, For ease of understanding, one displays contours of the coefficients such as those shown in figure 12.

Evaluation of CoMFA

The Abbott implementation of CoMFA (Martin et al. 1992) differs from that of Cramer and colleagues in that the molecular fields are calculated using the program GRID.

Martin and colleagues (1992) showed that CoMFA performs as expected. First, CoMFA fits and forecasts physical properties such as pKa's and linear free energy sterlc constants. Also, It provides a good fit for biological data that previously had been shown to be correlated with octanol-water IogP. For these three situations, we used different properties of the probe atoms. For pKa's, a positively charged probe with no hydrogen bonding character was used: for steric effects, a neutral probe with no hydrogen bonding character was used: and for IogP, a neutral probe that is both a hydrogen-bond donor and an acceptor was used.

3-D Searching and 3-DQSAR

We added an option to ALADDIN so that it now reads a set of CoMFA coefficients, a coordinate set that was part of the CoMFA, and the superposition rule (Y.C. Martin and E.B. Danaher, unpublished data). ALADDIN orients the designed molecule (and its enantiomer if requested) and marks atoms of the molecule that hit negative CoMFA coefficients. These atoms can be removed with the MODSMI routines.

As noted above, ALADDIN designed 508 compounds that match the D2 pharmacophore. Of these, 110 did not hit negative D1 steric contours. Thus, only 22 percent of the compounds designed to match a pharmacophore were forecast to be active. MODSMI was used on the remaining 398 compounds to remove the atoms that hit a negative D1 CoMFA steric contour. Of these redesigned compounds, 132 did not hit negative contours, and 26 of these were not in the first 110. Thus, ALADDIN designed 136 compounds that fit into the D1 steric contours.

The characteristics of the series of compounds tested will determine the information gained from a CoMFA analysis. Does the computer design a better set of compounds for CoMFA analysis than do chemists? A series of 20 chemist-designed D2 agonists were composed with a series of the same size selected from those designed by the computer. Shape was described by the steric energies as used in CoMFA. To choose the series of computer-designed compounds, a cluster analysis based on the 25 highest principal components of the steric fields was used. Compared with the chemistdesigned series, the computer-designed series shows a larger variation in steric properties and has less correlation between steric properties. it explores all space explored by the former series. The mean and range of the forecast D1 and D2 dopaminergic receptor-binding affinities for the two series are not different. Thus, multivariate statistical methods based on energy fields provide the tools to choose a good series of molecules for a CoMFA analysis. These methods also reduce a large set of suggested molecules to one that is reasonable to synthesise.

Toward the Design of New Inhibitors

There has been increased interest in the use of databases for the discovery of potential new lead compounds (Sheridan and Venkataraghavan 1987; Sheridan et al. 1989; Martin 1990). An excellent example of this effort is provided by ALADDIN, a computer programme that searches a database of three-dimensional structures for the design of new compounds with interesting biological properties. The author believes it is important to try to use more than one method in combination with a database of crystal structures for the design of new inhibitors. If one candidate is found with more than one method, this would enhance the possibility of its being a good template. This process is a distinct feature of this study. Initially, I focused my work on searches based mainly on shape properties, and thus I chose the following independent methods:

1. Docking techniques
2. CAVEAT analysis
3. QUEST programmes

The Cambridge Crystallographic Database (CCD) version 4.5 of July 1991, which contains 90,296 entries, was used in this work. What follows gives a succinct description of each of the methods used in combination with the CCD.

Docking Techniques

I have used DOCK versions 1.0 and 2.0 by DesJarlais and colleagues. These programmes use spheres to describe the active site of an enzyme, the structure of which is known from, for example, x-ray crystallography. The "negative" image of this receptor site is then used to test out compounds from the CCD. Using a score to rank these molecules docked onto the receptor site, one usually gets a family of compounds that fit well onto the receptor site.

Although many compounds of interest are rigid, this programme has been used for flexible molecules. An example of the use of DOCK forthe design of inhibitors is haloperidol, a compound that inhibits the human immunodeficiency virus 1 protease.

CAVEAT Analysis

The programme CAVEAT makes use of the CCD in a different way. For every molecule in the database, it stores the intramolecular bonds as vectors. This new database of vectors is stored independently from the original one, which contains atomic coordinates, and is then searched for vector matching. The approach is to start with the crystal structure of an inhibitor in complex with an enzyme and then search for new templates based on the spatial arrangements of the bonds of this known ligand. The user is then allowed to choose up to three vectors belonging to this ligand. The natural choice for these vectors are those along the bonds that make important chemical interactions with the target enzyme. It is then possible to search for molecules that could have a similar relative orientation of their bonds.

QUEST Programmes

These programmes supersede the querying codes that belong to older versions of the CCD. In particular, a similarity search and a powerful connectivity search are now an integral part of this package. It is also worth noting that a pharmacophore model for an inhibitor can be built easily using QUEST. The pharmacophore model, which is the set of distances and angles of a substructure that is important for a certain biological activity, can also provide new ideas for new templates.

Systems

There are two systems-papain and thrombin.

Papain

Cysteine proteases have been implicated in various pathological conditions, such as inflammation and malignancy. Papain belongs to the family of cysteine proteases, and it is isolated from the latex of tropical papaya fruit. Cathepsin B also is a cysteine protease found in, for example, human liver.

Mechanistic data gathered for cathepsin B suggest that it shares a common basic enzymatic mechanism with papain (Khouri et al. 1991). Papain, which has been extensively studied, can therefore serve as a template for the design of inhibitors aimed at related cysteine proteases of pharmacological importance such as cathepsins B, H, and L. From the known crystal structure of Bzo- Phe-Ala-CH2CI, an inhibitor, in complex with papain, three vectors were chosen along bonds that make, for example, hydrophobic interactions with papain.

The choice of vectors is important because the basic assumption of this method is that the shape of a compound can be described reliably by vectors along its bonds. This will, in turn, allow choosing other templates that interact with papain and, after some chemical modifications (e.g., introduction of a chloromethylketone group), show inhibitory properties. Using the CAVEAT analysis, I found two main classes of compounds.

The first family of compounds obtained with CAVEAT, panel A, had been suggested earlier by DesJarlais and colleagues in an attempt to find good inhibitors of papain using docking techniques. This is an interesting result because it shows that, by using different methods, families of compounds with similar geometrical features can be identified. The second class of compounds found using CAVEAT, panel B, had also been obtained independently by me with a similarity search available as part of QUEST.

Furthermore, within QUEST it is possible to search the CCD database using a model for the pharmacophore. This application has provided some ideas for new lead compounds, one of which is shown in panel B. This is a very promising candidate, not only because it is similar to the starting compound, but also because it has many hydrogen-bonding donor (acceptor) atoms. We at the Biotechnology Research Institute are in the process of synthesizing new compounds based on this template.

Thrombin

Thrombin is an important enzyme that initiates blood coagulation. Fibrinogen, thrombin's natural substrate, interacts strongly with two sites of thrombin, namely, the active site and the exosite. Because thrombus formation inside the vessels, started by the hydrolysis of fibrinogen, may lead to thromboembolic diseases, many scientists have been searching for new thrombin inhibitors to control blood coagulation. One of the most potent inhibitors of thrombin is hirudin, a 65-residue peptide from the salivary glands of the leech Hirudo medicinalis. A potent thrombin inhibitor based on hirudin's sequence has been synthesized and characterized at the Biotechnology Research Institute.

The high affinity and specificity of hirudin as a thrombin inhibitor are the result of its bivalent binding mode. In other words, in addition to blocking the active site, hirudin interacts with the exosite via its C-terminal undecapeptide fragment. Because the C-terminal hirudin fragment is available to digestion by many enzymes and its intactness is necessary for antithrombotic activity, a search for new analogs of the C-terminal fragment of hirudin, which are resistant to proteolysis, is necessary.

Cyclic peptides may enhance not only the biological activity but also the biological stability. Between residues Phe56 and IIe59 (hirudin's numbering is used), there is space to accommodate extra groups. Through the use of docking programmes, many aromatic compounds were successfully placed in this region. This suggests that aromatic rings in this position are well accepted by thrombin. This fact prompted me to design new inhibitors with an aromatic motif between the two residues mentioned above. The aromatic ring between these two residues was approximately in the same position as the best docked candidate extracted from the CCD. This constraint should allow the peptide to adopt the biologically active conformation even in solution, resulting in an increase of the activity because of the entropic gain during the interaction with thrombin.

Protein Sequence and Structure Databases

For the past several decades knowledge of cellular function has been growing rapidly. This rapid growth was caused by the introduction of many technological advancements in biology, which not only opened up a new field, biotechnology, but also brought an information explosion. To illustrate this growth of bioinformation, consider the basic constituent of all living organisms, a cell. Vast amounts of information have been gathered on various types of cells, their chromosomes, genes, nucleic acid, and protein. Most of this information has been accumulated as published literature, generated by different laboratories around the world. As this information began to flow, it was compiled into various databases that were circulated among only a few individuals. When the size of these databases started to increase, the need for quick archiving and retrieval became critical. This need was filled by the advent of fast computers and disk drives with large storage capacity, which in turn paved the way for the birth of a new field called bioinformatics. This field addresses the issues of access, update, and manipulation of various types of computer-based biological information.

The biological databases contain a wealth of information for understanding the structure and function of cells. The number of databases illustrates the current status of bioinformatics. The database Listing of Molecular Biology Databases (LiMB) contains various databases available in the field of molecular biology. There are more than 3,000 cultured cell lines available in the database maintained by American Type Culture Collection (ATCC). DNA and protein sequences are maintained, respectively, by Genbank and National Biomedical Research Foundation (NBRF). A protein threedimensional (3-D) structural data bank is managed by Brookhaven National Laboratory (BNL). When the sources of these databases are examined, it is clear that each database is managed by a different scientific agency.

An era of biological research is beginning in which scientists must rely on more than one of these databases. A major problem confronting modern research in bioscience is the availability and ease of utilisation of the biological databases. There is a need for either a certain uniformity among these databases, special tools to access the information across different databases, or both. Some earlier attempts in this direction were undertaken in Europe; OWL and SWISS-PROT are the outcomes of this attempt to integrate protein and nucleic acids sequence databases. It should be noted that a few in-house molecular modelling programmes are available to automatically search and extract the sequence and structure information from the Protein Data Bank (PDB). Often these programmes are found to be closely integrated with large onsite graphics or molecular modelling programmes and are not available for public use because of cost and hardware limitations.

Advancements in the fields of protein sequencing and genetic engineering will permit the addition of a large number of protein sequences to the Protein Identification Resource (PIR) sequence database. In addition, many 3-D structures of natural and genetically engineered proteins also will be determined to atomic resolution, Thus, a direct link between the primary sequence database (PIR) and the 3-D structure database (NBRF/PDB) becomes increasingly important in understanding the structure-function relationships of proteins. Prior to the author and colleagues' work these two important databases containing information about the structure and function of protein molecules did not have a direct link. Therefore, the authors created a sequence-structure database called NRL_3D derived from protein entries in PDB and searchable within the PIR environment.

As the number of databases pertaining to a certain scientific area increases, every effort should be made to cross-check and retrieve information. The most significant effort to integrate biological databases started with the establishment of the National Center for Biotechnology Information (NCBI) under the National Library of Medicine at the National Institutes of Health. In July 1990 NCBI announced a new database, Genlnfo Backbone Sequence Database. This new and integrated database includes the MEDLINE records that correspond to protein or nucleic acids sequences. Genlnfo will maximise the use of standard nomenclature and gene names from original sources. It is the first major database to use International Standard Organisation format for data representation, Genlnfo is implemented as a relational database offering a variety of advantages over other database systems. For the past few years, the authors have been interested in integrating databases on protein molecules.

Sequence-Structure Database, NRL_3D

PIR's protein sequence database contains most of the published protein primary sequences. PIR also provides a variety of software tools for protein sequence manipulation, sequence similarity searches, and sequence alignments.

Protein Sequences in PIR

BNL's PDB contains coordinates of 3-D structures of several proteins and other related biomolecules obtained using single crystal x-ray diffraction data. The growth is clearly exponential. In addition to x-ray diffraction data, PDB also contains coordinates obtained from nuclear magnetic resonance, modelling, and neutron diffraction data. A typical PDB entry for a biomolecule contains not only the 3-D atomic coordinates but also information such as sequence, bibliography, quality of the reported data, and secondary structure. However, because PDB uses a rigid, cryptic, and flat-file format for the distribution of these data, the general utility of this vast treasure of information has been restricted to a few scientists.

For example, the primary sequence of the protein is stored under the "SEQRES" record identifier. It may appear simple to construct a new sequence database similar to PIR by extracting the PDB protein sequences from these "SEQRES" records and then performing sequence similarity searches on them. However, this process is not straightforward for the following reasons. In PIR entries, the N-terminal residue is always the first residue and is identified by the number 1. The following residues are numbered contiguously.

In PDB entries, the residue numbers (residue identification scheme) may not be identified by contiguous numbers starting with 1 from the N-terminal residue. in some cases, the residue numbers also contain certain letters. The reasons for following this residue identification scheme in PDB are as follows. The residue identification was assigned according to the previously studied homologous protein. In cases where there is an insertion of amino acids, the sequence numbers of the inserted residues are the same as those of the homologous protein. in addition, an alphabetical designator (e.g., A, B, C) is attached to the sequence numbers of these inserted residues. If there is a deletion of amino acids, the residue numbers before and after the deletion will be the same as that of the homologous proteins. In other words, the residue numbers at the deletion site are not contiguous.

Finally, because of the quality of x-ray data and the nature of the structure refinement, it may not be possible to trace the backbone atoms of some of the residues. Hence, the 3-D coordinates for these residues are not reported in the PDB entry. Thus, using the primary sequence database derived from the "SEQRES" records alone, one cannot extract the 3-D coordinates for a given sequence. In short, when PDB sequences are reformatted, one has to keep track of the identification for each residue given in the "ATOM" record.

In the development of the NRL_3D database, Pattabiraman and colleagues extracted the sequence information from the "ATOM" records, based on the distance between two consecutive atoms. The sequences were then formatted according to PIR sequence database. In addition, the sequence identifications were extracted from the "ATOM" record, and a separate database file was created. NRL_3D database files for the alpha-lytic protein (PDB code is 2alp. In the current setup the NRL_3D database can be used interactively within PIR using the SCAN and MATCH commands. The authors and collaborators also developed a computer programme (PRENRL_3D) in C language that automatically creates NRL_3D database files from PDB protein entries.

Applications of NRL_3D

The authors' laboratory has been interested in the structure-function relationships of phospholipase A2 (PLA2) molecules. PLA2 catalyses specifically the hydrolysis of the ester bond at the C2 position of 3-snphosphoglycerides. PLA2 is a biologically important molecule involved in arthritis and wound healing. In addition, the activities of PLA2 found in snake venoms may be responsible for pharmacological effects such as myotoxicity, anticoagulant properties, and hemolytic effects. PLA2 includes a class of low molecular weight proteins composed of approximately 120 amino acids. In the current version of PIR, 53 primary sequences of PLA2 from different sources have been included. Six crystal structures of PLA2 are available in PDB. This was the first molecule of this class whose structure was determined. Secondary structures such as a-helix and · strand are held together by six disulfide bridges, which are shown as dashed lines. The structure of the PLA2 molecule is rigid because of these disulfide linkages.

Because of the linkage of PIR and PDB via the NRL_3D database, it is now possible to align the sequences of PLA2 of known 3-D structure with those of the sequences of unknown structure. The alignment of the sequences of pig, horse, and a snake venom PLA2 (C. Atrox) with that of bovine pancreas PLA2, whose 3-D structure is known. A star in the aligned sequences denotes that the amino acid is the same as that of the bovine pancreas PLA2. Shown within boxes of solid lines are the stretches of amino acids for which the aligned residue in the bovine PLA2 structure is an a-helix. Similarly, the -helices are represented by boxes with dashed lines. This gives an idea of possible secondary structures for the aligned sequences. Also, in the bovine pancreatic PLA2, the residues that are not solvent accessible are circled. This surface is computed by rolling a spherical "solvent" molecule around the exterior of the protein molecule, maintaining contact with the van der Waals' surface of atoms near the exterior. The locus of the points on the surface of the solvent molecule as it touches the protein during this journey generates the molecular surface. The molecular surface of the protein was calculated using the programme MS. This information will help to identify those residues that are buried inside the protein. The secondary structure and the solvent-accessible information described here will be useful to molecular biologists in their mutation experiments.

Now, let us examine another application of NRL_3D in the design of de novo metal-binding proteins. Arnold and coworkers have studied the characterisation of His-X3-His sites in -helices of synthetic metal-binding bovine somatotropin. Craik has demonstrated that changing the residue 97 in trypsin to a His and adding copper causes the activity of the protein to be shut down. In this process, a Cu^{+2} ion chelates to the residues His-57 and the nearby mutated His-97. To bind the metal, His-57, which is involved in the protein catalytic activity, must undergo a conformational change. Because of this metal-induced conformational change of His-57, the activity of the protein is lost. Once the CU^{+2} ion is removed, the catalytic activity can be restored. This is referred to as the active site "metal switch."

We were interested in deactivating the PLA2 enzyme using the metal switch mechanism as it was demonstrated in trypsin. In PLA2, His-48 is important for the activity of the protein. If one of the active site residues in PLA2 is replaced with a His, the modified residue and His-48 may bind to a Zn^{+2} ion. In PLA2, the residue His-48 is in the a-helix region. Hence, to create a metal binding site, there should be another His four residues away from His-48. To test this hypothesis, the NRL_3D database was used to extract sequences and 3-D coordinates corresponding to HXXXH (where X is any amino acid).

A ray-traced Corey-Pauling-Koltan surface of the 11 fragments is shown (a through k). The darker spheres are the atoms of the side chains of the His residues. The coordinates of atoms of the fragments were superimposed on the corresponding atoms of residues 48 to 52 of PLA2.

Fragments d, g, and h have a backbone conformation similar to that of residues 48 to 52. For fragment d, which was extracted from thermolysin crystal structure, the His residues at the N- and C-termini are found to interact with a zinc ion. With the use of this fragment, a zinc-binding site in PLA2 was built by replacing Tyr-52 with a His. In this model, the conformation of His-48 had to be significantly changed to chelate the Zn^{+2} ion. Because of the change in the conformation of His-48, we propose that the activity of PLA2 will be lost if a zinc ion happens to Interact wlth this modified protein. Mutation and metal-binding studies are needed to verify this model and to confirm the possibility of zinc-induced metal switching.

Chapter 7

Performance Evaluation Methods

Performance Evaluation of Phytopharmaceuticals

Plant-made pharmaceutical production has the potential to provide large amounts of protein for the pharmaceutical industry. The types of plants used for pharmaceutical protein production depend largely on their final application. To date, the plants that have successfully been transformed include tobacco, potato, tomato, corn, soybean, alfalfa, rice, and wheat. However, it is important to emphasize that no commercially available pharmaceutical products are currently produced in plants.

Tobacco was the first plant to be genetically engineered and has the advantage of being used as a plant biopharmaceutical for exactly that reason; the methods for gene transfer and expression are well established for this plant. Tobacco can also be cropped multiple times per year, giving it an edge over other plants in producing a large biomass. The protein of interest can also be targeted to the seed. In tobacco, up to one million seeds can be made on a single plant. One concern associated with using tobacco as a protein factory is that it has toxic alkaloids associated with it, which could be present in the final drug that is administered to the patient. Another concern is that if the protein is targeted for the leaf tissue, it must be frozen or dried and then processed immediately, making it difficult to harvest and store for preservation of the protein.

Legumes, such as alfalfa and soybean, and cereal crops, such as corn and rice, have been considered as ideal candidates for plant biopharmaceuticals because the protein can be targeted to accumulate in the seed and the seed can be harvested and stored for an extended amount of time. Legumes are good candidates because they naturally produce large amounts of protein in their seeds, making the final protein recovery much larger. When considering a cereal crop as a protein factory, yield is the main quality of importance, as well as ease of transformation and speed of production scale-up.

Application of the Protein

The application of the proteins made in plants includes antibodies, vaccines, hormones, enzymes, interleukins, interferons, and human serum albumins. Monoclonal antibodies have the potential to be among the first protein pharmaceuticals commercially produced in plants. Antibodies are produced in vertebrate immune systems to recognise and bind to antigens with amazing specificity. Because antibodies possess this specificity, they can be used as diagnostic tools as well as for prevention and treatment of diseases. There are more than 10 plant-derived recombinant antibodies that have been clinically validated and almost 1000 therapeutic antibodies being tested for various disorders and diseases.

A possible future use for monoclonal antibodies is to attach a chemotherapeutic agent onto the antibody and allow it to specifically bind to a tumor cell and eventually the chemotherapeutic agent will destroy the tumor cell. Another application for plant-made pharmaceuticals is the production of vaccines. Subunit vaccines are made up of specific macromolecules that induce a protective immune response against a pathogen. Subunit vaccine technology has increased the safety of administering vaccines because it does not involve the use of live or weakened viruses. Currently, it is very expensive to produce subunit vaccines as well as to store them because they are not heat-stable. Because the vaccines are not heatstable, this limits where they can be sent for use and unfortunately makes them unavailable in the developing countries where vaccines are needed the most.

Producing the vaccines in plants eliminates the heat-stability issue because the vaccinogenic plant tissue can be administered raw, dried, or in an encapsulated form; all of these forms can be stored and shipped at room temperature. The risk of contamination with animal pathogens during production is also eliminated. Oral delivery of the vaccine is another reason that vaccines produced in plants are an attractive possibility because they can eliminate injection-related risks. Overall, the fact that the vaccines can be stored as seeds are advantageous because large amounts of vaccines can be produced in limited time and storage is less of an issue because the seed is a stable form that will not degrade the protein over time.

The choice of the plant species will determine the way the vaccine is finally administered because only some plants can be consumed raw whereas others must be processed. With processing there is the potential that heat or pressure treatments could destroy the protein. Cereal crops are attractive species for expressing subunit vaccines because they can produce proteins in their seeds, which are stable for long storage periods. For animal vaccines, the plant could be chosen based on what is eaten as a major part of its diet, therefore eliminating the need to process the protein and the risk of destroying it as well.

Regulation

In the United States, the production of proteins in plants to be used in the process of creating a pharmaceutical product will follow the same regulatory requirements that have already been established for non-plant produced pharmaceuticals. However, there are unique aspects associated with producing drugs in plant systems. These unique aspects will involve the Food and Drug Administration (FDA), the United States Department of Agriculture (USDA), and to a lesser extent the Environmental Protection Agency (EPA). The FDA regulates the testing, manufacturing and sale of pharmaceutical products in the U.S., but the USDA will play a key role in the regulation of plant-made pharmaceuticals. The USDA regulates the production and distribution of transgenic plants, and is concerned with genetic containment and reducing the risk of gene transfer.

The agency is concerned with the transgenic plant's production process and also considers risk management strategies for the production of these transgenic plants. Overall the EPA is charged with ensuring environmental safety, but the USDA and FDA have the most regulatory responsibility associated with transgenic plants for protein production to be applied to pharmaceutical applications. The FDA and USDA regulate products that are registered, but also products under experimentation in the field, laboratory, and greenhouse environments. The challenges that arise with an open environment system and producing some of these pharmaceutical proteins in food-based crops create potential new risks to be considered by each regulatory agency.

Plant-Based Pharmaceuticals Advantages

Production of antigens in transgenic plants began in 1990, but to date there are still no vaccines for humans that have been produced using transgenic plants. The idea of producing vaccines in plants came about to improve current methods of vaccine production and advance the current immunisation programs. Plants as protein factories could reduce the cost of expanding production, potentially eliminating needles, and producing heat stable vaccines that would also eliminate the cold chain processes, which is a series of refrigeration steps en route from manufacturer to vaccination, currently in place for delivering vaccines.

Tobacco was the first plant transformed to produce Streptococcus mutans surface protein A and mice were successfully immunised with the plant material. Curtiss and his group were also able to create transgenic alfalfa for expression of the enterotoxigenic E. coli heat labile enterotoxin B-subunit (LT-B), and successfully induced both mucosal and serum antibody responses. Following these demonstrations of expression of vaccine antigen in plants was the Norwalk virus capsid protein, and the rabies virus glycoprotein expressed in transgenic tomatoes.

Not only would vaccine production in transgenic plants be helpful in developing countries, but it would also increase safety and reduce the cost of mass vaccination. Producing proteins in plants potentially is a safer alternative to mammalian and microbial cell cultures because they lack human pathogens, oncogenic DNA sequences, and endotoxins. The protein synthesis system pathway is also conserved between plants and animals and plants can fold and assemble recombinant human proteins efficiently. Bacterial systems sometimes fail to fold the proteins properly and then degrade or accumulate them as insoluble inclusion bodies.

Drug companies often spend $500 million to $700 million and it takes approximately five to seven years to build new vaccine-fermentation facilities. By using genetically engineered plants costs could be reduced by 50 percent and development times could be shortened by 3-4 months. The costs of processing are reduced when the product is more concentrated in the starting material. Expressing recombinant proteins in the seeds of transgenic plants allows high levels of the protein of interest to accumulate in a small volume. Scalability is relatively rapid when using plant-based systems versus cell systems because it is simply a matter of planting more seeds and retrieving more seeds or tubers for protein extraction and purification.

Production of Therapeutic Proteins

Recombinant proteins can also be transformed into plant-cell cultures. Plant cell suspension cultures produce recombinant proteins more rapidly than transgenic plants because testing time to ensure transgene expression stability and testing against adverse phenotypic changes in the host plant can take up to two years, whereas in plant cells the development and testing is much shorter.

Cell cultures also are contained in buildings rather than produced in the open environment thereby, reducing the risk of contamination to non-transgenic plants. Tobacco plant cell cultures are grown by disturbing the friable callus tissue that results in a homogeneous suspension of single cells. The cultures are maintained in conventional microbial fermentation vats and the system allows for fairly clean cultures (free of contamination) along with fairly straightforward purification protocols.

Plant-Based Pharmaceuticals Disadvantages

New technologies bring both risks and benefits and to protect the interest of people it is necessary to assess the risks before introduction into society. The risks associated with plants as protein factories include gene transfer through pollen dispersion to sexually compatible plants that are not genetically modified, and exposing the environment and its counterparts to antigens or selectable marker proteins. For instance, what happens to the insect or mammal that eats the plant? Risks are also associated with humans including oral tolerance, allergenic responses, inconsistent dosage, worker exposure and unintended exposure to antigens or selectable marker proteins in the food chain.

Plants have differences in their post-translational modifications with respect to glycan-chain structure. Plants lack the terminal galactose and sialic acid residues that are found on many native human glycoproteins. Therefore there are changes in the glycosylation pathway that are required to produce proteins with typical human glycan structures in plants.

One method to overcome this is to use purified human β(1,4)-glactosyltransferase and sialyltransferase enzymes for the in vitro modification of plantderived recombinant proteins. Another method is to express the human β(1,4)-glactosyltransferase in transgenic plants to produce recombinant antibodies with galactose-extended glycans.

Products, such as vaccines, are intended for healthy people and must be held to a high standard of safety assurance. Because vaccines are known to be among the safest medical interventions, many healthcare providers may not even entertain the idea that vaccination may be a potential cause of a post-vaccination deleterious event, thereby leading to substantial underreporting. Vaccine failure usually occurs because of inadequate storage or administration, or because of interference by related viruses.

Approximately 10,000 reports per year are submitted to The Vaccine Adverse Event Reporting System (VAERS). VAERS is a passive surveillance system for monitoring the safety of vaccines in the U.S. It began in 1990 and is managed by the Centers for Disease Control (CDC) and the Food and Drug Administration (FDA). About 15% of the 10,000 reports describe a serious event, defined for regulatory purposes as an event resulting in death, life-threatening illness, hospitalisation, prolongation of existing hospitalisation, or permanent disability. Vaccines are traditionally produced from the attenuated version of the virus itself and grown in cell cultures or hens' eggs. After a vaccine is given, it is rare that a severe side effect will occur. More often there is only redness or soreness from the injection. People rarely experience allergenic reactions to a vaccine and since it does not occur very often it is difficult to calculate the risk of a vaccine's allergic potential. There is sometimes more risk associated with not receiving the vaccine than receiving it because the disease itself could be fatal.

Bacterial Cell Culture Systems

Bovine cell culture systems or mammalian cell culture systems are the standard methods for producing glycosylated proteins (i.e. monoclonal antibodies). These culture systems may be able to offer properly folded and modified proteins, but the low yields per cost of production facility are a hindrance. Producing proteins in mammalian cell cultures poses the risk of infecting the batch with human pathogens and bovine viral diseases, such as bovine viral diarrhea, and also the degenerative central nervous system disease, bovine spongiform encephalopathy (BSE).

Microbial cell culture systems are also commonly used for the production of proteins. They are very efficient and offer a low cost of production, however they are limited to producing only simple non-glycosylated proteins because these do not require a sophisticated folding process. The downstream processing after the protein is produced in these systems is expensive. Scalability is difficult as well because it requires the production of new facilities with fermentation vats and also hiring skilled laborers.

The purpose of my project will be to assess specific ecological and human-health risks from the new technology platform of plant-cell derived and whole-plant derived pharmaceuticals and biologics. Quantitative human-health and ecological risk assessments will be conducted to characterise the risks associated with growing pharmaceutical proteins in crop-based plants. A comparative risk assessment will also be conducted on a poultry vaccine that is produced in a plant cell culture as well as a risk assessment on the conventional method of growing the virus for vaccine production in bacterial or mammalian cell cultures.

Reasonable worst-case scenarios will be assumed for each protein and virus being assessed and different exposure scenarios will be described and applied to each protein and virus. The three proteins of interest that are currently produced in wholeplant systems (corn) include aprotinin, gastric lipase and Escherichia coli heat-labile enterotoxin B subunit (LT-B). The virus that is grown in tobacco plant cell cultures and extracted for vaccine production is Newcastle disease virus. Newcastle disease vaccine is used as an example of a plant-cell cultured vaccine to show the differences of risks when compared to whole-plant systems, and microbial and bacterial systems.

Risk Assessment

Uncertainties in the evolving regulatory environment and the need to evaluate the human-health and environmental risks of plant-based pharmaceuticals on a case-by-case basis necessitate using a robust, transparent science-based approach. Risk assessment is a formal discipline that objectively evaluates risk in which assumptions and uncertainties are clearly defined. The process of risk assessment flows in a logical stepwise fashion that includes the following five steps:

— problem formulation;

— hazard identification;

— dose-response relationships;

— exposure assessment; and

— risk characterisation (Figure 1).

Hazard and dose are considered in relation to exposure to determine risk or what additional information is needed to calculate or refine risk estimates.

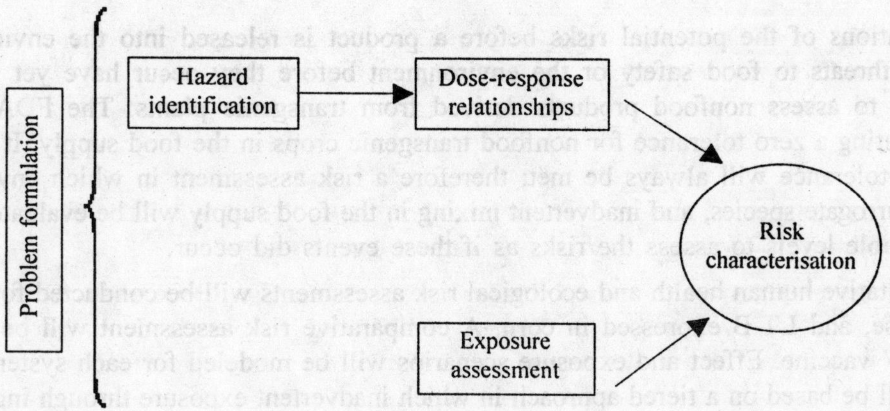

Figure 1. Risk Assessment Paradigm.

The problem formulation step sets the stage for the assessment establishing the goals and the focus of the assessment. In the next step, the analysis phase, the effects and exposures are characterised. The effects are any stressor that may affect the receptor and the exposures are the interactions of the stressor with the receptor. These are defined as reference dose, LD50's, NOEL's, and data assumptions based on time, place, and how much of the stressor is present.

The final step is risk characterisation. This phase is the consideration of the effects and exposures that were calculated previously to determine a final risk. This step states the probability of the risk and also determines if more data is needed to refine the risk assessment.

The problem formulation step might ask questions regarding the harm or impact the stressor or activity might have on the environment. There may be concern about human health effects from the stressor, or the route of exposure it is taking. These questions regarding a chemical or pesticide in the environment may be clearer and easily answered but when trying to answer these questions regarding therapeutic proteins that are inserted into crops and grown in the open environment, the actual hazard may not be evident.

A risk assessment utilises a tiered modeling approach beginning with a tier 1 assessment in which extremely conservative assumptions are used to screen out negligible risks. A tier 1 assessment is also deterministic, describing a single scenario, with high uncertainty and little data. However when moving up in the tiers the more refined the assessment becomes. In a tier 4 assessment (the highest) the uncertainties are addressed and the exposure scenarios are highly defined and often times multiple scenarios are used.

Probabilistic models are often used, and assumptions are typically verified by monitoring techniques making higher tiered approaches more expensive to conduct. A higher tiered assessment typically means a closer-to-reality description of the hazard or stressor that was defined. Even though a tier 1 assessment may not give a complete understanding of the system it does help to provide information for regulators to make decisions and communicate to the public.

Evaluations of the potential risks before a product is released into the environment to understand threats to food safety or the environment before they occur have yet to be used consistently to assess nonfood products derived from transgenic plants. The FDA drafted a guidance stating a zero tolerance for nonfood transgenic crops in the food supply. It is unlikely that a zero tolerance will always be met; therefore a risk assessment in which environmental impact to surrogate species, and inadvertent mixing in the food supply will be evaluated at levels above tolerable levels to assess the risks as if these events did occur.

Quantitative human health and ecological risk assessments will be conducted for aprotinin, gastric lipase, and LT-B expressed in corn. A comparative risk assessment will be conducted on the NDV vaccine. Effect and exposure scenarios will be modeled for each system and each scenario will be based on a tiered approach in which inadvertent exposure through ingestion will be examined to determine a risk characterisation of the plant-based pharmaceuticals.

The therapeutic proteins and vaccine we have chosen for this project are significant because they have been expressed in whole-plant systems or in the case of NDV it has been expressed in a plant-cell culture. By already being expressed in plant systems it provides information for each therapeutic to conduct a risk assessment. Even though some of the information will have to be assumed we have some starting points with these proteins to conduct a formalised risk assessment. The risk assessment will be useful for future proteins that have the potential for expression in plants and grown in cell cultures in a closed system or in the whole plant and grown in the open environment. It may provide a model to evaluate future plant-based proteins and assess them on a case-by base basis. Evaluation of acute ingestion toxicity endpoints will be obtained based on information from known toxicological endpoints. The expression of each therapeutic protein expressed in the maize kernels will be obtained through current literature sources and will be equated with the toxicity endpoint values to determine potential human and ecological acute risks from each pharmaceutical protein. The poultry vaccine expressed in plant-cell cultures will be evaluated qualitatively because quantitative information is not available to determine risk quotient values. The exposures will be compared to corresponding effect levels and to the risk quotients of aprotinin maize, gastric lipase maize, and Lt-B maize. The exposures for plant-cell derived NDV will be compared qualitatively to the exposures of conventionally derived NDV.

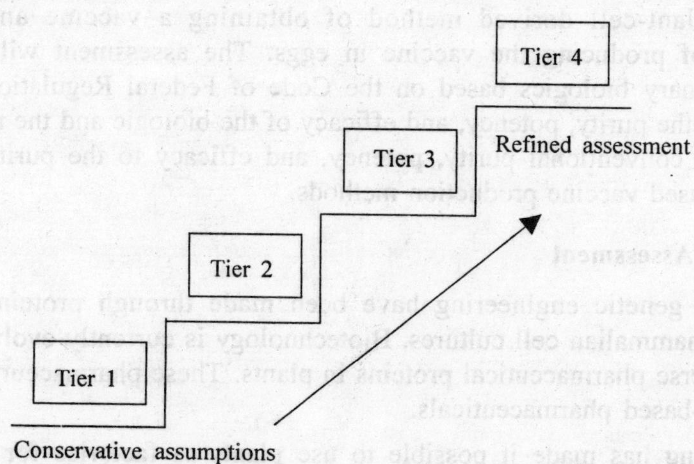

Figure 2. Tiered Approach to Risk Assessment.

The Food Commodity Intake Database (FCID) will be used with the Continuing Surveys of Food Intake by Individuals (CSFII) to determine the exposure and dietary consumption of individuals consuming maize products. The FCID is a database that was developed by the USDA for use by the EPA and other organisations when conducting exposure components of dietary risk assessments. The CSFII was created by the USDA and it measures the foods actually eaten by individuals.

The survey collects data that include demographics such as household size, income, race, age, sex, and where the food was purchased, how it was prepared, and where it was eaten. The Dietary Exposure Evaluation Model (DEEM) uses the information from the CSFII; therefore this project will use DEEM to estimate the inadvertent dietary intake of the therapeutic proteins in food. The goal of using this model is to determine the exposure of the population of concern and identify the variability in that exposure. The model includes an adjustment factor in which percentage of the crop (maize in this case) can be entered according to how much will reach non-transgenic maize though pollen flow.

The ecological risk assessment for aprotinin, gastric lipase, and LT-B will use surrogate species to determine dietary risk while employing the same exposure scenarios. The four species will include an ungulate species (deer), a rodent species (vole), an avian species (bobwhite quail), and a ruminant species (feeder and slaughter cattle). The species were chosen based on the ability to extrapolate effect data to these species and as a result successfully conduct an ecological risk assessment. These are all vertebrate species and information gained from this risk assessment will correlate nicely with the human dietary risk assessment. Effect information is not currently available for insects, fish, and soil dwelling organisms (earthworms, microorganisms).

A comparative risk assessment for NDV will be conducted by examining the risks to chickens through a plant-cell derived method of obtaining a vaccine and through the conventional method of producing the vaccine in eggs. The assessment will focus on the requirements for veterinary biologics based on the Code of Federal Regulations (CFR). The CFR is concerned with the purity, potency, and efficacy of the biologic and the risk comparison can be made based on conventional purity, potency, and efficacy to the purity, potency and efficacy to plant-cell based vaccine production methods.

Human Dietary Risk Assessment

Pharmaceuticals using genetic engineering have been made through protein expression in bacterial, fungal, and mammalian cell cultures. Biotechnology is currently evolving to produce more complex and diverse pharmaceutical proteins in plants. These pharmaceuticals are known as plant-made or plant-based pharmaceuticals.

Genetic engineering has made it possible to use plants as factories for pharmaceutical protein production. Plant-based pharmaceuticals are made by inserting a segment of DNA that encodes the protein of choice into the plant cells. The plants or the plant cells are essentially factories used to produce the desired proteins and are only grown for the purpose of pharmaceutical applications.

Many people suffer from infectious, inflammatory, and cardiovascular diseases—and these numbers are growing. Protein-based drugs are the fastest growing class of drugs for the treatment of these diseases in humans and other animals. However, the current method of producing proteins for pharmaceutical application is predicted to fall short in the years to come because of population growth and demographic trends.

Maize is an attractive vehicle for cloned vaccine antigens and other pharmaceutical proteins because it is capable of being processed into several palatable forms. Maize-based antigens are also inexpensive to produce and scale up. The distribution of the cloned antigen within the maize kernels is homogeneous, allowing for a reproducible dose. Maize is also free of human and veterinary disease agents. Maize-based vaccines would be well suited for developing nations where refrigeration during storage and distribution is often difficult, and syringes and other supplies for immunisation are expensive and unsafe. The proof-of-concept for transgenic plant vaccines has been demonstrated in animal models and extensive trials are underway with promising results.

Plant-based pharmaceutical production has created public concerns about humanhealth and ecological risks from exposure in the open environment and contamination of the food supply. The traditional method of vaccine production includes containment in facilities where cell cultures are grown and not exposed to the open environment. With this new method of growing transgenic crops expressing proteins for pharmaceutical production, those proteins will be exposed to the environment. However, in a field there are special containment practices that can be employed to reduce the risk of contamination from the transgenic plants to non-transgenic plants. Risks pertaining to this method of producing pharmaceutical proteins will need to be evaluated to ensure proper precautions are taken before cultivating these plants in the environment.

Pharmaceutical proteins have different structures, stabilities, and toxicities, and, because of this, regulatory guidelines should address each plant and protein combination on a case-by-case basis. "The route and frequency of administration should be as close as possible to that proposed for clinical use," but the clinical use of the protein may not result in the same toxicity of indirect exposure through adulterated food consumption. By using a risk-based approach to address these concerns, and others, many of the implications can be resolved or managed by knowing where the risk occurs in the system.

Risks can be understood using the science-based paradigm of risk assessment. Risk assessment is a formal discipline that objectively evaluates risk, in which assumptions and uncertainties are clearly defined. The process of risk assessment flows in a logical stepwise fashion. Hazard and dose are considered in relation to exposure to determine risk or what additional information is needed to calculate or refine risk estimates.

The problem formulation step sets the stage for the assessment, establishing the goals and the focus of the assessment. Effects (hazard identification and dose-response relationships) are the ways in which a stressor (hazard) affects a receptor (e.g., human). Exposures are the interactions of the stressor with the receptor and depend on the frequency and degree of contact between the two. Effects typically are expressed as quantified toxicity endpoints, such as reference doses, LD50's, or no-observed-effectlevels (NOEL's). Exposures are quantified based on considerations of time, place, and how much of the stressor is present. The final step is risk characterisation. This phase is the consideration of the effects and exposures that were calculated previously to determine a final risk. This step states the probability of the risk and also determines if more data are needed to refine the risk assessment.

A risk assessment utilises a tiered modeling approach beginning with a tier-1 assessment in which extremely conservative assumptions are used to screen out negligible risks. A tier-1 assessment is also deterministic, describing a single scenario, with high uncertainty and few data. Even though a tier-1 assessment may not give a complete understanding of the system, it does help to provide information for regulators to make decisions and communicate to the public. When progressing to higher tiers, the risk assessment becomes more refined, meaning a more realistic estimate of hazard and exposure. Probabilistic models are often used in higher tiers and may be verified by monitoring techniques, which often causes these higher tiered approaches to be more expensive.

Materials and Methods

Quantitative dietary risk assessments were conducted to characterise the risks associated with inadvertent consumption of pharmaceutical proteins in food as a result of production of those proteins in transgenic maize. The three proteins were aprotinin, gastric lipase, and Escherichia coli heat-labile enterotoxin B subunit (LT-B). Three dietary exposure scenarios of varying conservatism were evaluated. Percentiles of dietary exposure and risk were determined for demographic groups such as toddlers, children, and seniors.

Aprotinin is a polyvalent protease inhibitor that has been in clinical use since the early 1960's. Manufactured and sold by Bayer as Trasylol, aprotinin is supplied as a solution containing 10,000 kallikrein inactivation units per milliliter (KIU/ml), which equals 1.4 mg/ml.

Aprotinin has been shown to decrease protease activity when administered in conjunction with proteins and peptides. The coagulation activity of aprotinin led to the recommendation on the product label to not be used on normally clotting patients due to the risk of thrombosis, but recently this risk has been discounted. In rare first use cases, aprotinin has caused life threatening anaphylactic reactions, and this risk increases with re-exposure. Currently aprotinin is used intravenously mainly in cardiac surgery for its beneficial effect on the reduction of the perioperative blood loss. It is also referred to as "bovine pancreatic trypsin inhibitor," which affects known serine proteases such as trypsin, chymotrypsin, plasmin, and kallikrein.

Aprotinin was traditionally extracted from bovine lungs and is used mainly for medicinal purposes, but also is used in laboratory research and development for controlling degradation of proteins. Some of the medicinal applications include minimisation of blood loss during cardiac surgery to reduce the amount of transfusions needed. It can also be used to reduce blood loss in orthopedic surgeries as well as in pediatric patients undergoing cardiopulmonary bypass surgeries and organ transplantation. Following surgery, aprotinin has been observed to reduce systemic inflammation. Acute pancreatitis is a disease that has benefited from the effects of aprotinin by inhibiting the pancreas from producing enzymes.

Therapeutic administration and dosage

Aprotinin is administered via IV (intravenous route) because it is not bio-available (inactive) after oral administration. To increase the clinical use of aprotinin and decrease the protease activity, oral dosage with other drugs is required. Soybean trypsin inhibitors and gel-forming polymers such as plycarbophil are drugs than can be given in conjunction with aprotinin to improve bioavailability.

Stability

Aprotinin is quite stable due to its compact tertiary structure. Because of this structure it can withstand high temperatures, pH extremes, acids, alkalies, organic solvents, or proteolytic degradation. Only thermolysin has been found capable of degrading aprotinin after heating to 60-80 °C. Aprotinin is soluble in water and in aqueous buffers of low ionic strengths.

The protein is highly basic and will adhere to dialysis tubing and gel filtration matrices (Sigma, Technical Bulletin). It has been tested against kunitz-trypsin inhibitor and against peptic digestion (pH 1.2) and found to be stable for greater than 60 minutes. Aprotinin can form stable complexes and block active sites of enzymes, but binding to the active site by most aprotinin-protease complexes can be reversed and dissociated at pH greater than 10 or less than 13 .

Respiratory and skin reactions

Respiratory effects or bronchospasms have been reported rarely with aprotinin as a result of IV injection. Hypersensitivity reactions by IV injection have been reported as skin rash, acute uritcaria, and anaphylaxis. Vucicevic and Suskovic reported a case in which a 24-year-old man received aprotinin therapy to control bleeding after a tonsillectomy and, two days after the surgery, he was readmitted and received a constant infusion of aprotinin at a 20 mg dose to stop capillary bleeding. Two hours after the infusion of aprotinin, the patient had hypotension and collapsed peripheral veins, and the aprotinin was discontinued.

The man was discharged six days later. The promoter for aprotinin is expressed in organs of maize other than grain. This could potentially mean a route of exposure to people via pollen or contact with other plant parts. Inhalation of pollen could potentially result in exposure of the nasal mucosa and upper airways with aprotinin. This route of exposure has not been studied.

Allergic reactions

Allergic reactions to primary exposure are rare. However, adverse reactions after repeated applications, especially within a few weeks, have been reported. Life-threatening anaphylactic reactions increase by 5% of cases upon re-exposure. Patients with a history of allergic reactions to drugs may be at greater risk of developing a hypersensitivity or anaphylactic reaction upon exposure to aprotinin.

Hypersensitivity reactions can range from skin eruptions, itching, dyspnea, nausea, and tachycardia to fatal anaphylactic shock with circulatory failure. Because of concerns over allergenicity, a test is recommended for all patients before aprotinin treatment. A 1.4 mg (10,000 KIU) test dose is administered intravenously at least 10 minutes before the loading dose. With patients who have already been exposed, an intravenous dose of H1-histamine antagonist (antihistamine) is recommended before the loading dose. For some patients with a high risk of bleeding that have been exposed to aprotinin, re-exposure to aprotinin may outweigh the risk of serious allergic reactions.

Pregnancy

There has been no evidence of teratogenic or other embryotoxic effects of aprotinin treatment in animal studies. Only limited amounts of aprotinin penetrate the placental barrier and no studies are available on the passage of aprotinin into the mother's milk. Because aprotinin is not bio-available after oral administration, the drug would have no effect on the baby. Aprotinin should only be used in the first three months of pregnancy and only after careful risk/benefit assessment.

Urogenital effects

Kidney toxicity has been observed in patients and in clinical trials. Acute renal dysfunction is among the more serious complications after cardiac surgery and causes the need for dialysis in patients, which is associated with a high mortality rate. In a study of 60 patients undergoing coronary artery bypass grafting surgery with cardiopulmonary bypass (CPB), the patients were randomised into three groups: placebo, low-dose aprotinin, and high-dose aprotinin. The placebo group received 280 mg of saline, the low-dose group received 280 mg of aprotinin, and the high-dose group received a loading dose of 280 mg, a constant infusion dose of 70 mg/h, followed by 280 mg of a pump prime dose. Aprotinin caused a significant increase in α 1- microglobulin excretion but not in Nacetyl-β-D-glucosaminidase (β-NAG) excretion during CPB, which may be interpreted as a renal tubular overload without tubular damage.

The rate of acute kidney failure was 0.5% for aprotinin compared to 0.6% for placebo. The rate of tubular necrosis was 0.8% for aprotinin compared to 0.4% for placebo. Aprotinin showed a high affinity for renal tissue and pre-clinical studies have shown deposits of proteins in the phagosomes of the epithelial cells for the proximal renal tubules that are not metabolised or excreted until after the seventh day after intravenous administration of the drug.

Thromboembolism

Thromboembolism is the formation in a blood vessel of a clot (thrombus) that breaks loose and is carried by the blood stream to plug another vessel. The clot may plug a vessel in the lungs (pulmonary embolism), brain (stroke), gastrointestinal tract, kidneys, or leg. Thromboembolism is an important cause of morbidity and mortality, especially in adults. Treatment may involve anticoagulants (blood thinners), aspirin, or vasodilators (drugs that relax and widen vessels).

Obstruction of blood vessels, or thromboembolism, can occur with aprotinin treatment. Early signs of blood vessel blockage were observed on the pulmonary artery catheter of 3 cardiac surgery patients who were receiving a high-dose of aprotinin. The obstruction was observed 45-55 minutes after the catheter was inserted. A case of a 69 year old woman had a thrombotic event after cardiopulmonary bypass surgery and the event was attributed to aprotinin in which the woman had received a total dose of 6×10^6 KIU before and during the surgery.

Cardiovascular effects

Tachycardia has been observed in some patients treated with intravenous aprotinin. Tachycardia is a rapid heartbeat initiated within the ventricles, characterised by three or more consecutive premature ventricular beats. Ventricular tachycardia is a potentially lethal disruption of normal heartbeat (arrhythmia) that may cause the heart to become unable to pump adequate blood through the body. The heart rate may be 160 to 240 (normal is 60 to 100 beats per minute). Mangano et al. conducted a comparative risk assessment by assessing three agents commonly given to patients undergoing revascularisation.

The three agents were aprotinin, aminocaproic acid, and transexamic acid, and all were compared to using no agent during surgery. A group of surgeons monitored 3,000 patients who had been administered the three agents and 1,374 patients who had been given no agent at all. It was found that aprotinin was associated with an increased risk of death compared to the other two agents (2.8% vs. 1.3%, $P = 0.02$), cardiovascular events (20.4% vs. 13.2%, $P<0.001$), cerebrovascular events (4.5% vs. 1.6%, $P<0.001$), and renal events (5.5% vs. 1.8%, $P<0.001$). Aprotinin was associated with a 48 % increase in risk of myocardial infarction ($P<0.001$) and a 109% increase in the risk of heart failure ($P<0.001$).

Sedrakyhan et al. argued that the observational study conducted by Mangano et al. contradicted the conclusions of the meta-analysis of 35 randomised trials—3,879 patients undergoing coronary-artery bypass grafting—whichshowed no increased risk of myocardial infarction, renal failure, or stroke, an was in line with results of previous meta-analysis. Mangano et al. reported cardiac, renal, and cerebral complications to be almost double in frequency in patients treated with aprotinin as compared to patients not receiving antifibrinolytics.

Pancreatic disease from ingestion of protease inhibitors

There are two classes of protease inhibitors in plants. Serine protease inhibitors that inhibit proteases, trypsin and chymotrypsin, and cysteine protease inhibitors that inhibit enzymes with a cysteine in their active site. Both classes of protease inhibitors have been shown to have a growth retardant effect on insect pests and fungi. The protease inhibitors inhibit the digestive enzymes in the gut of insects. The proteases in the plant raise the question of any possible health hazards they pose to humans.

Animal experiments have shown that protease inhibitors decrease growth by interfering with protein digestion and lead to hypertrophy and hyperplasia of the pancreas. The pancreas reacts to this interference by enlargement and abnormal secretory activity. Aprotinin could potentially cause pancreatic disease in animals upon ingestion because it is a serine protease inhibitor. It is unknown if the same effects would be observed in humans after ingestion. However, introduction of soybean-derived serine protease inhibitor into the duodenum of humans caused a significant increase in the ability of the pancreas to secrete trypsin, chymotrypsin, and elastase. This demonstrates in humans that the pancreas responds negatively to the effects of a protease inhibitor.

Dlugosz et al evaluated the effects of aprotinin on tryptic activity by mixing a 1:1 ratio of duodenal juice samples from the pancreas with either saline solution or with aprotinin solution (25000 KIU/ml). The mixtures were incubated for 10 minutes at 37°C, and kept on ice for 1 hour to simulate the fate of aprotinin infused introduodenally, and aspirated together with bile-pancreatic juice. The tryptic activity was inhibited from aprotinin by 91 ± 2.6%. In both insects and mammals, protease inhibitors may inhibit digestive enzymes and consequently stimulate over-secretion of these same enzymes in a negative feedback loop. In mammals, this leads to pancreatic disease. In insects, this triggers a third effect, depletion of essential amino acids, which may be the chief mechanism of toxicity. It is unknown in humans if it could deplete amino acids, causing nutritional deficiencies.

Glycosylation

The carbohydrate sequence used in plant glycosylation is slightly different than that produced in mammals. In most cases this difference does not lead to any functional differences in the proteins, with one notable exception. Plants have differences in their post-translational modifications with respect to glycan-chain structure. Plants lack the terminal galactose and sialic acid residues that are found on many native human glycoproteins. Therefore, there are changes in the glycosylation pathway that are required to produce proteins with typical human glycan structures in plants.

Aprotinin produced in transgenic maize seed is not glycosylated, and its structure-function characterisation does not include glycosylation. The sequence of aprotinin was entered into a database to predict glycosylated residues. According to the results, the sequence may not contain a signal peptide. Proteins without signal peptides are unlikely to be exposed to the Oglycosylation machinery and thus may not be glycosylated (in vivo), even though they contain potential motifs. So far there is no evidence that such differences cause adverse reactions in human patients.

Effects on pediatric patients

The effects of aprotinin on pediatric patients undergoing cardiopulmonary bypass surgeries are controversial. Costello et al. administered aprotinin to children six months of age or younger and showed that aprotinin reduced operative closure time and blood transfusion and reported no observed allergic reactions. Jaquiss et al. reported no long-term ill effects of aprotinin reactions in children. It was reported that the risk for hypersensitivity reactions to aprotinin is low in young children undergoing cardiothoracic surgery, even with multiple exposures to the medication.

Reactions are more likely with re-exposure, and risk increases with multiple exposure. Aprotinin seems to be beneficial in pediatric organ transplantation, and repeat use of aprotinin appears to be safe and does reduce blood loss in retransplantation patients, but allergy to aprotinin is a concern. However, according to the Trasylol label, safety and effectiveness in pediatric patients have not been established.

Aprotinin toxic endpoints

The toxicity endpoints for the human health risk assessment for aprotinin were based on the dose regime that is administered to patients undergoing cardiopulmonary bypass surgery. The loading dose for patients was chosen as the toxic endpoint over the dog NOEL determined by Trautschold et al., because the dog NOEL did not seem appropriate for a human toxic endpoint. Adverse events have been observed in patients who received the loading dose during surgery, and it is a more conservative value than the dog NOEL. The loading dose was then divided by the body weight of an average adult male (70 kg), which gave the endpoint value (280 mg aprotinin ÷ 70 kg = 4 mg/kg body weight (BW)).

Assessment of Gastric Lipase Effects

Gastric lipase is a protein that was developed as a pharmaceutical to aid in the treatment of exocrine pancreatic insufficiency (EPI), which is an incapacity in the human body to send digestive enzymes to the gut to assimilate food particles. The absence of lipase in the body does not allow digestion of food lipids, which leads to a condition known as steatorrhea, which means there are excess fatty deposits in feces. This disease (EPI) mainly affects cystic fibrosis patients. Lipases are produced naturally in many animals, plants and microbes, and have been consumed for many years without any adverse effects.

Acute oral toxicity

Two groups of five female and five male rats in each group were orally administered once via gavage with recombinant lipase expressed in Aspergillus oryzae. The rats weighed 70-76 g and were given 5 g/kg BW of lipase. The rats were observed for 14 days and then necropsied. All survived the 14-day treatment and showed no clinical signs of toxicity. Therefore, the LD50 and NOEL exceeded 5 g/kg BW.

Flood and Kundo studied groups of 12 male and 12 female Sprague-Dawley SPF (specified pathogen free) rats at six weeks of age that were dosed with Lipase D (activity 3,170,000 U/g, defined as the activity of one gram of pure enzyme protein) by gavage at levels of 0, 500, 1,000, and 2,000 mg/kg BW/day for 13 weeks with a dose given everyday. Additional groups of six males and six females received 0 or 2,000 mg/kg BW/day during the treatment period (13 weeks) and a four-week recovery period.

Animals were observed three times daily and body weights and food consumption were recorded twice weekly. No adverse clinical signs or ophthalmologic abnormalities or deaths were observed, and food consumption and body weights did not differ significantly from the controls. There were no ocular changes or changes in hematology parameters. Even though there was reduced urinary pH and histopathological effects observed in the male rats at the highest dose of 2000 mg/kg BW they were not considered to be toxicologically significant, just an increase in metabolites. The NOEL for males was 1,000 mg/kg BW, and the NOEL for females was 2,000 mg/kg BW.

Acute inhalation toxicity

Five male and five female Sprague-Dawley rats weighing 115-142 g were confined in a nose-only inhalation chamber and exposed for four-hours to an atmospheric concentration of 0.74 +/ - 0.1 mg/liter. This is the highest concentration that was maintained over the four-hour period. The inhalation median lethal concentration (LC_{50}) was not demonstrated in this limit test other than an indication that the value exceeded 0.74 mg/liter.

Skin irritation

The backs of 12 albino rabbits were shaved, and 0.5 g of test material was introduced under gauze. The test materials (batch C and batch A) used was from batches of Humicola lanuginose lipase expressed in Aspergillus oryzae. The skin was abraded in one area and intact in the other. Patches were secured onto the test sites for four hours and then removed with water after the four-hour period and skin reactions were evaluated at 1, 24, 48, and 72 hours after removal. A primary irritation index from test batch C was classified as a mild irritant, and a non-irritant was classified from test batch A.

Eye irritation

Test batch C was used for an eye irritation study in which three albino rabbits were administered 0.1 ml of test material into the conjuctival sac of the left eye. The eyes were evaluated at 1, 24, 48, and 72 hours. No corneal or iris reactions were observed.

Skin sensitisation

Berg used test batch C to test for induction and challenge procedures on groups of 20 guinea pigs to determine whether sensitisation occurred. The induction test required injection of 20 guinea pigs four times with 0.1 ml of test material at a concentration of 500 LU/g, or 500 lipase units per gram. Ten guinea pigs were injected with 0.9% sterile saline as negative controls. They were also challenged epicutaneously 13 days later with a six-hour patch containing the test material (30,000 LU/g). A week later all the animals were challenged intradermally in the flank with 0.1 ml test material (200 LU/g). One week after the intradermal challenge they were all challenged epicutaneously to confirm the first epicutaneous challenge.

Gene mutation

Pederson used test batch A to examine mutagenic activity by using various bacterial strains. Bacteria were exposed to five doses of test material in a phosphate buffered nutrient broth for 3 hr (0.1 to 10 mg/ml incubation mixture at halflog intervals). The test was conducted in the presence and absence of metabolic activation by a liver preparation from male rats. It was concluded that there was no mutagenic activity in the presence or absence or metabolic activation.

Chromosome aberrations

Marshall used test batch A to observe mitotic inhibition at specific dose levels, in an in vitro assay of human lymphocyte cultures from a male and a female donor. Treatments were done on the presence and absence of metabolic activation by a rat liver post-mitochondrial fraction (S-9) from Aroclor-1254 induced animals. The test material was unable to induce chromosome aberrations in human lymphocytes when tested up to 5,000 µg/ml in either the absence or presence of S-9. There was no evidence of treatment-related mitotic inhibition at any of the analysed dose levels.

Toxicity of Lipase from Genetically modified Aspergillus oryzae

The enzyme lipase is currently permitted for use as a processing aid, including when sourced from a genetically manipulated strain of *A. oryzae*. To approve the use of lipase from a genetically modified microorganism involves the use of two organisms: *A. oryzae* (the source organism) and *F. oxysporum* (the donor organism). *A. oryzae* is currently listed in Standard 1.3.3 Processing Aids as a microorganism permitted for use in the production of certain enzymes, and has a history of safe use.

The genetic modification process involves the transfer of the lipase gene from *F. oxysporum* to *A. oryzae*. The recombinant organism was found to be stable during production fermentations. Southern blotting technique was used to investigate the stability of the integration of the lipase gene after large-scale fermentation, and found that the DNA was stably integrated into the host genome.

Three toxicological studies were done to test the safety of lipase from the source organism (*A. oryzae*) carrying the gene from *F. oxysporum*. The studies consist of a 13-week oral toxicity study in rats, a bacterial mutagenicity assay (Ames test), and a human lymphocyte cytogenetic assay. The 13- week oral toxicity study administered lipase by gavage to three groups of rats (10/sex/group) at doses of 0.083, 0.249, and 0.830 g TOS (total organic substance)/kg/day using a constant dose volume of 10 ml/kg BW/day for 13 weeks. The control group received tap water. The daily treatment with test substance at concentrations of up to 0.830 g TOS/kg/day for 13 weeks resulted in no treatment related effects. Therefore, the NOEL for lipase is 0.830 g TOS/kg/day, which was the highest dose in the study.

A test for mutagenic activity examined strains of Salmonella typhimurium (TA 98, TA 100, TA 1535 and TA 1537) and *Escherichia coli WP2uvrA.* A liquid culture assay was applied, and bacteria were exposed to six doses of test substance in a phosphate buffered broth for three hours with 5 mg/ml as the highest concentration. After incubation, the number of revertants to prototrophy and viable cells was estimated. The study comprising *E. coli* used the direct plate incorporation assay.

The test was carried out both in the presence and absence of metabolic activation, with 5 mg/plate as the highest dose level, followed by bi-sections between doses. No dose-related or reproducible increases in revertants to prototrophy were obtained with any of the bacterial strains exposed to lipase. The study also confirmed that lipase did not exhibit any mutagenic activity under the conditions of the tests. The third study, concerned with the potential of lipase to damage the chromosomal structure in human lymphocytes, tested human lymphocyte cultures from a female donor. The first experiment in the absence and presence of metabolic activation in the form of S-9 lasted 3 hours with 17 hours recovery prior to harvest. The highest concentration chosen for analysis was 5,000 μg/ml and induced at approximately 12% and 42% mitotic inhibition in the absence and presence of S-9, respectively.

The second experiment was continuous for 20 hours in the absence and presence of S-9. Treatment in the presence of S-9 was for 3 hours, followed by a 17-hour recovery period. The concentrations for this experiment, 5000 μg/ml and 1638 μg/ml, induced approximately 0% and 53% mitotic inhibition in the absence and presence of S-9, respectively. The treatment did not produce biologically-or statistically-significant increases in the frequency of aberrant chromosomes at any concentration tested when compared to control values.

Positive controls (4-nitroquinoline-1-oxide and cyclophosphamide) gave the expected increases in frequency of aberrant metaphases. The enzyme activity was found to be 4,000 LU/g (defined as the activity of one gram of pure enzyme protein), and the total organic substance (TOS) content was 3%. The enzyme preparation complies with the JECFA (Joint Expert Committee on Food Additives) specifications, and the enzyme preparation causes no mutagenic or cytogenic effects in in vitro studies. The NOEL from sub-chronic rat feeding studies was 0.830 g TOS/kg/day.

Because the genetic modifications were well characterised, well-known plasmids were used for the vector constructs, and the introduced genetic material did not encode and express any toxic substances, it was concluded that the use of this genetically modified lipase as a processing aid in food would pose no significant risk to human health.

Toxicity of lipase derived from rhizopus oryzae

A lipase enzyme from Rhizopus oryzae produced by fermentation was subjected to a series of toxicological tests to document the safety for use as a food additive. The enzyme was examined for acute, subacute, and subchronic oral toxicity, as well as mutagenic potential. Lipase enzyme from *R. oryzae* has been consumed for many years as a digestive aid without adverse effects.

Acute oral toxicity

Five male and five female rats were given a single oral dose by gavage of the lipase enzyme in the tox-batch at 5,000 mg/kg BW and were observed for 14 days. The rats were killed and autopsied, and it was found that there was no mortality and no clinical signs during the study. The LD50 of the tox-batch in rats of either sex was established as exceeding 5000 mg/kg BW.

Subchronic 14-day oral toxicity

A 14-day study with four groups of five male and five female young SPF (specified pathogen free) rats were given the lipase enzyme in the tox-batch in purified water by oral gavage at doses of 0, 20, 100, 500, and 1,000 mg/kg BW/day. There were no changes in clinical appearance, body weight gain, food consumption, efficiency of food utilisation and organ weight. Only minor changes in two males receiving 1000 mg/kg BW/day in their stomach walls were observed. The stomach walls were thicker when the rats were autopsied.

Subchronic 90-day oral toxicity

The lipase enzyme in the tox-batch was administered to SPF-free rats by oral gavage. There were four groups with 20 males and 20 females. The doses were given with purified water, and administered daily. The dose concentrations were 0, 50, 200, and 1,000 mg/kg BW/day. There were no changes in body weight, food consumption, food conversion efficiency, opthalmoscopic examination, macroscopic examination, organ weights and microscopic examination. The NOAEL of the tox-batch in this study was 1,000 mg/kg BW/day.

Lipase Capsules

Pancrease capsules are a pancreatic enzyme supplement for oral administration. Pancrelipase is the active ingredient in the capsule and is harvested by extraction from the pancreas of the hog. The lipase enzyme concentration in one capsule is 4,500 U.S.P. units (United States Pharmacopia unit) (equal to an international unit IU).

Nursing mothers

Pancreatic enzymes act locally in the gastrointestinal tract and are not likely to be systemically absorbed. Some of the constituent amino and nucleic acids are likely to be absorbed along with dietary proteins. Thus, there is a possibility of the protein being in the breast milk.

Pediatric use

Colonic strictures, in children with cystic fibrosis, have been associated with doses above the recommended dosing range. Patients currently receiving doses >2,500 lipase units/kg/meal or 4,000 lipase units/gm fat/day should be re-evaluated and the dosage immediately decreased to the lowest effective clinical dose, as assessed by three-day fecal fat excretion.

Adverse reactions

The most frequently reported adverse events resulting from the post-marketing experience with Pancrease (gastric lipase) were gastrointestinal and included diarrhea, abdominal pain, intestinal obstruction, vomiting, flatulence, nausea, constipation, melena, and perianal irritation. Other adverse reactions included weight decrease and pain and hyperuricemia and hyperuricosuria with non-coated formulations. Some cases of fibrosing colonopathy have been reporting in cystic fibrosis patients.

Dosage

Dosage should be based on the individual and determined by the degree of steatorrhea and fat content of the diet. The lowest possible dose should be given first and then gradually increased until the desired level of steatorrhea is obtained. Children less than four years of age can begin with a dosage of 1,000 U.S.P. lipase units/kg/meal to a maximum of 2,500 lipase units/kg/meal, and children greater than four years old can begin with a dosage of 400 U.S.P. lipase units/kg/meal to a maximum of 2,500 lipase units/kg/meal. Doses are higher in infants because on average infants ingest five grams of fat per kilogram of body weight per day, whereas adults ingest approximately two grams of fat per kilogram of body weight per day. There have been no reports of acute over dosage.

Meristem Therapeutics

Recombinant mammalian gastric lipase

The first clinical trial conducted in healthy patients and in adult cystic fibrosis patients showed that maizederived gastric lipase was well-tolerated and that it resulted in improved assimilation of lipids when combined with high doses of porcine pancreatic extracts. Meristem's gastric lipase is currently in phase II clinical trials to define the dosage of lipase necessary to substitute porcine pancreatic extracts completely. Meristem reported up to 5,000 mg/kg BW acute toxicology in mice and rats. For dogs and monkeys, the dose was up to 2,500 mg/kg BW. A single IV dose in rats was reported to be up to 450 mg/kg/day. A four-week toxicology study on gastric lipase reported rats could receive up to 500 mg/kg/day and micro pigs could receive up to 150 mg/kg/day. The expected active dose in cystic fibrosis patients is 10 mg/kg BW/day. There were no observed allergenic effects in the animals and humans after these studies.

Gastric lipase toxic endpoints

The ingestion NOEL for gastric lipase is 1000 mg/kg BW in rats. Lipases are produced naturally in many animals, plants and microbes, and the rat NOEL is the only known NOEL for this protein. Because of its ubiquitous nature, this known NOEL may be extrapolated for a human dietary risk. Therefore, the toxicity endpoints were based on this value.

E. coli *Heat-labile Enterotoxin B Subunit Effects Assessment*

Escherichia coli heat-labile enterotoxin (LT-B) is made up of five "B" subunits and one "A" subunit. The "A" subunit is an active protein that causes adverse effects in the small intestine by entering the epithelial cells and causes water loss from the cells. The "B" subunit is harmless by itself but will provoke an immune response to the entire enterotoxin. LT-B is a non-toxic subunit that is part of the heat-labile toxin produced by enterotoxigenic strains of E. coli, which is the leading cause of diarrhea in developing countries. LT is an 84-kilodalton oligomeric protein composed of two major noncovalently linked immunologically distinct peptides called LT-A and LT-B. LT-B is a 55-kilodalton homopentamer of 11.6 kDa peptides responsible for binding of the toxin to the host-cell receptor galactosyl-N-acetylgalactosaminyl-sialyl galactosyl glucosyl ceramide, which is found on the surface of eukaryotic cells.

Therapeutic administration and dosage

The antigen, *E. coli* heat-labile enterotoxin B sub-unit (LT-B), induces an immune response when orally administered and enhances immune responses to conjugated and co-administered antigens. LT-B also has potential to be used as an oral vaccine against E. coli induced diarrhea. A human clinical trial was designed to demonstrate that transgenic potato could induce an immune response in humans.

The trial involved 14 healthy adults, and all of the adults ate a dose of raw potato. Three subjects were given ordinary potatoes, and the other eleven subjects were given a potato expressing the LT-B antigen. Ten out of the eleven who ate transgenic potatoes had a four-fold increase in the amount of antibodies to E. coli in their blood. Six out of the eleven subjects showed a four-fold increase in the amount of mucosal antibodies. A dose is equal to one raw potato, and each subject ate a total of three doses (potatoes) in a four week period.

Stability

Transgenic corn expressing LT-B is stable to high temperatures that are typical in food processing, especially wiih the antigen expressed in the kernel. However, LT-B is degraded in simulated gastric fluids in less than five minutes.

Equivalence

For safety reasons, it is important that the antigen expressed in plants is equivalent to the antigen derived from the original source. For corn expressed LT-B, established equivalence to the microbial forms of LT-B in terms of activity and physical characteristics is important as well as following the guidelines of the United States Food and Drug Administration (FDA) of establishing equivalence of the transformed host plant as part of the manufacturing process. Maize expressed LT-B has been shown to be equivalent to the microbial forms in terms of activity and physical characteristics.

Glycosylation

Post-translational glycosylation for LT-B expressed in maize has not been reported.

Oral feeding study

Feeding experiments in mice showed that transgenic corn meal expressing LT-B was capable of inducing strong serum and mucosal antibodies and protected mice from the E. coli labile toxin. Chikwamba et al. showed that four doses of 10 μg LT-B/g of corn meal pellet were adequate to induce an immune response in mice. Using the gamma zein promoter, LT-B levels of up to 350 μg/g of dry kernel tissue were attained. The expression level was more than required to induce a protective immune response in mice. Mason et al. suggested that up to 1.1 mg would be required to induce a protective immune response in humans, and this dosage requirement could be met in 3 grams of dry maize meal from P77-7 R3 kernels. Lamphear et al. further investigated the immunogenicity of LT-B transgenic maize by examining defatted germ fraction in which the concentration of antigen is increased over whole kernels. Lamphear et al. also delivered the antigen to mice over a wider range of doses and included very small doses.

The mice were fed defatted LT-B maize germ meal or defatted wild type maize germ meal (negative control), and serum and fecal samples were collected and analysed. They found serum IgG responses after the first dose and after the second dose for the lowest dose levels given to the mice. The serum IgG response increased throughout the study with continued doses. All the mice (10 out of 10) fed 3.3 or 33 μg of LT-B and the mice fed 0.33 μg responded (8 out of 10) with LT-B specific serum IgG assay values exceeding twice the average value for pre-immune serum. These data show that even 0.33 μg of LT-B antigen is sufficient to give a serum IgG response. The amount of maize material fed in this case was only 0.7 mg.

Transgenic maize expressing 1 mg of E. coli LT-B was fed to adult volunteers in three doses, each consisting of 2.1 g of plant material. Seven of the nine volunteers developed increases in both serum IgG anti-LT and numbers of specific antibody secreting cells after vaccination. Four of nine volunteers also developed stool IgA. This showed the LT-B in the plant material was an effective agent for an oral vaccine antigen. Tacket et al. showed no adverse effects in a human clinical trial in which the subjects ingested up to 1.1 mg LT-B (0.016 mg/kg BW for a mean adult body weight of 70 kg) from transgenic potato.

E. coli heat-labile enterotoxin B subunit and four other antigens have been successfully expressed in vegetables. Animal studies have been conducted for transgenic potatoes containing LT-B, Cholera toxin B subunit (CT-B), and the Norwalk virus capsid protein. The "B" subunit of E.coli was the protein expressed in potatoes. The transgenic potatoes were fed to mice and the mice were exposed to the entire heat-labile enterotoxin.

The mice that consumed the transgenic potatoes showed less fluid secretion in their intestines than the mice that had not eaten the transformed potatoes. The interaction of LT-B with the immune system is not presently well understood. Ongoing research is seeking to determine whether indirect toxicity through an adjuvant effect on a toxic protein is possible. Until the nature of LTB effects is better understood, it is necessary to be cautious when considering unintended occurrence of LT-B in food.

Human clinical trial

The "B" subunit of E. coli heat-labile enterotoxin has been tested in human clinical trials to show that the transgenic potatoes could induce an immune response in humans. Fourteen healthy adults were chosen for the trial and ate a dose of raw potato at the beginning of the study, and as the study progressed they consumed two more doses. Three of the individuals were given non-transgenic potato and the other 11 were given the transgenic potato expressing the LT-B antigen. The results showed that 10 of the 11 individuals had a four-fold increase in the amount of antibodies to E. coli in their blood, and six of the 11 had a four-fold increase in the amount of mucosal antibodies. There were no serious side effects reported from this trial.

Allergic reactions

Homology with a known allergen is an indicator of a potential allergen for a transgenic protein. A transgenic maize variety expressing LT-B was screened against a database of known protein allergens and showed no matches for 35% or greater homology over an 80 amino acid window and no match of any eight contiguous amino acids.

Enterotoxin B subunit toxic endpoints

In a clinical trial in which humans ingested up to 1.1 mg LT-B from transgenic potato, no adverse effects were identified. The NOEL, with an average adult male human body weight of 70 kg, was reported as 0.016 mg/kg BW. Therefore, this endpoint (NOEL) will be used for the human dietary risk assessment.

Exposure Assessment

Aprotinin expression in maize

The company, ProdiGene, began commercial scale-up of aprotinin in field-grown maize in 2003-2004. Aprotinin traditionally has been extracted from bovine lungs. ProdiGene's recombinant aprotinin is equivalent to bovine aprotinin. Zhong et al. found that aprotinin was at a higher concentration in maize embryonic tissue than in endosperm tissue. Azzoni et al. reported the expression level of aprotinin produced from transgenic maize seed to be 0.17%; Zhong et al. observed an expression level of 0.1%.

Gastric lipase expression in maize

The company, Meristem Therapeuticas, is developing a recombinant mammalian gastric lipase. Recombinant gastric lipase is grown in maize and then purified and extracted and used in pre-clinical studies. The mammalian lipase from porcine tissue was selected because it is naturally resistant to digestion by stomach acids and maintains a high enzymatic activity after passage through the stomach. The expression level is approximately 1 mg/g kernel and there is no expression in other plant organs. The expression was observed to be stable over 11 generations.

LT-B expression in maize

Chikwamba et al. produced the B sub-unit of the enterotoxin *E.coli* heat-labile enterotoxin in transgenic maize seed. In their study, the LT-B gene was regulated by a 27-kDa gamma zein promoter, a seed-specific promoter and no LT-B expression was detected in callus tissues. For analysis of the LT-B protein levels in R1 seed, proteins from 20 kernels per ear representing each event were extracted separately and assayed for LT-B expression by ELISA. Data from all LT-B positive kernels in each ear were pooled to determine the mean and standard deviation for each ear. Levels of LT-B accumulation in P77 (one ear per event) and P112 (two ears per event) were shown. Of 19 LT-B expression P77 events, 11 had LT-B protein levels higher than 0.01% of total aqueous-extractable protein (TAEP).

Two events (P77-2 and P77-3) had LT-B levels of up to 0.07%. P112 transgenic events showed the highest level of LT-B accumulation in R1 seeds. P112 events carry the construct pRC4-1, in which the endoplasmic reticulum-retention signal sequence SEKDEL was included in the Cterminus of LT-B gene. Inclusion of the SEKDEL motif in the LT-B gene under the regulation of the seed-specific promoter greatly enhanced the LT-B level in P112 events. Compared to transgenic maize plants carrying CaMV 35S promoter/LT-B constructs, plants carrying zein promoter/LT-B constructs (P77 and P112) were more vigorous in overall performance.

Chikwamba et al. showed that LT-B protein was detected internally and externally in starch granules of maize. The strong association between the starch granules and the protein gives an effective co-purification of the antigen in the processing of the starch fraction of the corn kernels, thermostability, and resistance to peptic degradation in simulated digestion fluids. The strong association would help to understand and monitor for any chance of inadvertent occurrence, whereas the thermostability and resistance to peptic degradation indicates the antigen would be stable after ingestion and might be a concern if the LT-B maize is inadvertently mixed with food. Maize-derived LT-B has been extracted to reveal kernel expression levels of 9.2% of total soluble protein, and 3.7% of total soluble protein has been achieved by using seed specific promoters. As much as 350 μg/g LT-B could be expressed in kernels with the seed specific promoters.

Protein expression assumptions

Information on expression levels and protein distribution within various parts of the plant is needed to determine potential dietary exposure. Protein expression levels are not known for all of the proteins, but the expression of LT-B is typically 35-50 μg/g of dry seeds (about 4-5 kernels). Improvements in transformation and translation will be made over time and likely increase expression levels. Therefore, for this human-health risk assessment, 100 mg/kg (ppm) and 1000 mg/kg (ppm) are used as point-estimate expression levels for all three proteins. Expression of 100 mg/kg represents what is currently being achieved, and 1000 mg/kg represents the potential protein expression in the near future.

Human Dietary Exposure Scenarios

Scenario 1. The first, and most conservative, exposure scenario for this risk assessment assumed that the transgenic maize expressing the therapeutic protein was harvested and accidentally taken to a specialty food processing facility. The specialty food processing facility makes tortilla chips, and the transgenic maize was made directly into the tortilla chips with no dilution from non-transgenic maize. During the food preparation process, the protein was not denatured. The tortilla chips were then eaten by individuals in a variety of age ranges. The expression level of the proteins was calculated by multiplying the weight of a bag of Tostitos® tortilla chips (0.3827 kg) by each expression level (100 ppm and 1000 ppm).

The exposure was calculated by multiplying the estimated protein expression levels by the consumption (assuming consumption of the entire bag of chips in one day) and then dividing that product by the appropriate agespecific body weights (Table 1). This exposure scenario was similar to Wolt et al. in that the transgenic maize was harvested and made directly into tortilla chips with no loss of protein function. However, their scenario assumed a dilution with non-transgenic maize. Also, this risk assessment was conducted on a variety of demographic groups rather than just a high-end consumer group.

Scenario 2. The second exposure scenario assumed that there was a harvest of pharmaceutical maize. The recombinant maize was accidentally taken to a food manufacturing facility. However, unlike Scenario 1, the recombinant maize was diluted with non-recombinant maize, and the protein in the maize was not degraded during processing. This scenario assumed the same dilution factors as Wolt et al.

Protein expression level in maize kernel was assumed to be 100 mg/kg and 1000 mg/kg of dry grain. For this scenario, it is assumed that one hectare of transgenic maize will yield 5 Mg or 5 metric tons. The one hectare field was harvested and taken to a dry mill with a daily milling capacity of 2000 Mg where the maize was processed into dry-milled food products. Therefore, the percentage of the protein adulterating the maize processed into food products was 0.25% (99.75% dilution). All dry-food products derived from maize (e.g., chips, flour, bran, and starch) from this manufacturing facility were assumed to have the potential to contain transgenic maize and could be eaten by any age group (infant to elderly).

Scenario 3. The third, and least conservative, exposure scenario assumed that the edge of a field expressing transgenic, pharmaceutical-maize pollen drifted to a neighboring non-pharmaceutical maize field (kernels have not been formed yet, fertilisation happened when the maize pollen drifted from the transgenic maize field), and the protein was then expressed in 8% of the non-transgenic maize (92% dilution). The 8% expression of transgenic maize in non-transgenic maize was derived from a study conducted by Pla et al. They determined that gene flow frequency was a function of the distance between the donor transgenic maize and non-transgenic maize in fields adjacent to each other.

The assumptions were that the transgenic maize was planted with no distance between itself and the receptor (non-transgenic) field. The normal distance required between receptor (non-transgenic) maize and source maize (transgenic) is 0.8 km to 1.6 km and a 15.24 m fallow zone around the entire source maize field. However, this risk assessment does not include any of the required precautions for potential pollen flow. No border rows around the source field site were planted to minimize pollen flow.

The neighboring maize that was assumed to express both transgenic and nontransgenic maize was harvested and taken to a food manufacturing facility. The original dilution factor of

99.75% from Scenario 2, and the second dilution factor of 92% from pollen fertilisation to the non-transgenic field were used for this scenario. The two dilution factors were multiplied together for a dilution product that was used in the dietary risk model. The "non-transgenic" field was harvested and taken to a food manufacturing facility and made into dry-milled maize products. All food products derived from maize (e.g., chips, flour, bran, and starch) from this manufacturing facility were assumed to have the potential to contain transgenic maize and could be eaten by any age group (infant to elderly).

Demographic groups

Five subgroups were used for Scenario 1: adult males (71.8 kg), adult females (60 kg), youth 10-12 years old (40.9 kg), children 5-6 years old (21.1 kg), and toddlers 2-3 years old (14.3 kg). Body weights were obtained from USEPA Exposure Factors Handbook. Six subgroups were selected for Scenarios 2 and 3: total U.S. population, non-nursing infants, children 1-6 years old, females 13+ (pregnant/not nursing), males 20+ years old, and seniors 55+ years old.

Food consumption assumptions

Acute dietary exposures were defined as a single-day event. The Food Commodity Intake Database (FCID) was used with the Continuing Surveys of Food Intake by Individuals (CSFII) to determine the dietary consumption of individuals through consumption of food products containing maize for Scenarios 2 and 3. The FCID is a database that was developed by the USDA for use by the EPA and other organisations when conducting exposure components of dietary risk assessments.

The CSFII was created by the USDA and it measures the foods actually eaten by individuals. The survey collects data that include demographics such as household size, income, race, age, sex, and where the food was purchased, how it was prepared, and where it was eaten. The Dietary Exposure Evaluation Model (DEEM) uses the information from the CSFII; therefore, DEEM was used to estimate the inadvertent dietary intake and risk of the therapeutic proteins in food.

Scenario 1 did not use DEEM because only one food item (tortilla chips) was included in the exposure estimate, and DEEM cannot calculate dietary exposures based on one single, branded food item. Scenario 1 assumed that each individual consumed an entire bag of Tostitos tortilla chips in one day, regardless of body weight. For Scenarios 2 and 3, data on body weights and consumption patterns for these demographic groups were part of the algorithms within the DEEM software. DEEM calculated dietary exposures to each protein by multiplying the protein expression level (100 or 1000 ppm) in maize kernels by the dilution factors and by records of consumption of food products containing maize. Then, DEEM determined percentiles of dietary exposure to the protein within each demographic subgroup.

Ecological Risk Assessment

Pharmaceuticals using genetic engineering have been made through protein expression in bacterial, fungal, and mammalian cell cultures. Genetic engineering has made it possible to use plants as factories for pharmaceutical protein production. Plantbased pharmaceuticals are made by inserting a segment of DNA that encodes the protein of choice into the plant cells. The plants or the plant cells are essentially factories used to produce the desired proteins and are only grown for the purpose of pharmaceutical applications.

Plants expressing pharmaceutical proteins are currently being grown in field environments (although on few hectares) throughout the United States and other countries. Plant-based pharmaceuticals have the benefits of being less expensive to produce and potentially being more readily available to individuals in remote locations. It is also a cleaner method of producing a protein for drug manufacturing because plants are free of mammalian and avian infectious agents.

Maize is an attractive vehicle for cloned vaccine antigens and other pharmaceutical proteins because it is capable of being processed into several palatable forms. Maize-based antigens are also inexpensive to produce and scale up. The distribution of the cloned antigen within the maize kernels is homogeneous, allowing for a reproducible dose. Such a vaccine would be well suited for developing nations where refrigeration during storage and distribution is often difficult, and syringes and other supplies for immunisation are expensive and unsafe. The proof of-concept for transgenic plant vaccines has been demonstrated in farm animal models and extensive trials are underway with promising results.

However, there are concerns about growing therapeutic proteins in the open environment. Plant-based pharmaceuticals in the environment have the potential for intra-and inter-species gene flow, protein exposure to the public and non-target organisms, contamination of livestock feed, and water contamination.

Plant-based pharmaceutical production requires regulatory involvement of both the U.S. Department of Agriculture (USDA) and the U.S. Food and Drug Agency (USFDA), and this often involves risk assessment approaches. A risk assessment ensures a robust, transparent, and science-based process in which the assumptions and uncertainties associated with the assessment are considered and presented.

Ecological risk assessments evaluate the likelihood that adverse ecological effects may occur or are occurring as a result of exposure to one or more stressors. Much attention 73 has been directed toward the use of probabilistic risk assessment techniques that statistically quantify ecological risks as well as the associated uncertainty and variability in the subsequent risk conclusions.

Risk assessment paradigms for genetically engineered plants do not differ in principle from those for other technological risks. Therefore, probabilistic approaches to quantify risks for crop biotechnology should be used for conducting ecological risk assessments, where appropriate.

The objective of this study was to use probabilistic approaches to quantify the ecological risks associated with three pharmaceutical proteins produced in field-grown maize. Ecological dietary risks from three proteins occurring in field-grown maize were evaluated based on a single exposure scenario, and the potential risks were compared between species and proteins.

Materials and Methods

Problem formulation

The ecological risk assessment for plant-based pharmaceuticals was conducted for four receptor species used as surrogates for a wider range of species. The four receptor species chosen were vole (Microtus pennsylvanicus), bobwhite quail (Colinus virginianus), whitetail deer (Odocoileus virginianus), and feeder and slaughter cattle (Bos taurus). Body weights and maize consumption rates for each species were modeled from currently available information and used to calculate the exposure based on different expression levels of the proteins.

The two expression levels were 100 mg/kg dry kernel weight (ppm) and 1000 ppm for all three proteins (aprotinin, gastric lipase, and LT-B). The acute dietary exposure for the receptor species was a single-day event, where the total maize consumption came from the recombinant maize. Body weights, consumption rates, protein expression levels, and total protein exposures were determined using probabilistic, quantitative methods.

Effects Assessment

Aprotinin

Toxic endpoint: Acute LD_{50} values for mice, rats, dogs, and rabbits have been determined. Each study group received IV injections of aprotinin. LD_{50} values were 910 mg/kg body weight (BW) for mice, 700 mg/kg BW for rats, 190 mg/kg BW for dogs, and 70 mg/kg BW for rabbits. The toxicity endpoint for the ecological risk assessment was based on the no-observed-effect-level (NOEL) for dogs injected with aprotinin at 140 mg/kg BW.

Gastric lipase

Toxicity of Lipase from Genetically Modified Aspergillus oryzae Aquatic Organism Toxicity: Five waterfleas (Daphnia magna) were put in a test tube with an aqueous solution of test material at 1 g/L to test the solution's ability to immobilise the Daphnia over a 24-hr period under static conditions. No immobilisation was seen after the 24-hr exposure. Acute toxicity was also studied in carp (Cyprinus carpio). Ten carp were put in an aquarium of an aqueous solution of test material at 1 g/L, with the solution renewed every 48 hours. No mortality was observed after 96 hours.

Algal Growth Inhibition Test. An algal growth inhibition test was conducted to observe if there was any inhibitory effect on green algae (Scenedesmus subspicatus) when exposed to the test material. The algae were exposed to five concentrations (10-160 mg/L) of test material. The EC_{50} for inhibition of growth after 72 hours was 97 mg/L and the EC_{50} for inhibition of maximum growth rates (24-72 hr) was 99 mg/L. The NOEL was 40 mg/L.

Biodegradability. The biodegradability test recorded dissolved organic carbon of 250 mg of test material in sealed flasks. Gastric lipase was tested for its biodegradability in the closed bottle test at concentrations of 5 and 25 mg/L. The material was not readily biodegradable in the closed bottle test, but was not toxic to the microbes present in the medium.

Toxic Endpoint. The ingestion NOEL for gastric lipase was 1000 mg/kg BW in rats. After a 13-week oral toxicity study in rats by ANZFA, an ingestion NOEL of 830 mg/kg BW was determined. Greenough et al. also support the 1000 mg/kg BW ingestion NOEL. The maximum NOEL used in their 13-week oral toxicity study in rats was 1350 mg/kg BW. The toxicity endpoint for this risk assessment was 1000 mg/kg BW.

E.coli Heat-Labile Enterotoxin B Subunit (LT-B)

Toxic Endpoint: When LT-B was administered to adult female mice (30 g) through intragastric administration, Guidry et al. observed a NOEL of 125 μg of LT-B. Therefore, a NOEL of 4.2 mg/kg BW was used for the ecological risk assessment.

Exposure assessment

Aprotinin Expression in Maize. ProdiGene began commercial scale-up of aprotinin in field-grown maize in 2004. Aprotinin traditionally has been extracted from bovine lungs. ProdiGene's recombinant aprotinin is equivalent to bovine aprotinin. Zhong et al. found that aprotinin was at a higher concentration in maize embryonic tissue than in endosperm tissue. Azzoni et al. reported the expression level of aprotinin produced from transgenic maize seed to be 0.17%, the study by Zhong et al reported an expression level of 0.1%.

Gastric Lipase Expression in Maize. Meristem is developing a recombinant mammalian gastric lipase. Recombinant gastric lipase is grown in maize and then purified, extracted, and used in pre-clinical studies. The mammalian lipase from porcine tissue was selected because it is naturally resistant to digestion by stomach acids and maintains a high enzymatic activity after passage through the stomach. The expression level is approximately 1 mg/g kernel, and there is no expression in other plant organs. The expression was observed to be stable over 11 generations.

LT-B Expression in Maize. Chikwamba et al. produced the B subunit of the enterotoxin E.coli heat-labile enterotoxin in transgenic maize seed. In their study, a seed-specific promoter regulated the LT-B gene, and no LT-B expression was detected in callus tissues. Data from all LT-B positive kernels in each ear were pooled to determine the mean and standard deviation for each ear. P112 transgenic events showed the highest level of LT-B accumulation in R1 seeds. P112 events carry the construct pRC4-1, in which the endoplasmic reticulum-retention signal sequence SEKDEL was included in the C-terminus of LT-B gene. Inclusion of the SEKDEL motif in the LT-B gene under the regulation of the seed-specific promoter greatly enhanced the LT-B level in P112 events. Compared to transgenic maize plants carrying CaMV 35S promoter/LT-B constructs (P51 and P65), plants carrying zein promoter/LT-B constructs (P77 and P112) were more vigorous in overall performance.

Chikwamba et al. showed that LT-B protein was detected internally and externally in starch granules of maize. The strong association between the starch granules and the protein gives an effective co-purification of the antigen in the processing of the starch fraction of the corn kernels, thermostability, and resistance to peptic degradation in simulated digestion fluids, which could be a concern if the LT-B maize is inadvertently mixed with food.

Maize-derived LT-B has been extracted to reveal kernel expression levels of 9.2% of total soluble protein, and 3.7% of total soluble protein has been achieved by using seed specific promoters. As much as 350 µg/g LT-B could be expressed in kernels with the seed specific promoters.

Protein Expression Assumptions

Expression levels and protein distribution within various parts of the plant is needed to determine potential dietary exposure. Protein expression levels are not known for all of the proteins, but the expression of LT-B is typically 35-50 µg/g of dry seeds (about 4-5 kernels). Improvements in transformation and translation will be made over time and will increase expression levels. Therefore, for this ecological risk assessment, 100 mg/kg and 1000 mg/kg are used as the expression levels for all three proteins. Expression of 100 mg/kg represents what is currently being achieved and 1000 mg/kg represents the potential protein expression in the near future (K. Wang, Iowa State Univ., personal communication).

Exposure Assumptions for the Ecological Risk Assessment

Choice of surrogate species

The surrogate species were chosen to represent a relatively broad range of species that could potentially ingest the pharmaceutical protein expressed in maize kernels. The surrogate species included: feeder and slaughter cattle, whitetail deer, voles, and bobwhite quail.

Pathways and duration of eposure

The exposure assumptions for the ecological risk assessment were that the entire daily food intake for each receptor species came from the transgenic maize kernels expressing the therapeutic protein and that this was their sole source of food. The exposure duration was acute, occurring only over one day. Other exposure routes, such as inhalation of pollen and ingestion of leaves, stalks, and roots were not considered because it was assumed that each pharmaceutical protein would be produced only in the kernels. For cattle and whitetail deer, it was assumed that individuals entered the field and fed on the kernels, as they were mature or maturing while still on the ears. For voles and quail, it was assumed that individuals fed on kernels that may have dropped from the ears during or just before harvest.

Table 1. Human dietary risk assessment results from exposure scenario 1.

Subgroup (age in years)	*Aprotinin RQ (100 ppm)*	*Aprotinin RQ (1000 ppm)*	*Gastric Lipase RQ (100 ppm)*	*Gastric Lipase RQ (1000 ppm)*	*LT-B RQ (100 ppm)*	*LT-B RQ (1000 ppm)*
Adults - males; 73.8 kg	0.13	1.3	0.001	0.01	32.44	324.38
Adults - females; 60.6 kg	0.16	1.58	0.001	0.01	39.5	395

Youth (10-12); 40.9 kg	0.23	2.34	0.001	0.01	58.5	585
Children (5-6); 21.15 kg	0.45	4.52	0.002	0.02	113.06	1130.63
Toddlers (2-3); 14.3 kg	0.67	6.69	0.003	0.03	167.25	1672.5

Assessment of Probabilistic Exposure

A Monte Carlo simulation model was used to determine protein exposures to surrogate species. The simulation was set to perform 5,000 iterations for distributional analysis using several input assumptions (Table 1). Monte Carlo simulation uses random numbers to measure the effects of uncertainty and variability in a spreadsheet format. The simulation uses a probability distribution function from each input variable to randomly select values and repeatedly selects values based on their frequency of occurrence in the distribution.

The variability for each input is taken into account in the output of the model so that the output is itself a distribution and reflects the probability of values that could occur. The animal body weights and food consumption rates for each surrogate species were defined with a probability distribution based on the most relevant data. To calculate the protein exposure for each surrogate species the following equation was used:

$$IE = (PE * FC) \div BW \tag{1}$$

where IE = Ingestion Exposure (mg protein/kg body weight/day), PE = Protein Expression (mg/kg kernel), FC = Food Consumption (kg dry weight of kernels/day), and BW = body weight (kg).

Protein Expression

Protein expression was the amount of protein expressed in the maize kernels. Two mean expression levels, 100 mg/kg and 1000 mg/kg, were used for each protein. Expression levels were assumed to be normally distributed with a standard deviation of 20%.

Feed Consumption Rate

The cattle weights used for both feeder and slaughter cattle were derived from individual weight records separated by state. The states chosen for this ecological risk assessment were located in the Midwestern US and included Illinois, Nebraska, South Dakota, Missouri, Oklahoma, Kansas, and Iowa. There were no data for slaughter cattle for South Dakota, but all other states were included in the slaughter cattle calculation. A weighted mean and a standard deviation were calculated for both feeder and slaughter cattle.

The weighted mean for body weight was calculated by dividing the number of cattle measured in each state by the total number of cattle measured in all states, and then multiplying this value by the average weight from each state. The final mean was obtained by adding the values. The feeder cattle weight mean was 293.31 ± 3.31 kg, and the slaughter cattle weight mean was 570.43 ± 15.68 kg. The weights for both were normally distributed (Table 1). The feed consumption rate was determined for both feeder and slaughter cattle by calculating a weighted mean based on values from a corn feeding study. The same equation used to calculate body weight was used to calculate a weighted consumption mean. The feed consumption rate mean was 7.03 ± 0.1 kg for both feeder and slaughter cattle and the data were normally distributed.

Vole weight was derived from Krol et al. by calculating a weighted mean, as described above. The mean weight was 25.6 ± 3.7 g. Food consumption rate was also determined by calculating a weighted mean from the values presented in Krol et al. The weighted food consumption mean was 6.1 ± 0.8 g. Data for both food consumption rate and body weight were normally distributed (Table 1). The weight and food consumption rate of the bobwhite quail were obtained from the USEPA Wildlife Exposure Factors Handbook. The mean body weight was 191.26 ± 4.27 g, and the food consumption rate mean was 14.842 ± 0.0139 g. Data for both food consumption rate and body weight were normally distributed. Body weights for whitetail deer were calculated from a range of 40 to 136.36 kg (90 to 300 lbs). The range of distributions for body weight was obtained from Alabama Land Trust (2005) and Sedgwick County Zoo. Weight was modeled as a triangular distribution with 88.64 kg as the likeliest weight. Consumption rate was also modeled as a triangular distribution with 2.02 kg as the minimum rate, 2.27 kg as the likeliest rate, and 2.52 kg as the maximum rate. These values were obtained based on the observed 2.27 kg/day food consumption rate.

Risk Quotient (RQ)

Risk quotients (RQ's) were calculated for all three scenarios to integrate exposure and effect (toxicity). The dietary exposure values were determined probabilistically by Monte Carlo analysis. The exposure values were then divided by the toxic endpoint for each protein to determine the RQ. Therefore, the RQ, as used here, was the ratio between dietary exposure and the toxic endpoint.

Recent Advances and Applications of Flow Injection-Capillary Electrophoresis (FI-CE)

Capillary electrophoresis (CE) offers a number of advantages as a separation technique:

i) it requires only small quantities of material;

ii) it is applicable to watersoluble, high molecular-weight species in aqueous buffer solution, and;

iii) various separation modes make it applicable for the analysis of a variety of biological and nonbiological species.

CE, however, suffers from a number of limitations including discontinuous and biased sample introduction, fouling of the capillary walls and limited amount of sample introduced in the capillary resulting in low concentration limits of detection. The majority of these limitations can be reduced or completely eliminated upon coupling CE to a flow injection (FI) front end. This coupling allows enhanced sample throughput and reproducibility as well as the ability to introduce modern preconcentration techniques. In addition, enhanced detection schemes including electrogenerated chemiluminescence (ECL), amperometry and fluorescence using liquid core waveguides can be easily incorporated. Other inherent advantages of coupling FI and CE include high separation efficiency, low reagent consumption, ability to analyse small molecules in complex matrices and overall cost and simplicity.

Principles and Concepts

Flow Injection (FI)

FI was first introduced in the mid-seventies and continues to be a very useful and versatile tool in modern analytical chemistry. FI has many unique features including limited sample/reagent consumption, short analysis time, and on-line separation, preconcentration and physicochemical conversion of analytes into detectable species. FI is based on three principles:

i) reproducible timing;

ii) reproducible sample injection, and;

iii) partial and controlled dispersion of the sample zone.

In FI, the length of the manifold tubing remains constant and carrier and reagent flow rates vary little during transport of the sample zone from injection to detection, thus allowing proper sample zone transport and mixing. As the injected zone advances, it broadens forming a dispersed form as it moves downstream and changes from an asymmetrical to a more symmetrical shape. This continuum of concentrations can be viewed as being composed of individual elements of fluid, each having a certain concentration (Fig. 3).

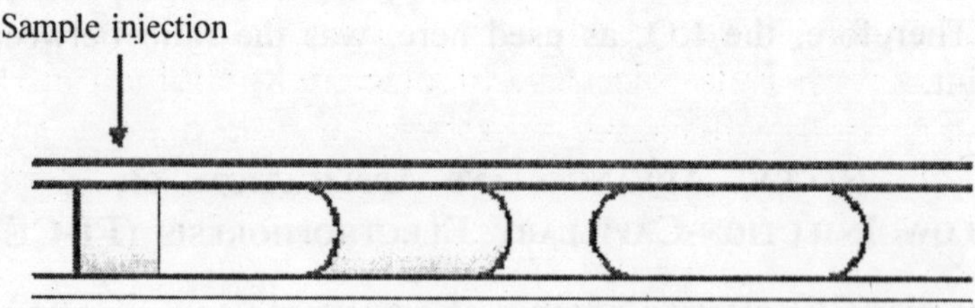

of the movement of molecules are determined by the sum of two vector components, the migration and the electroosmotic flow (EOF). Molecules migrate through the capillary column based on their charge-to-mass ratio. In addition, the mobility (μ) of ionic species is directly proportional to the ratio of charge to radius (q/r) and reciprocal to the viscosity (η) of the solution. Thus, small, highly charged ions have high mobilities, whereas large, less charged species have low mobilities. EOF is a bulk hydraulic flow of liquid in the capillary driven by the applied electric field and is a consequence of the surface charge of the capillary. In a capillary column filled with buffer a double layer is formed due to electrostatic forces. This double layer can be described by the zeta (x) potential. The EOF results from the movement of the layer of electrolyte ions near the capillary wall under the force of the electric field. The basic CE instrument set-up consists of a high-voltage power supply, two buffer reservoirs, a capillary and a detector.

Coupling of the two techniquesis not without its technical challenges. The FI-CE combined system is based on electrokinetic sample splitting with the bias effect inherent in this type of introduction unavoidable. Proper calibration measures or use of a non-pressurised sample introduction approach should help minimise such bias. The introduction of air bubbles in the reservoirs and capillary is also of concern in the combined approach. Upon construction, it is important to position the platinum electrode with its end to the right of the separation capillary to avoid interferences from electrolytically generated gas bubbles. The construction of a vertical flow cell has been reported to limit the air which can interfere with the electric current and/or flow conditions. In addition, external high-voltage power sources are used and every effort must be made to effectively ground the instrument through an appropriate earth contact.

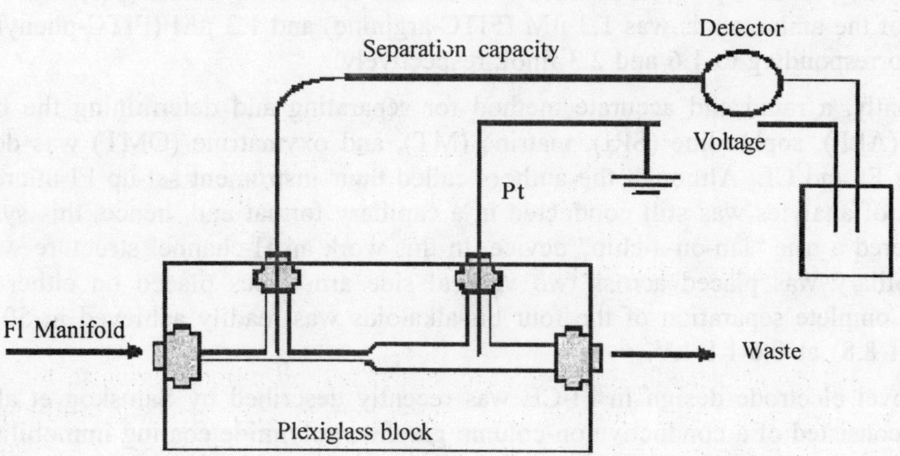

Figure. 4. A basic FI-CE interface set-up.

Applications

The coupling of CE with FI has resulted in enhanced separation techniques with advanced sample introduction/pretreatment capabilities of a wide range of analytes.

Biological laboratories and food samples

Over the past two decades CE has become a must technique in many biological laboratories and, in some cases, is the technique of choice when analysing small quantities of materials. Because of the versatility afforded by the CE format, it was a natural choice for coupling to other analytical techniques. Mass spectrometry (MS) and nuclear magnetic resonance (NMR) are but two techniques, that when coupled to CE, have yielded critical data on biological species and their physicochemical properties. This examination of biomaterials has continued with the recent coupling of FI and CE.

Simonet et al. coupled FI to a commercial CE instrument with indirect photometric detection to examine myo-inositol phosphates in food samples. The FI system served to clean-up and preconcentrate myo-inositol phosphates while the commercial instrument allowed for increased selectivity and programmability. The lower limit of detection for myo-inositol phosphate ranged from 11-26 μM with a coefficient of variation of 3.9-5.0%. The method determined the content of myo-inositol hexakisphosphate in nuts to be 2-3 times higher than that found in legumes. Kubán et al. showed that small inorganic cations in proteinaceous samples could be directly determined using FI-CE. Using a buffer containing 4-aminopyridine (PAP) and cetyltrimethylammonium bromide (CTAB) at pH 4.5 potassium, sodium calcium, magnesium, and lithium could be detected in milk and blood plasma samples.

Wang et al. described a low cost FI-CE system with fluorometric detection using light emitting diodes (LED). Continuous introduction of 30 μL samples containing fluorescein isothiocyanate (FITC)-labeled amino acids was conducted with a throughput rate of 144 samples/hour and good precision (3.2% RSD). Baseline resolution was achieved for FITC-arginine, phenylalanine, glycine, and FITC in sodium tetraborate buffer (pH 9.5). The limits of detection of the amino acids was 1.3 μM (FITC-arginine) and 1.3 μM (FITC-phenylalanine and glycine) corresponding to 1.6 and 2.3 fmol, respectively.

Recently, a rapid and accurate method for separating and determining the bis-alkoloids aloperine (ALP), sophordine (SRI), matrine (MT), and oxymatrine (OMT) was developed by combining FI and CE. Although the authors called their instrument set-up FI-microfluidic CE, separation of analytes was still conducted in a capillary format and, hence, this system cannot be considered a true "lab-on-a-chip" device. In this work an H-channel structure was produced and a capillary was placed across two vertical side arm tubes placed on either side of the channel. Complete separation of the four bis-alkaloids was readily achieved in 50 mM borate buffer (pH 8.8) at 0.6-1.8 kV.

A novel electrode design in FI-CE was recently described by Samskog et al.. Here, the electrode consisted of a conductive on-column graphite/polyimide coating immobilised onto the CE column inlet. The on-line FI-CE system was coupled to electrospray ionisation (ESI)-time of flight (TOF)-MS detection. The authors demonstrated separation of three peptides (methionine-enkephalin, neurotensin, and substance P) in an electrolyte consisting of 50% formic acid/ ammonia and 50% acetonitrile. This electrode configuration shows a high mechanical and electrochemical stability and performance comparable to normal platinum electrodes.

Environmental appplication

Timerbaev et al. extensively reviewed the growing acceptance of using CE technology for environmental analysis. This trend has continued over the past five years with major improvements in sample introduction and preconcentration by incorporating FI technology. Kubán et al., for example, developed a novel FI-CE on-line flow stacking system for use in the detection of eleven US Environmental Protection Agency priority pollutants. This unique system continuously delivered low concentrations of phenols dissolved in distilled water to the capillary by means of a peristaltic pump. This innovative delivery system, one in which the sample temporarily replaced the electrolyte solution forming a water pre-plug, allowed optimised stacking conditions and achieved a 2000-fold preconcentration of phenolic pollutants.

Huang et al. enhanced the monitoring capabilities of FI-CE by incorporating chemiluminescence (CL) detection on a chip platform for the determination of Co2+ and Cu^{2+}. A falling-drop interface was applied for FI split-flow sample introduction and the CE microchip approach further enhanced sample throughput efforts. The performance of the system was studied using the luminal-hydrogen peroxide CL reaction and achieved overall detection limits of 1.25×10^{-8} and 2.3×10^{-6} mol dm^{-3} for Co^{2+} and Cu^{2+}, respectively. More recent advances by Kubán et al. paved the way for a fully automated field-based FI-CE system for the determination of inorganic ions (e.g., Cl^-, NO_3^-, SO_4^-, K^+, Ca^{2+}, Na^+, Mg^{2+}). This system employed dual injection at opposite ends of the separation capillary which allowed concurrent anion and cation determinations at 10 min intervals with detection limits in the range of 20-200 µg L^{-1} for all ions.

Medicinal and pharmaceutical industries

The application of CE to the medical and pharmaceutical industries has burgeoned in recent years with a diversity of applications including the analysis of protein-based pharmaceuticals, drug analysis and design and routine quality control. Coupling with FI has further expanded the medicinal and pharmaceutical applications of CE by providing ultrasensitive, high-throughput analysis capabilities. Chen et al., for example, developed an online FI conversion method for the determination of the antimalarial agent artemisinin.

The coupling of FI allowed rapid analyses (less than 12 min after the conversion of artemisinin to a strongly UV-absorbing compound) with a sampling frequency of 8 h^{-1}. More recent work by Cheng et al. led to an improved FI-CE method for artemisinin determination incorporating the use of an orthogonal design in investigating experimental factors. Cao et al. achieved high separation efficiency (8 mm plate height) and sample throughput (48 h^{-1}) analysis for the determination of sulphamethoxazole and trimethoprim in sulphatrim tablets. In this study, a miniaturised CE system incorporating a modified falling-drop interface was employed for detection limits of 1 µg L^{-1} and 0.5 µg L^{-1} for sulphamethoxazole and trimethoprim, respectively.

A novel FI-CE system was also developed for the kinetic study of aspirin hydrolysis in aqueous solutions. This system employed a split-flow interface for on-line electrokinetic injection and a knotted reactor for on-line quenching reactions. Overall, the FI-CE system achieved a sampling rate of 20 h^{-1} with a detection limit of 1.0 µg mL^{-1}. Cheng et al. developed a novel FI-

CE system for the determination of aspartic acid (Asp) enantiomers by on-line derivatisation with o-phthalaldehyde and mercaptoethanol. The enantiomers were converted to UV-absorbing diastereoisomer derivatives, which were reproducibly separated by micellar electrokinetic chromatography (MEKC). Detection limits were 0.11 and 0.12 μg mL^{-1} for D-Asp and L-Asp, respectively.

Further applications and advances in miniaturisation and automation will continue as technology progresses. For example, have recently developed a block FI-CE system incorporating a miniature charge-coupled device (CCD) spectrometer employing 200 mm fiber optic cables and an inhouse written graphical programming environment for full data acquisition and instrument control. Figure 5 shows an electropherogram of four injections of 1 mM vancomycin and nicotinamide adenine dinucleotide reduced form (NADH). This graph shows the applicability of our system for model separations. Continued efforts like this will likely lead to commercially available FI-CE systems with a variety of laboratory and field-based applications.

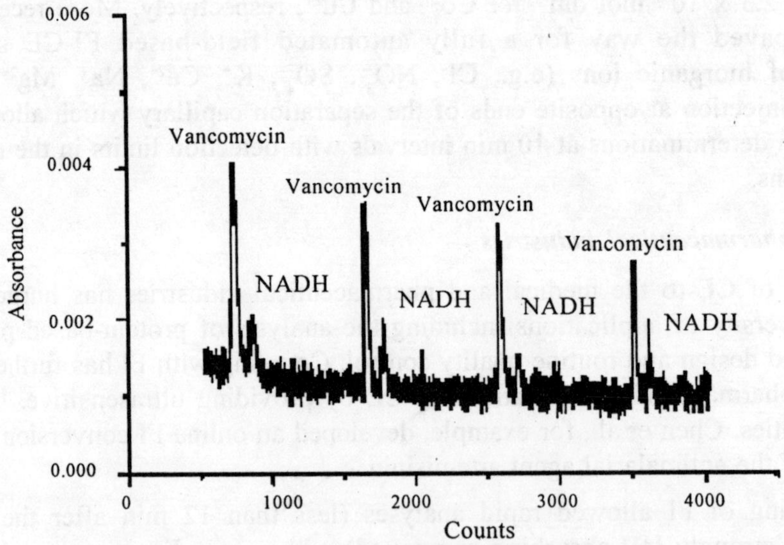

Figure 5. A representative electropherogram of four direct injections of vancomycin (1 mM) and NADH (1 mM) in 192 mM glycine-25 mM Tris buffer (pH 8.3). The total analysis time in each experiment was 20 min (200 counts equal to one min) at 10 kV using a 36 cm (inlet to detector), 50-μm I.D. open, uncoated quartz capillary. Flow rate of the combined sample and buffer line was 1.3 mL min-1.

Application of Streptomycin Materials

Although streptomycin was not the first antibiotic (penicillin, a fungal product, had been isolated some years earlier), its discovery was a landmark in antibiotic history. It was the first effective therapeutic for tuberculosis, a disease that had terrorised humans for centuries and a cause of human morbidity and mortality unmatched by wars or any other pestilence. Streptomycin was the first aminoglycoside to be identified and characterised and is noteworthy in being the first useful antibiotic isolated from a bacterial source. At the present time, the use of streptomycin in infectious disease therapy has largely been replaced by less toxic and equally effective compounds, but it still has significant applications as a second-line treatment for TB and occasionally for the treatment of nosocomial multidrug-resistant gram-positive infections. Streptomycin's preeminent place in the history of antibiotics is assured!

Selman Waksman's commitment to the isolation and screening of soil bacteria in the search for bioactive small molecules, especially potential antibiotics, was validated by the discovery of streptomycin. This led to the creation of the modern biopharmaceutical industry and the subsequent isolation of tens of thousands of bioactive small molecules from soil bacteria and other environments. A proportion of these compounds have become highly successful therapeutics, not only for all types of infectious diseases, but also in the treatment of many other human and animal ailments and as anticancer, immuno-modulatory, and cardiovascular agents. Waksman and Fleming could be considered the fathers of chemical biology (Figure 6).

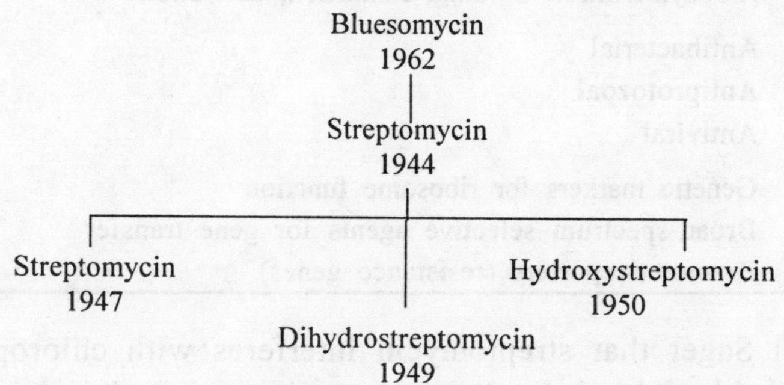

Figure 6. The structural relationships of the streptamine family of antibiotics.

Following on the discovery of streptomycin and its streptamine-based relatives, a new generation of the aminoglycosides derived from 2–deoxystreptamine (DOS) was not long in coming (Figure 6). For a variety of reasons, many of these compounds have not been employed as human therapeutics; for example, neomycin has rarely been used in the clinic because of its extreme toxicity. Surprisingly, paromomycin, a naturally occurring 6-desaminoderivative of neomycin, is receiving increasing interest in the treatment of a variety of tropical diseases, including leishmaniasis and certain types of fungal infection. This serves to illustrate that the aminoglycosides (and the related aminocyclitols, such as spectinomycin) have a broad range of biological activities and have found use in a wide variety of applications as indicated in Table 2. In addition to these compounds, there is a large group of atypical aminoglycosides, compounds that are of diverse microbial origin, structure, and biological activity (Table 3).

Many applications of the aminoglycosides have been of historical significance in genetics and microbiology. For example, mutations to streptomycin resistance were employed as counterselective genetic markers in the historic experiments of William Hayes that demonstrated the existence of bacterial conjugation and the requirement of donor (Hfr or F^{+}) and receptor

(F^-) species. These experiments showed that conjugal gene transfer occurs with directional polarity and led to the subsequent characterisation of sex factors that were ultimately shown to be extrachromosomal DNA elements, or plasmids.

Table 2. Some of the Myriad Properties and Applications of the Aminoglycosides

Protein synthesis inhibition—prokaryotes
Protein synthesis inhibition—eukaryotes
Mistranslation on ribosomes
Nonsense mutation suppression
DNA translation
Phenotypic suppression
Membrane leakiness
Nucleic acid binding/precipitation
Probing ribosome structure
Allosteric activation of enzyme activity
Ribozyme/intron binding, inhibition, activation
Antibacterial
Antiprotozoal
Antiviral
Genetic markers for ribosome function
Broad-spectrum selective agents for gene transfer
Promoter-reporters (resistance genes)

The finding by Ruth Sager that streptomycin interferes with chlorophyll production in Chlamydomonas and that high-level streptomycin resistance mutants exhibit cytoplasmic rather than Mendelian inheritance (due to alteration of the chloroplast genome)provided evidence in support of the bacterial (endosymbiotic) origin of chloroplasts in Chlamydomonas and plants. In the early 1970s, kanamycin resistance (encoded by a resistance plasmid) was used as a dominant selective genetic marker for heterologous gene transfer in the seminal recombinant DNA studies of Herbert Boyer, Stanley Cohen, and their colleagues.

Table 3. Other Classes of Aminoglycoside-Aminocyclitol Antibiotics

Ashimycin
Astromicin/Istamycin
Boholmycin
Kasugamycin
Myomycin
Spectinomycin
Trehalosamine
Validamycin

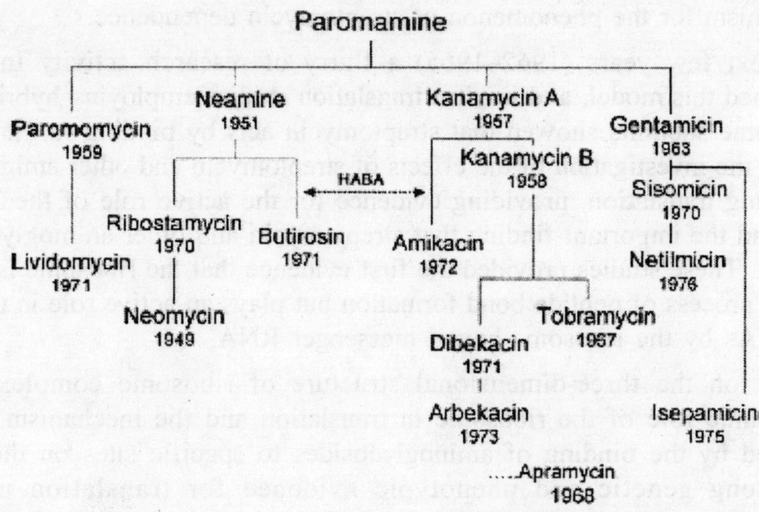

Figure 7. The structural relationships of the 2-deoxystreptamine family of antibiotics.

The later observation that kanamycin and certain other aminoglycosides have inhibitory activity against some types of eukaryotic cells led to their application in the genetic manipulation in higher organisms, including plants. In particular, two antibiotics have been widely used for eukaryotic gene cloning: G-418 (Geneticin™)and hygromycin B. G-418, related to gentamicin, has become the preferred selective agent for mammalian cell studies, and large amounts of the compound are currently employed for this purpose. The neomycin phosphotransferase gene was the first bacterial gene approved in tests of human gene therapy in 1982 and remains the genetic marker of choice for all types of eukaryotic cloning.

Biochemical Mode of Action

The biochemical mode of action of the aminoglycosides as antibacterials has long been a topic of great interest. Early experiments carried out soon after the introduction of streptomycin suggested a variety of modes of action, but these conclusions were based largely on symptomatic analyses of antibiotic-treated bacterial cultures. One important experiment done in 1948 showed that streptomycin blocks enzyme induction in susceptible bacteria; this was the closest that anyone came to identifying the mechanism of action at the time.

A series of genetic and biochemical studies in the late 1950s and early 1960s led to the definitive identification of protein synthesis as the primary target for the antibacterial action of streptomycin. Initially, Erdos and Ullmann employed the incorporation of radioactive amino acids to show that production of labeled protein by cell-free extracts of Mycobacterium tuberculosis is effectively blocked by streptomycin. The results of these experiments were subsequently confirmed by others, using defined cell-free translation systems from other bacteria and with synthetic polynucleotides as messenger RNAs. A seminal paper by Spotts and Stanier proposed the ribosome as the probable target for streptomycin action and came up with a plausible biochemical mechanism for the phenomenon of streptomycin dependence.

Within the next few years (1962–1965) a flurry of research activity in a number of laboratories confirmed this model, and in vitro translation studies employing hybrids of sensitive and resistant ribosome subunits showed that streptomycin acts by binding to the 30S ribosome subunit. This led to the investigation of the effects of streptomycin and other aminoglycosides on coding fidelity during translation, providing evidence for the active role of the 30S subunit in protein synthesis and the important finding that streptomycin and other aminoglycosides induce errors in translation. These studies provided the first evidence that the ribosome is not simply an inert support in the process of peptide bond formation but plays an active role in the selection of aminoacylated tRNAs by the ribosome-bound messenger RNA.

Current work on the three-dimensional structure of ribosome complexes has amply confirmed the dynamic role of the ribosome in translation and the mechanism by which this process is perturbed by the binding of aminoglycosides to specific sites on the 30S subunit. There is now strong genetic and phenotypic evidence for translation misreading by aminoglycosides in living cells. While it has been shown that a number of other translation inhibitors also provoke mistranslation, this may be a symptom of protein synthesis inhibition and not a direct effect on codon reading, as with the aminoglycoside antibiotics.

Surprisingly, in the presence of some aminoglycosides, DNA can be accurately read as a messenger on the ribosome and to generate polypeptides in vitro; it is not known if this occurs in vivo. Parenthetically, the ability of aminoglycosides to cause mistranslation has itself been applied recently to an "indirect" form of gene therapy; the administration of gentamicin or related compounds to patients with hereditary diseases such as severe hemophilia or cystic fibrosis can result in partial suppression of the disease. Aminoglycoside-induced read-through of nonsense mutations leads to the production of small amounts of the missing protein and prevents nonsense-mediated decay of messenger RNA.

As is the case with most antibiotics, at subinhibitory concentrations the aminoglycosides induce significant changes in the transcription of some 5% of the genes in susceptible bacteria. The mechanism responsible is not known but may be due to some form of coupling between translation and transcription not previously identified. We can assume that transcription modulation is associated with antibiotic activity in therapeutic use and may contribute to some of the side effects. On the other hand, at low concentrations in the environment, the aminoglycosides and other antibiotics may be acting as cell-signaling molecules.

The use of streptomycin or spectinomycin resistance as a genetic marker was critical to the cloning and identification of the gene clusters encoding structural elements of the ribosome in bacteria. Once it had been demonstrated that resistance to streptomycin and spectinomycin is associated with amino acid changes in ribosomal proteins, bacteriophage P1 transduction studies showed that the associated genes are linked in clusters on the bacterial chromosome. Masayasu Nomura and others then used disruption and reconstitution of ribosome particles from 16S rRNA and isolated R proteins to demonstrate the roles of the proteins RpsL (str) and RpsE (spc) in the determination of antibiotic resistance; this confirmed the earlier genetic and phenotypic studies and ratified the role of R proteins in ribosome function.

There followed a decade of argument as to the relative importance of ribosomal RNA versus ribosomal proteins in the structure and function of the particle, and a paradigm change occurred when it was shown by numerous sequence and functional studies that the two major rRNA molecules are the structural basis of ribosome function in translation. The fact that these RNA molecules are the targets for the binding and interaction of different antibiotics on the ribosome, resulting in interruption of the translation process, provides strong confirmation of their roles in translation. The spectacularly successful rRNA footprinting studies and X–ray structure analyses carried out by the groups of Noller, Ramakrishnan,and others have amply confirmed this dominant role of rRNA and the consequences of antibiotic binding to the ribosome, initially with the aminoglycosides but subsequently with most ribosomal inhibitors. However, although the primordial template for peptide bond formation is likely to have been RNA alone, the involvement of both RNA and protein is essential in the dynamic role of the "modern" ribosome in translation; this is a topic of continuing interest. To date, it is only in the case of streptomycin that three-dimensional structure analysis of the antibiotic/ribosome complex identifies an interaction of the drug with both R proteins and rRNA. There is increasing evidence for the existence of nonribosomal functions of the protein components of the ribosome. Studies using antibiotics such as the aminoglycosides will undoubtedly continue to play important roles in developing this story.

During these years of exciting revelations concerning aminoglycoside activity and the ribosome, one question relative to the therapeutic use of aminoglycosides has remained unsolved. Unlike most antibiotic inhibitors of protein synthesis in bacteria that lead to bacteriostasis, the aminoglycosides are rapidly bactericidal. The ability of the aminoglycosides to kill bacterial pathogens is an important attribute in their therapeutic use. This action is somewhat surprising when we consider that most inhibitors of ribosome function act in a similar fashion to the aminoglycosides, by binding to target sequences within the 16S or 23S rRNAs. For example, the aminocyclitol spectinomycin is bactericidal in action. The difference between cidal and static action has been the topic of much discussion and many publications; this work has been largely physiological in nature, and a satisfactory biochemical explanation for the lethal action of the aminoglycosides still eludes us. The possibility that aminoglycosides (as distinct from other translation inhibitors) induce a process of programmed cell death (apoptosis) in bacteriacould provide an explanation.

Antibiotic Resistance and Aminoglycoside Evolution

Antibiotic resistance (both endogenous and acquired) is an important determining factor in the historical development of the aminoglycosides as therapeutic agents. After streptomycin was introduced for the treatment of tuberculosis, it was found that bacterial resistance to the drug often developed; this was shown to be due to spontaneous mutants arising during the course of therapy with the antibiotic, although the biochemical mechanism was not known at the time. Kanamycin, the first useful DOS aminoglycoside, was isolated in Japan in 1957 and rapidly became an antibiotic of choice in that country. However, the appearance of strains resistant to both streptomycin and kanamycin increasingly interfered with their therapeutic use; in addition, hospital infections of Pseudomonas aeruginosa, a bacterium that is naturally less susceptible to antibiotics, were on the rise. A major breakthrough came with the discovery of a novel class of 2–DOS compounds, the gentamicins. These are extremely effective antibiotics with good activity against the pseudomonads and other problem pathogens, such as Proteus and Serratia species, that were being increasingly encountered as nosocomial infections.

Gentamicin and related compounds lack the 3′ OH group, and the absence eliminates the modification by phosphorylation at this site and confers activity against pathogens possessing aminoglycoside 3′ OH phosphotransferases; gentamicin, being a mixture, contains one component with a modified 6′ amino group and has reasonable potency against strains harboring plasmid-encoded 6′ acetytransferases that inactivate kanamycin. By this time it was known that resistance to antibiotics by enzymic modification could be acquired by plasmid transfer. Gentamicin was also effective for the treatment of staphylococcal and enterococcal infections, frequently being used in combination with a α-lactam antibiotic in these circumstances.

In spite of its nephrotoxicity, gentamicin was the treatment of choice for gram-negative nosocomial infections for many years, and its success led to the introduction of tobramycin, a related compound. However, novel antibiotic resistance mechanisms began to appear on the scene; of particular concern was the adenylylation of the 2′ OH of gentamicin and related compounds that appeared on the scene in 1971 and conferred high-level resistance to the newest generation of aminoglycosides. The increasing, worldwide use of different aminoglycosides led to the appearance of many different types of resistant strains; the local use of specific classes of aminoglycoside often led to the selection of distinct local classes of resistance.

Fortunately, the discovery of a novel DOS derivative in 1971 provided the next breakthrough. This compound, butirosin, related to ribostamycin and produced by a Bacillus species (not an actinomycete), inhibits a variety of aminoglycosideresistant hospital pathogens, including those inactivating the drugs by 3′ phosphorylation and 2" adenylylation. This property is due to the presence of a 4-hydroxy-2-aminobutyric acid (HABA) substituent on the 1-position of the DOS of butirosin. The latter antibiotic lacked good pharmaceutical properties, but synthetic insertion of a HABA or related group on the 1-position of the DOS of kanamycin (and subsequently of gentamicin-derived compounds) provided a novel series of potent semisynthetic aminoglycoside antibiotics with improved activity against a number of types of resistant strains. In particular, amikacin, a kanamycin derivative with a broad spectrum of activity against resistant strains, has had considerable clinical and commercial success. Since its discovery in 1976, no chemical modifications of substance have been reported, in spite of the fact that the spread of resistance has continued unabated and new resistance enzymes and efflux systems have appeared,in particular a great variety of 6acetyltransferases. Effort has been channeled primarily to tinkering with the DOS core.

A variety of bacterial genera have been shown to produce aminoglycoside–aminocyclitol antibiotics. These include *Streptomyces, Micromonospora, Bacillus,* and so on. Only those compounds emanating from Streptomyces are named "-mycins" (e. g., tobramycin) while others are "-micins" (gentamicin), "-osins," "-asins," or "-acins. " The biosynthetic pathways for the aminoglycosides and the control of their expression are not well-studied. Streptomycin is the exception, and Piepersberg's group has contributed significantly to this effort. The intricacy of the biosynthesis is evident from the fact that upwards of 30 enzymatic steps are required for the formation of streptomycin from d-glucose.

The therapeutic use of aminoglycosides has diminished somewhat, but they are still important potent and widely used antibiotics in hospitals; most of the class are now generics. There is no question that a novel aminoglycoside derivative with demonstrated activity against the current generation of resistant pathogens, and preferably with reduced toxicity, would be a welcome addition for the treatment of infectious diseases. Attempts have been made to produce inhibitors of one or more of the aminoglycoside-modifying enzymes, and a number of different small molecule inhibitors have been described. In principal, such inhibitors could be used in combination with an aminoglycoside for the treatment of resistant infections, much like the successful combination of a β-lactam antibiotic with a lactamase inhibitor. However, none of the inhibitors of aminoglycoside resistance enzymes have been employed in serious clinical trials. Given the increasing problems of antibiotic resistance in hospitals worldwide, it is surprising that this approach has not been pursued with more purpose.

Toxicity of Aminoglycosides

As previously mentioned, another drawback limiting an expanded therapeutic use of the aminoglycosides is their toxicity, which varies in form and intensity with the different types of molecules; the main toxic responses are ototoxicity and renal toxicity. Streptomycin and other aminoglycosides target sensory hair cells of the inner ear and can lead to hair-cell degeneration and permanent loss; this occurs by an as yet undetermined mechanism and leads to irreparable hearing loss in up to 5% of patients on extended treatment with aminoglycosides. A variety of dosing regimens have been employed and shown to reduce the incidence of toxicity. On the positive side, significant advances in understanding of the general mechanisms of drug-induced ototoxicity in recent years have provided important information on the genetic and structural elements of hearing loss in humans; it would appear that mutations affecting mitochondrial rRNA predispose to aminoglycoside ototoxicity.

From a therapeutic point of view, however, relatively little effort has been put into attempts to redesign aminoglycoside structure to reduce toxic responses, probably because good in vitro testing models have not been available. The largely random analyses of structure–activity relationships between the inhibitory and toxicity responses of the aminoglycosides have provided few significant insights into the problem. One has the impression that, because the two responses are so closely related in structure–activity terms, a less toxic, equipotent aminoglycoside is unattainable! An interesting series of experiments on the relationship between activity against eukaryotic cells and the role of the various functional groups of the DOS aminoglycosides has provided some valuable clues concerning antibiotic/ ribosome/rRNA interactions,but this work has not yet been exploited with reference to toxic responses during aminoglycoside therapy. Obviously, such information would be of great value in the design of new aminoglycosides for use as antimicrobials or in other therapeutic applications. To date, the development of semisynthetic aminoglycosides has been largely driven by the goal of finding compounds active against evolving resistant or recalcitrant bacterial pathogens.

Chapter 8

Computer-aided Drug Design

All the world's major pharmaceutical and biotechnology companies use computational design tools. At their lowest level the contributions represent the replacement of crude mechanical models by displays of structure which are a much more accurate reflection of molecular reality, capable of demonstrating motion and solvent effects. Beyond this, theoretical calculations permit the computation of binding free energies and other relevant molecular properties. The theoretical tools include empirical molecular mechanics, quantum mechanics and, more recently, statistical mechanics.

DNA Astarget

The sequencing of the human genome represents one of the major scientific endeavours of this century. A major aspect of the utilisation of this information will be the provision of small molecules which will recognise selected sequences, perhaps with the goal of switching off particular genes as in cancer chemotherapy.

For some time antibiotics such as netropsin have been known to bind preferentially to sequences rich in A-T pairs. A variant based on this research has been to try to design a bioreductive ligand based upon netropsin. The idea of bioreductive anti-cancer agents statts with the fact that tumours receive less blood and hence less oxygen than normal tissue. Thus it becomes possible, at least in principle, to contemplate having a ligand which can exist in two forms, oxidised and reduced, and if the redox potential is appropriate to be in the oxidised form in normal tissue but reduced in tumours. If only the reduced form will bind to the macromolecular target and cause cell death, then differentiation in action between cells which it is desirable to desttoy and normal cells is achievable, with concomitant reduction in side-effects.

A second starting point for sequence selective ligands is an organometallic molecule with chiral properties. The propeller- like ruthenium tris-phenanthroline complexes do show differential binding between A-T and G-C sequences and moreover may exhibit a preference for purine 3', 5' pyrimidine sites in DNA. Perhaps the most intriguing starting point for a molecule upon which to build nucleic acid selectivity is the ubiquitous spermine. It has been proposed that spermine can bind to DNA in a cross-groove manner, with relatively non-specific interactions between the positive nitrogens of the spermine and the negatively-charged phosphate backbone.

In addition there is a highly specific binding down the major groove of poly(dG-dC) involving hydrogen bonds to N7 and 06 of guanine. This latter interaction could be an aspect of the property of spermine in inducing conformational changes in DNA including the B-Z transition. It is then possible to speculate that the role of spermine as a messenger may be to control which portions of a DNA sequence are readable by altering the coiling of the nucleic acid.

PROTEIN ASTARGET

If an enzyme structure is known then designing inhibitors which will block activity in the test-tube should be a relatively straightforward problem. The binding free energy of the inhibitor to the enzyme is a crucial quantity: strong binding is essential. Computationally it is possible to calculate differences in the binding free energies of two ligands A and B to an enzyme E, using the cycle.

$$\begin{array}{ccc} & \Delta G_1 & \\ E + A & \rightarrow & EA \\ \downarrow \Delta G_3 & & \downarrow \Delta G_4 \\ & \Delta G_2 & \\ E + B & \rightarrow & EB \end{array}$$

The desired (ΔG_i - ΔG_2) is equated to (ΔG_3 - ΔG_4). These latter free energy charges are non-physical but may be computed using free energy perturbation techniques.

The transformation ΔG_3 represents the molecule A being changed into molecule B in aqueous solution. This may be simulated either by using Monte Carlo techniques or by molecular dynamics. The other perturbation, ΔG_4, is more readily followed by molecular dynamics since with protein involved, most Monte Carlo moves are not accepted. With care, however, relative binding free energies can be computed 1 to an accurqcy approaching 1 kcal mol^{-1}.

This same free energy perturbation approach can also yield the redox potentials which are fundamental to the bioreductive idea. In this case the thermodynamic cycle is a little more complex and it is also necessary to calculate a gas-phase energy difference between pairs of oxidised and reduced molecules. High quality ab initio molecular orbital methods including electron correlation effects provide those energy differences.

DRUG TRANSPORT

Sceptics quite rightly point out that designing an enzyme inhibitor which will work in the test-tube is one thing; getting a compound which will work in a cell is another. Transport across the biological membrane is essential. Compounds must be soluble enough in the lipid to get into the membrane, but not so soluble that they remain there. Within the pharmaceutical industry the partition coefficient between water and n-octanol is used as a guide to membrane transport. The free energy perturbation technique just described can also be adapted to compute partition coefficients.

More excitingly, however, it is becoming possible to model biological membranes. Starting with crystal structures of membranes involving DMPC (1,2-dimyristoyl-sn-glycero-3-phosphoryl choline) a highly realistic simulation is possible, involving a hydrated lipid bilayer. After very long molecular dynamics simulations the resulting membrane model is in agreement with all the available experimental data; lead p u p separation; order parameters and diffusion coefficients. This model can be used as the 'solvent' in calculations of partition coefficients which should be considerably more realistic than experimental values in n-octanol. Furthermore it will be W b l e to introduce cholesterol and protein into the model membrane to produce a truer simulation of how a given drug is transported into a cell.

Predicting Protein Structure

One of the major contempomy scientific aims is to use the abundance of gene and hence protein sequences to predict the three-dimensional structure of proteins: going from primary to tertiary structure. Were this routinely pwsible the choice of drug target where the architecture of the binding site is known would increase from a handful of cases to many thousands. The currently favoured and only successful methods are all based upon finding similarities and homologies between the protein of known sequence but unknown topology and known structures from three-dimensional databases.

Generally sequences are compared with scoring matrices being used to ascertain just how similar a short length of polypeptide in the unknown is in comparison with a known case. One successful prediction, that of the important small protein big endothelin, was made using not the identities of amino acids in the sequence, but their properties, notably their hydrophobicities. The property profile is smoother than an identity specification where each amino acid can be one of twenty.

Where the similarity is low the use of colour graphics to permit the human eye to detect similarities has many advantages although it is inevitably subjective. This approach, using the computer program CAMELEON, has recently been used to predict the structure of the interleukin-4 receptor. It is believed that the folding topology of the beta sheets of IL4R is the same as that seen in the crystal structure of CD4, despite sequence identity being low. Each domain of the IL4R monomer was aligned with CD4 using single residue hydropathy properties. Loops were added from a database of immunoglobulins so as to connect the sheets; side-chains were added using a side-chain rotamer library and the unsolvated structure energy-minimised using molecular dynamics. The whole structure was thus placed in an 8Å shell of water and unconstrained molecular dynamics canied out for 60 ps. Finally the whole structure was minimised.

Assuming that the IL4 receptor acts in the same way as growth hormone receptor as a dimer, one molecule of IL4 was docked to a pair of receptor proteins. The docking shows which portion of IL4 binds to the receptor: in this prediction notably the D helix. On the basis of this it should be possible to design mimetics of the crucial parts of the IL4 D helix which would interfere with the biochemical consequence of the cytokine binding to its receptor, leading to antagonists with potential medicinal applications.

Transition State Mimetics

Where no knowledge about the macromolecular target in atomic detail exists, then it is still possible to utilise computer-aided design techniques. A popular idealised approach would be to compute the energy profile of a biochemical transformation which it would be desirable to inhibit; locate the transition state or intermediate and then create a stable mimic of these unstable transients. Such a mimic should be recognised by the enzyme responsible for catalysing the reaction and would hence act as an inhibitor.

Only two logical steps are necessary: find the transient structure and secondly design a stable mimic. The former task is probably best achieved by using a combination of quantum and molecular mechanics. A recent review suggests that the combined potential method used by Bash et a1 for the triosephosphate isomerase reaction is probably the technique likely to be followed in the future.

The second stage of the process invokes the introduction of the idea of molecular similarity, a quantitative measure of just how similar one molecule is to another. Perhaps the most important aspect of similarity is similarity of shape and secondly similarity of molecular electrostatic potential, both of which can be represented by gaussian functions which introduce major computational gabiS in the calculation of similarity indices, of which several different types may be defined. Despite the simplicity of the logic this method of designing novel pharmaceutical products has not as yet had any major successes.

Similairity in Activity Relationships

Much more striking has been the achievement of similarity measures in structure-activity relationships and in quantitative structure-activity relationships. Good et a1., considered the series of steroids for which binding affinity data are available and which was the set studied in the earliest comparative molecular field three-dimensional structure-activity work. Every molecule in the series was compared in terms of shape and electrostatic potential similarity with every other member of the series yielding an n by n matrix for each property. The columns of these matrices were then used as input to a symmetrical neural network with number of nodes being n; n/3; 2; n/3 and n. The output was trained to be identical to the input and the values of the two central nodes (labelled x and y) noted. If one then plots x against y, clear structure-activity correlations emerge: strongly binding and weakly binding compounds cluster in different parts of the x/y plot.

The same matrices can be subjected to partial least squares analysis. The cross validated correlation coefficients obtained from the statistical analysis compare well with those obtained using the more commonly used matrices of similarities at grid points in the space surrounding the molecules which of coume demand massive matrices of perhaps thousands of points. In addition there is no need for arbitrariness about the extent of molecular 'surface' or the size of the three-dimensional box into which the molecules have to be placed. Although in its infancy molecular similarity matrices to seem to have a lot to offer in QSAR and in the optimisation of molecular structures for particular biological effects.

Molecular Dissimilarity

The molecular dissimilarity between a pair of molecules can be defined as (1 - Similarity). Similarity has a range of values 0 to 1 with unity representing identity. The interest in dissimilarity is in the comparison of chiral forms of the same molecule. The dissimilarity can be used as a 'chirality coefficient', a number which gives a range of values of chirality rather than this being an all-or-none property. Currently there is a great deal of research into producing pure chiral forms of compounds for use as pharmaceutical agents: the more active form being termed the eutomer and the less active the distomer, with their ratio being the eudismic ratio. For an homologous series of compunds we have shown that their is a direct correlation between the eudismic ratio and the chirality coefficient. An example is shown in Figure 1.

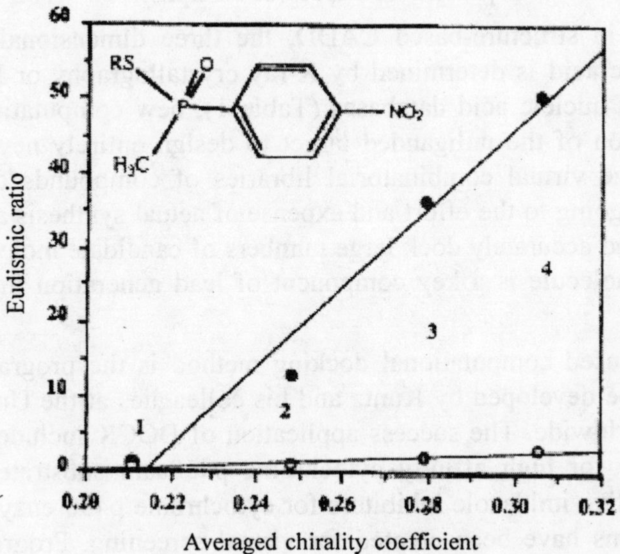

Figure 1. The linear correlation between the eudismic ratios and chirality coefficients of muscarinic 1,3 dioxalone (R = (1) isopropyl; (2) ethyl; (3) methyl; (4) hydrogen)

This type of correlation should assist in the prediction of eudismic ratios prior to synthesis and provide a rational basis upon which to decide whether the production of a single optical form is important or not.

Proteomics in Computer-Aided Drug Design

In principle, the drug discovery process involves three pre-clinical stages before clinical trials, namely target selection, lead identification, and clinical candidate selection (Fig. (2)). Due to rapid advances in structural biology and computer technology, structure-based computer-aided drug design (CADD) using docking techniques, virtual screening and library design, along with target/structure focusing combinatorial chemistry, has become a powerful tool in the multi-step process of drug discovery.

As an emerging technology, CADD accelerates drug development by making use of the accumulated information of existing drugs and diseases, combined with inter-disciplinary inputs from other fields. This process extensively uses mathematical models and simulation tools based on the evaluation of potential risks from drug safety and the experimental design of new trials. During the early 1980s, structural biologists began to design rational drugs based on protein structures. The first projects were underway in the mid-1980s, and the first successful stories, computer-aided rational design of peptide-based HIV-proteinase inhibitors, were published by the early 1990s. From then on, CADD has become a vital technique in drug candidate screening. The most recent example includes the structure based design of anti-SARS drug, a proteinase inhibitor of viral main proteinase Mpro (or 3CLpro).

As the first step in structure-based CADD, the three dimensional (3D) structure of a target protein or nucleic acid is determined by X-ray crystallography or NMR. Using recently constructed protein and nucleic acid databases (Table 1), new computational methods use the 3D structural information of the unliganded target to design entirely new lead compounds de novo. In this way, large virtual combinatorial libraries of compounds can then be screened computationally before going to the effort and expense of actual synthesis and biological studies. The ability to rapidly and accurately dock large numbers of candidate molecules into the binding site of a target macromolecule is a key component of lead generation in structure-based drug design.

The most widely used computational docking method is the program DOCK which has been and continues to be developed by Kuntz and his colleagues at the University of California and other scientists worldwide. The success application of DOCK includes the in silico virtual high throughput screen for high affinity cytochrome p450cam substrates and the computer-assisted design of selective imidazole inhibitors for cytochrome p450 enzymes. Besides DOCK, numerous other programs have been created for virtual screening. Programs such as ADAM, AutoDOCK, FlexX, and SLIDE, and other dock databases of compounds can score candidate molecules according to their interactions with the selected site of target protein. De novo generation of ligands can be performed with computer programs including 3D-QSAR, DISCO, GRID, LUDI, MCSS, and PASSA.

With the rapid accumulation of biological and chemical information, CADD has been dramatically reshaping research and development pathways in drug candidate identification.

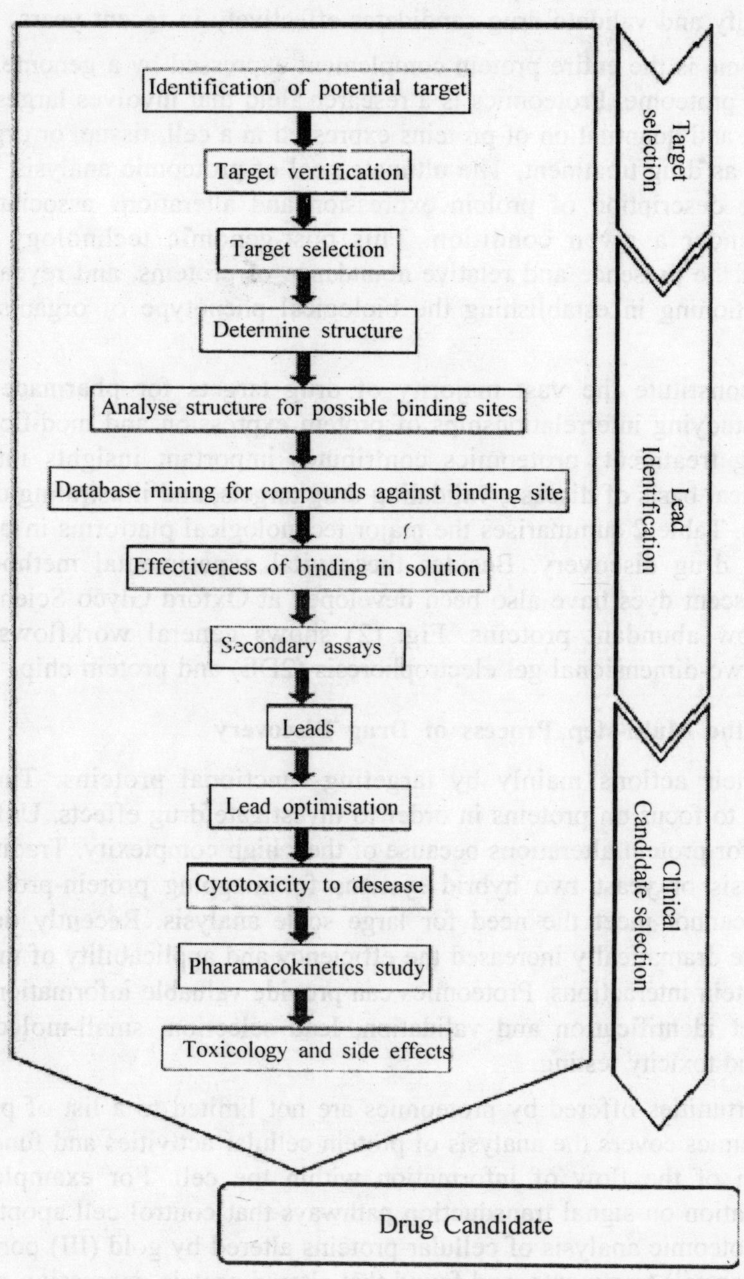

Figure 2. Schematic flow diagram of drug design and screening process.

On the other hand, the escalating number of therapeutic candidates are increasing demand on new technologies and strategies to streamline the process of screening for safe and effective therapies. This has inspired the application of molecular approaches including proteomics in an attempt to identify and validate drug candidates effectively in recent years.

The proteome is the entire protein complement expressed by a genome, and proteomics is the study of the proteome. Proteomics is a research field that involves largescale identification, characterisation, and quantitation of proteins expressed in a cell, tissue, or organism under given conditions such as drug treatment. The ultimate goal of proteomic analysis is a comprehensive and quantitative description of protein expression and alterations associated with biological perturbations under a given condition. This post-genomic technology provides a direct measurement of the presence and relative abundance of proteins, and reveals the consequence of protein functioning in establishing the biological phenotype of organisms in healthy and disease states.

Proteins constitute the vast majority of drug targets for pharmaceutical drug design processes. By studying interrelationships of protein expression and modification in health and disease or drug treatment, proteomics contributes important insights into determining the pathophysiological basis of disease, validating drug targets, and illustrating drug action, toxicity and side effects. Table 2 summarises the major technological platforms in proteomics and their applications in drug discovery. Besides these vital experimental methods for proteomics, sensitive fluorescent dyes have also been developed at Oxford Glyco Sciences (OGS, UK) for detection of low abundant proteins. Fig. (2) shows general workflows of the proteomic approaches of two-dimensional gel electrophoresis (2DE) and protein chip.

Proteomics in the Multi-step Process of Drug Discovery

Drugs exert their actions mainly by targeting functional proteins. Therefore, it appears straightforward to focus on proteins in order to investigate drug effects. Unfortunately, it is not easy to screen for protein alterations because of their high complexity. Traditional methods such as NMR analysis or yeast two hybrid systems for mapping protein-protein interactions are laborious and cannot meet the need for large scale analysis. Recently developed proteomic approaches have dramatically increased the efficiency and applicability of mapping drug-protein and protein-protein interactions. Proteomics can provide valuable information for drug discovery including target identification and validation, lead selection, small-molecular screening and optimisation, and toxicity testing.

The opportunities offered by proteomics are not limited to a list of proteins. Instead, the scope of proteomics covers the analysis of protein cellular activities and functions, including the characterisation of the flow of information within the cell. For example, protein networks provide information on signal transduction pathways that control cell apoptosis. We performed comparative proteomic analysis of cellular proteins altered by gold (III) porphyrin and cisplatin (as a positive control) treatments, and found that altered protein expression provided information on the mechanism of gold (III) porphyrin as a potential anticancer lead. Another proteomic analysis demonstrated that high levels of arsenite target oxidativestress pathways leading to apoptosis in rat lung epithelial cells.

Besides drug target identification, validation and lead selection, proteomics can also be used in toxicity testing. The Early Detection Research Network in the National Cancer Institute is employing proteomics in the discovery and evaluation of biomarkers for cancer detection and for the identification of high-risk subjects. Combined with traditional biochemical methods, proteomics has been used to elucidate mechanisms of toxic damage in several model systems. Bandara et al. have found several markers correlated to kidney toxicity of 4-Aminophenol, D-serine, and cisplatin by proteomic evaluation. Using proteomic analysis combined with Western blot, Zhang et al. identified that the increased levels of heat shock protein 70 was involved in estrogen and androgen protection of human neurons against intracellular amyloid b_{1-42} toxicity.

Sub-disciplines of Proteomics

Recognised for their special contribution in drug discovery, a series of sub-proteomic technologies, including computational proteomics, chemical proteomics, structural proteomics, and topological proteomics, are increasingly integrated into emerging drug design research fields.

Computational proteomics

Computational proteomics refers to the large-scale generation and analysis of 3D protein structural information. Accurate prediction of protein contact maps is the beginning and essential step for computational proteomics. The major resources for computational proteomics are currently available protein and nucleic acid structures. The 3D-GENOMICS and PDB, and other databases (Table 1) provide a broad range of structural and functional annotations for proteins from sequenced genomes and protein 3D structures, which make a solid foundation for computational proteomics.

Chemical proteomics

Chemical proteomics makes use of synthetic organic chemistry, cell biology, biochemistry, and mass spectrometry to design specific protein-modifying reagents that can be used for functional studies of distinct proteins within a certain proteome.

Table 1. Useful Websites in Computer-Aided Drug Design and Proteomics

Database Description	*UTL*
Ontario Center for Structural Proteomics	http://www.uhnres.utoronto.ca/proteomics/
Network service for comparing protein structures in 3D	http://www.ebi.ac.uk/dali/
Databases and Tools for 3-D Protein Structure Comparison and Alignment	http://cl.sdsc.edu/ce.html
Integrated Sequence—Structure Database	http://www.protein.bio.msu.su/issd/
PROCAT 3D enzyme active site templates	http://www.biochem.ucl.ac.uk/bsm/PROCAT/PROCAT.html
Structural Classification of Proteins	http://scop.mrc-lmb.cam.ac.uk/scop/

Topology of Protein Structure	http://www.tops.leeds.ac.uk/
TopNet for Topological Proteomics	http://networks.gersteinlab.org/genome
Biolmolecular interaction network database	http://www.blueprint.org/bind/bind.php
Protein Data Bank	http://www.rcsb.org/pdb/
Protein sequence analysis and structure prediction	http://www.embl-heidelberg.de/predictprotein/predictprotein.html

Table 2. Major Technological Platforms for Proteomics

Technique	*2DE (Two-Dimensional Electrophoresis)*	*Protein Chip Array*	*ICAT (Isotope-Coded Affinity Tags)*
Separation based on:	Molecular weight and isoelectric point	Surface affinity and molecular weight	Chemical labeling and relative abundance
Protein ID identified by:	MALDI-TOF MS MS/MS	SELDI-TOF MS MS/MS	LC-ESI MS/MS
Applications in drug	Biomarker discovery discovery Drug screening Action mechanisms Toxicity	Biomarker discovery Drug screening Diagnosis	Biomarker discovery Diagnosis
Remarks	Suitable for cell line, tissue, serum etc.; Identification of over 1000 proteins at the same time; Wide detection range (6-200kDa); Not suitable for low abundant proteins, and very alkaline or very hydrophobic proteins; Affected by post-translational modifications, including pohosporylation, *glycosylation, etc.*	Capture, detect and analyze proteins directly from crude biological samples; Low limit of detection (< fmole of protein); Small sample size (< 5 μl); Rapid results; Significant result; Wide detection range (0-300 kDa); *More automated.*	Labled with biotinylated tags before analysis; Detection and quantitation of lowabundance regulatory proteins; Suitable for abundances of light and heavy proteins; Not suitable for post-translational modified proteins; *More automated.*

The most important tool of this field is carefully designed chemical probes that can specifically target diverse sets of enzyme families. A chemical probe contains three parts, a reactive ligand that can covalently bind to the target protein/enzyme, a linker region modulating the reactivity and specificity of the reactive ligand, and a tag for identification and purification of the target protein/enzyme. Several kinds of chemical probes have been used in proteomics studies, for example, serine hydrolase probes, S-transferase probes, and phenyl sulfonate probes.

Structural proteomics

Structural proteomics is the determination of the relationship of all the proteins or protein complexes in a specific cellular organelle and the establishment of the relationship of these proteins in a proteome-wide scale. Combining structural biology with computational and medicinal chemistry, structural proteomics can help design drugs effectively. The major goal of structural proteomics is to determine the 3D structures of as many as possible proteins, so that other proteins in an organelle can be computationally modeled on the basis of similarity of their amino acid sequences.

Topological proteomics

Topological proteomics aims at localising and characterising entire protein networks within a single cell, providing quantitative insights into their basic organisation, which are valuable information in identifying new drug targets and selecting potential lead compounds. The proprietary technology, Multi-Epitope-Ligan Kartographie (MELK), is an ultra-sensitive topological proteomics technology for analysing proteins on a single cell level. MELK can trace out large scale subcellular protein patterns simultaneously within a cell, hence unravelling hierarchies of proteins related to a particular cell function or dysfunction. Another topological proteomic program, TopNet, is an automated web tool designed to facilitate the analysis of interaction networks, which is available from TopNet (Table 1).

Current Achievements and Application of Proteomics

Identification of drug targets

Drug target discovery, which involves the identification and early validation of disease-associated targets, is the first step in the drug discovery pipeline. Disease involves alterations in protein expression and modification and thus offers a basis for detection of drug targets through examining the protein expression profiles. Altered proteins in disease are candidates of drug targets that can be validated by modulating the proteins' activities in a model system to determine the outcome on disease phenotype (target validation). Proteomics is an effective means to globally view and detect protein expression alterations in disease and drug treatment and thus serves in both processes of target identification and validation.

Examples using proteomic approaches for target protein discovery include the identification of transforming growth factor-beta in lung epithelial cells and pancreatic carcinoma cells, plasma membrane proteins in breast cancer, BCNP1 and MIG2B in chronic lymphocytic leukemia, and heat shock protein 90 alpha for tumor cell invasiveness. Others have applied preprecipitation steps prior to the proteomic approach to identify targets in signaling pathways or certain cellular reactions. By using tandem affinity purification and nanospray microcapillary tandem mass spectrometry together with two-dimensional electrophoresis, Kumar et al. has reported their comprehensive analysis of thioredoxin-targeted proteins in *Escherichia coli*. They found a number of proteins associated with thioredoxin that either participate directly (SodA, HPI, and AhpC) or have key regulatory functions (Fur and AcnB) in the detoxification of the cell. The thioredoxin targets in the unicellular photosynthetic eukaryote Chlamydomonas reinhardtii have also been identified by proteomics approaches. With an efficient proteomics method, Godl et al. have identified the cellular targets of protein kinase inhibitors, and this target may have significant implications on the development of p38 inhibitors as inflammatory drugs.

Proteomics can also be used to validate potential protein targets for those highly effective, widely used or newly available drugs with unknown action mechanisms. For instant, heat shock protein 70 has been reported as a target of farnesyl transferase inhibitor in ovarian cancer 2774 cell line and heat shock protein 90 as a direct target of the antiallergic drugs disodium cromoglycate and amlexanox. Cellular response of yeast cells to lithium and the enzyme active sites through labeling enzyme targets by sulfonate ester probes have also been investigated by proteomic approaches.

Functional proteomics is particularly useful for mapping protein-protein interactions and for identifying potential targets. Protein-protein interactions, or receptor-ligand interactions, play a critical role in cellular processes such as signal transduction, and thus are essential for the understanding of basic biological processes. In this regard, proteomics is often combined with other methods to study protein-protein interactions in developing suitable drug targets.

Serebriiskii et al. used an enhanced Dual Bait two-hybrid system together with proteomic approaches to detect peptides, proteins and drugs that selectively interact with protein targets. Other researchers applied luciferase complementation imaging together with proteomics to study kinetic regulation of protein-protein interactions. Rodriguez and his colleagues reported an oriented peptide array library (OPAL) approach to facilitate high throughput proteomic analysis of protein-protein interactions. The interaction of the SCF-like ubiquitin ligase was demonstrated as a potential target of drugs to control differentiation.

Drug mechanism of action

Once a target protein is validated, the task of identifying chemical compounds that can appropriately modulate the target can be performed by proteomic techniques, and the cellular mechanisms of drug candidates can also be examined through proteomic analysis. Action mechanisms are the biochemical basis of drug activity. Understanding drug action modes provides valuable insights for drug modification and new drug design. Investigation of altered protein expression in response to drug treatment in established model systems is a commonly used strategy to examine drug action mechanism.

There are numerous examples of research aimed at mapping signaling pathways that are involved in disease processes. A group of researchers investigated apoptotic pathways involved in the selection of inhibitors of fatty acid synthase. LAF389, a synthetic analogue of bengamides, has been found to directly or indirectly inhibit methionine aminopeptidases (MetAps) by a proteomics-based approach. Additionally, a structural study revealed that three key hydroxyl groups on the inhibitor coordinate the di-cobalt center in the enzyme active site. MacKeigan et al. found that taxol activated the pathways of mitogen-activated protein kinase (MEK)/extracellular signal-regulated kinase by implementing a proteomic approach. By combining with MEK inhibition, taxol synergistically enhances apoptosis by altering the expression of the proteins RS/DJ-1 (RNAbinding regulatory subunit/DJ-1 PARK7) and RhoGDIalpha (Rho GDP-dissociation inhibitor alpha). RhoGDI alpha.

Oxidative stress is a major area of drug treatment. Our proteomics analysis revealed that arsenite induced apoptosis by stimulating the oxidative stress pathway. Young and his collaborators showed that Ras-mediated oncogenic transformation of ovarian epithelial cells was through activation of antioxidant pathways. The effect of a novel drug lead, IBTP (4-iodobutyl triphenylphosphonium), for ovarian cancer treatment was found to mainly act on mitochondria through oxidative stress. Further proteomics analysis reported that a major cellular response to oxidative stress was the modification of several peroxiredoxins.

Apoptosis, or programmed cell death, is a tightly controlled multi-step cellular event. Proteomic approaches have been increasingly employed in mapping out the apoptosis pathways involved in chemotherapy. Trichostatin-A (TSA) was found, through proteomic profile analysis, to cause apoptosis in a pancreatic adenocarcinoma cell lines (Paca44) at G2 arrest. Combining proteomic approaches together with other biological tests, McJilton et al. demonstrated that protein kinase cepsilon interacted with Bax and promoted survival of human prostate cancer cells. Ueda's results of two-dimensional immunoblots suggested that the p38 MAPK-MAPKAP kinase 2- BAG2 phosphorylation cascade may be a novel signaling pathway for response to extracellular stresses. Research data from a proteomic-based screening suggested that protein turnover inhibition of caspase-dependent proteolysis by the degrading proteasome was a general event in programmed cell death from Drosophila to mammals.

Considering the molecular complexity of entire proteomes in tissues and cells, more researchers have applied proteomic analysis to sub-cellular fractions. A group of scientists in the Sidney Kimmel Cancer Center (San Diego, California) used subtractive proteomics and bioinformatics to analyse endothelial cell surface proteins, and found two of these proteins, aminopeptidase-P and annexin A1, as selective in vivo targets for antibodies in lungs and solid tumours respectively. Such sub-cellular analysis has also been performed on mitochondria, and S-nitrosylation of cysteine thiol was shown to be a significant part of nitric oxidation mediation. Other scientists have reported that mitochondrial translocation of the actin-binding protein, cofilin, was an early step in apoptosis induction. The signaling pathways of membrane proteins, endoplasmic reticulum, and golgi apparatus have also been investigated by proteomics.

Drug toxicity and side effects

Given the low success rate in drug development, detection of potential toxicity and side effects in early stages of drug candidate identification can save money and time by focusing resources on those safe drug leads and candidates. By establishing a database that defines the response of a tissue proteome to specific drugs, comparative proteomics can be used to determine the propensity for a new compound. Proteomic signatures can also be constructed based on the toxicity responses previously observed with known agents. This can provide information to screen similar compounds for modification and improvement in drug design.

Currently, many studies focus on the mechanism of toxic damage by existing drugs, especially in the liver, kidney and cardiovascular system. Venkatraman et al. have identified the modification of mitochondrial proteins in response to ethanol-dependent hepatotoxicity, and demonstrated that chronic ethanol consumption extended to a modification of the mitochondrial proteome much broader than realised previously. Meneses-Lorente et al. reported a proteomic signature associated with hepatocellular steatosis in rats after dosing with a compound in preclinical development. Evaluation of drug toxicity to kidney was also performed by proteomic approaches.

Studies of drug toxicity related biomarkers are also of great importance for drug screening. Proteomic and immunological techniques were used to identify in vitro protein biomarkers of idiosyncratic liver toxicity by Gao and his colleagues, and revealed that BMS-PTX-265 and BMSPTX- 837 were potential toxic biomarkers for up to twenty drugs. Human aldose reductase-like protein-1 (hARLP-1) was the most prominent tumor-associated AKR member detected by proteomic approaches as a strong candidate for immunohistochemical diagnostic marker of human HCC.

Besides toxicity, drug resistance is another important reason for the failure of chemotherapies. A systematic proteomic approach for the study of chemoresistance mechanisms of vindesine, etoposide and cisplatin was first undertaken by Sinha et al. Differential proteomic analysis of vinca alkaloid-treated drug-sensitive human leukemia cells (CCRF-CEM) showed that numerous proteins were involved in drug resistance, and some of them could be novel targets for elucidation of resistance mechanisms. Comparative proteomic analysis revealed that methionine adenosyltransferase and Sadenosylmethionie played unique roles in methotrexate resistance in leishmania.

Bernstein et al. found that resistance to deoxycholate-induced apoptosis was modulated by over-expression of multiple anti-apoptotic proteins and under-expression of multiple pro-apoptotic proteins. By proteomic analysis, landmark proteins for insulin resistance and protozoan parasite leishmania resistance have also been reported. In mapping out mechanisms of drug resistance, one important issue is to differentiate adaptive and acquired resistance. By using proteomic analysis associated with cadmium adaptation in U937 cells, Jeon and his collaborators found that a newly identified protein, calbindin-D28k, is the secondary cadmiumresponsive protein that conferred resistance to cadmiuminduced apoptosis. The rich information obtained from proteomic study will accelerate lead identification and drug modification and improve drug efficacy and safety in preclinical and clinical studies.

Proteomic Signatures or Biomarkers

Biomarkers are usually proteins that have their expression altered in response to a disease condition. Biomarkers can be used as signatures to determine drug efficacy and clinical effects. Biomarkers can also be drug targets for further development. In proteomics, the challenge is to identify unique molecular signatures in complex biological mixtures that can be unambiguously correlated to biological events in order to validate novel drug targets and predict drug responses.

Proteomics has emerged to be a powerful approach for directly identifying highly predictive pharmacogenomic markers in blood or tissues. Previously, we have reported the proteomic analysis of oral tongue carcinoma to globally search for tumor related proteins. A number of tumorassociated proteins were consistently found to be significantly altered in their expression levels in tongue carcinoma tissues, compared with their paired normal mucosae. These proteins are potential biomarkers for tongue carcinoma diagnosis and therapeutic monitoring. A similar analysis for buccal squamous cell carcinoma also produced biomarker candidates that can be the proteomic signature for diagnostic and treatment. Hepatocarcinoma is another cancer that received much attention recently. Several biomarkers have been identified by proteomic approaches, such as aldose reductase-like protein (ARLP), cytokeratin 19, and ferritin light chain. Proteomic approaches have also been applied to biomarker or antigen identification for other cancers, including prostate cancer, bladder cancer, and ovarian cancer.

Advances of proteomic technology also hold great promise for improvements in the understanding, diagnosis and therapy of central nervous system disorders. Jin et al. revealed a role of stathmin in adult neurogenesis by proteomic and immunochemical characterisation. Others have reported that collapsin response mediator protein (CRMP-2) was a marker of changes developed in rat hippocampus. Great efforts have been made in searching for new and accurate biomarkers for cardiovascular system disease, HBV and HCV, and arthritis.

Biomarker discovery could make great contributions to the characterisation of the pharmacology of drug candidates and to the understanding of diseases subtypes to which a therapeutic intervention applies. Proteomic approaches have been proved to be promising techniques in the process of biomarker discovery.

Protein-Protein Interactions

Protein-protein interactions are extremely important in a wide range of biological processes. Currently, the development of drugs that target such interactions is a very active research field. Upon completion of this lecture the students will be aware of the general role of protein-protein interactions, including some illustrative examples. In addition, the student will be aware of drug design approaches in these systems, focusing on peptidomimetics and target-based virtual screening.

Roles of protein-protein interactions (PPI):

— cellular structure

— immune response

— signal transduction

— apoptosis (cell death)

PPI result in complexes of two or more proteins. PPI arise from (1) noncovalent interactions between the amino acids of each protein and (2) the drive to bury hydrophobic surfaces on the proteins.

— noncovalent interactions: hydrogen bonding, p-p interactions between aromatic residues, cation-π interactions between positively charged residues (Arg, Lys) and aromatic residues (Phe, Tyr, Trp)… These noncovalent interactions involve mainly electrostatics, van der Waals forces and charge transfer interactions.

Binding

— proteins that structurally exist as homodimers (e.g. in multimeric subunit enzymes) bind strongly (K_D=10^{-9}-10^{-12}M) through a large contact area containing many hydrophobic interactions. Homodimers, (e.g. dimers, tetramers, quadromers) are associations of the same proteins. Many proteins exist as multimers: acetylcholinesterase, alcohol dehydrogenase, citrate synthase, estrogen receptors, hemoglobin...

— proteins that associate and disassociate in response to their environment, such as the PPI biological functions listed in section A, have less favorable binding constants (K_D=10^{-6}-10^{-9}M). In general, PPI contact sites (~800 Å2) are similar in amino acid content to other protein surfaces (hydrophilic residues), but have a slightly higher content of Trp, Tyr and Arg. Mutations of surface amino acids to alanine revealed the existence of 'hotspots', small patches of amino acids which might contribute significantly to the binding through long range electrostatic interactions. Some proteins expose hydrophobic 'sticky patches' after undergoing a conformational change.

Relationship of inhibitor binding affinity to the PPI affinity- It is not necessary for the inhibitor to have the same or more favorable binding affinity as the 'substrate protein' if its concentration is higher. The ratio between concentration and binding constant determines if the inhibitor (I) will successfully compete with the protein substrate (P_2) as seen in figure 3.

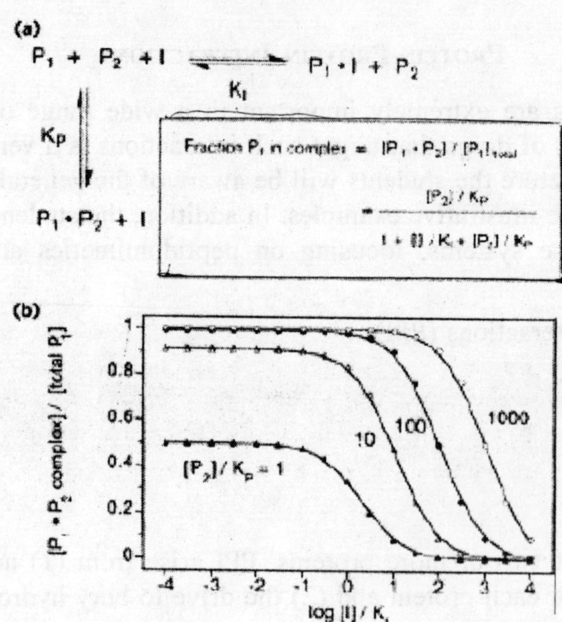

Figure 3. (a) Competition binding equilibrium. P1 and P2 are proteins that associate as the complex $P_1.P_2$. I is an inhibitor that binds to P_1. The boxed equation relates the fraction of P_1 in the complex to the concentrations and dissociation constants of the competitors P_2 and I. (b) The fraction of P_1 in the complex is plotted as a function of added inhibitor for several concentrations of P_2.

A. Inhibition of enzymatic active sites vs. inhibition of PPI:

— *enzymes:* knowing the substrate chemical structure provides a starting point for drug design without further structural knowledge of the protein.

— *PPI:* even after knowing the 3D structure of the individual proteins, it is necessary to identify the key amino acids involved in the PPI, which is currently done by point mutation experiments.

Active sites in enzymes are highly conserved, and often enzymes with different functions have the same substrate (i.e. kinases / ATP). A drug that binds to the active site could also bind to the active site for the same substrate in a different enzyme! Targeting PPI inhibition over enzymatic inhibition in such cases might resolve this problem.

Drug design approaches

General assumption: only a few of the many residues involved in the PPI contact site are energetically important (i.e. they stabilise the complex).

1. Inhibitors by experimental screening (competitive binding, enzyme assay, fluorometry) and computational (i.e. target-based) screening.

2. Inhibitors based on primary or secondary structure of the protein in the region where the PPI occur (peptidomimetics).

— *Peptidomimetics:* nonpeptide molecules that mimic peptides. Peptidomimetics are designed to mimic short peptide sequences taken from the 'substrate' protein ; several have been shown to be inhibitors. The PPI contact area can contain β-sheets, α-helices and turns. Many peptidomimetics have been developed that imitate β-turns (figure 4) and α-helices (figure 5).

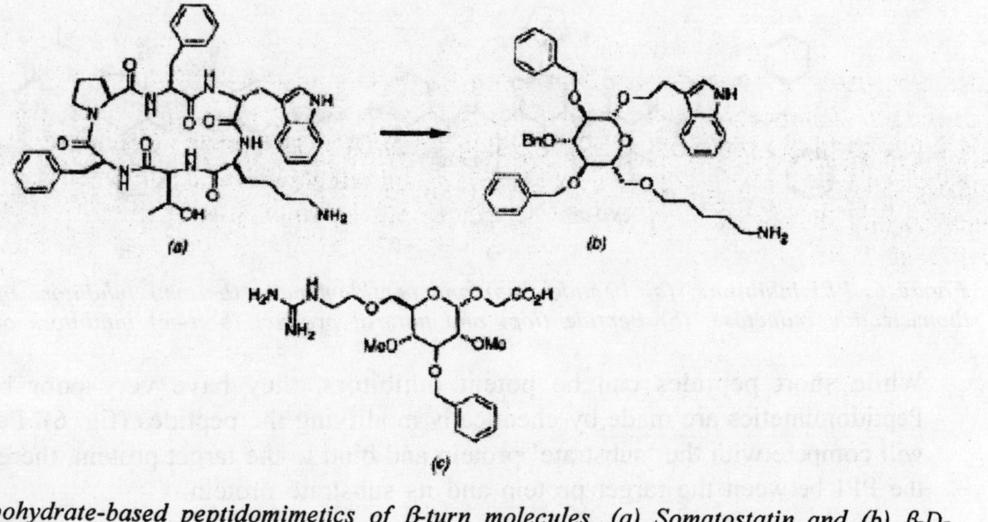

Figure 4. Carbohydrate-based peptidomimetics of β-turn molecules. (a) Somatostatin and (b) β-D-glucose-derived mimetic of somatostatin. (c) Representative mimetic of a cRGDFV turn.

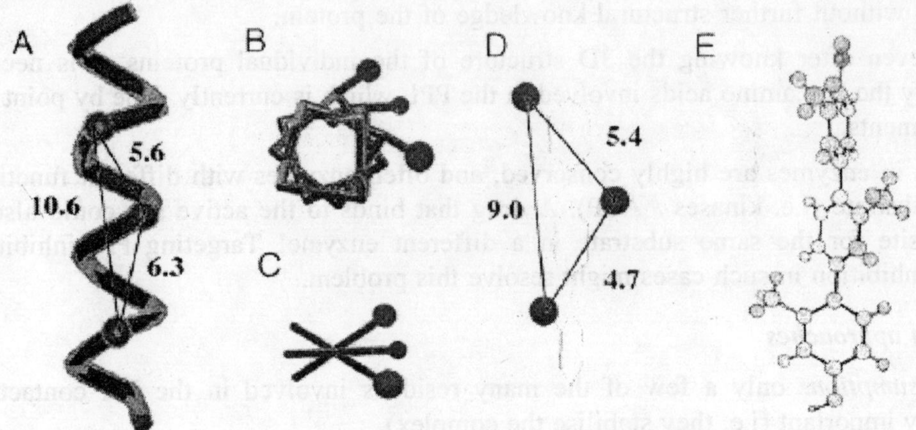

Figure 5. (A) Schematic representation of an α-helical 12-mer peptide with i, i + 3, and i + 7 substituents, side view; (B) top view; (C) 3,2',2"-trisubstituted terphenyl, top view; (D) side view; (E) X-ray crystal structure of 1.

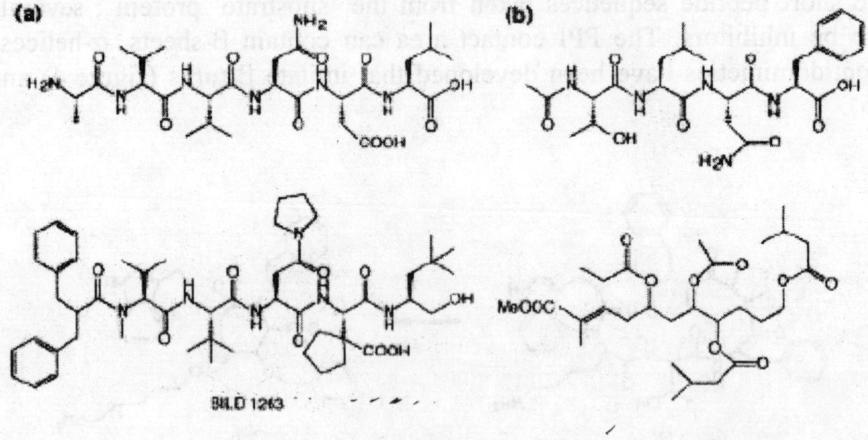

Figure 6. PPI inhibitors. (a) Peptide (top) and peptidomimetic (bottom) inhibitors of herpes virus ribonucleotide reductase. (b) Peptide (top) and natural product (bottom) inhibitors of HIV protease

While short peptides can be potent inhibitors, they have very poor bioavailability. Peptidomimetics are made by chemically modifying the peptides (fig. 6). Peptidomimetics will compete with the 'substrate' protein and bind to the target protein, therefore inhibiting the PPI between the target protein and its substrate protein.

Which groups were changed? Why?

Challenges to developing medicines that inhibit PPI:

Antagonism of intracellular PPI has been limited to antisense therapies that block the expression of the targeted protein(s), not the actual PPI itself.

1. Natural small molecules known to bind at protein - protein interfaces are rare → no template available for designing antagonists.

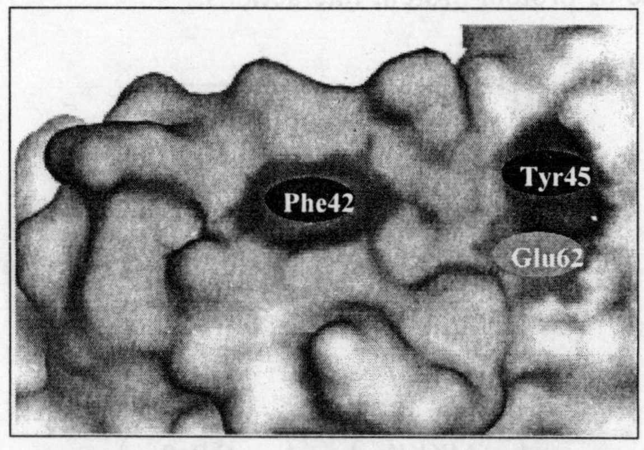

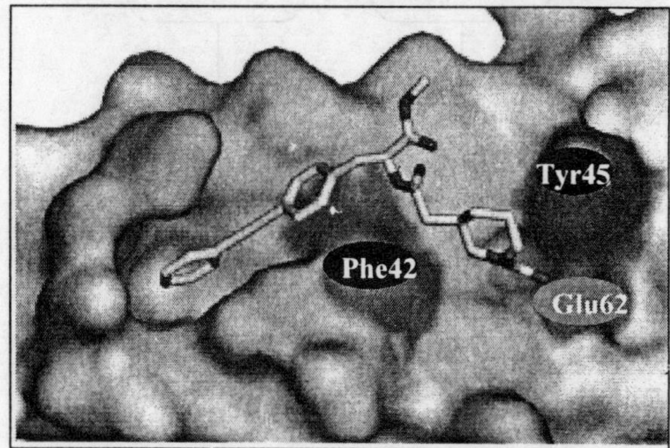

Figure 7. Structures of (a) unliganded IL-2 and (b) Ro26-4550 bound to IL-2.

2. X-ray structures do not show small, deep cavities that could make good smallmolecule binding sites.
3. Assaying inhibition is difficult in contrast to enzyme inhibition (recall Michaelis-Menten: competitive vs. allosteric antagonists of enzyme activity)
4. Therapeutic antibodies are an effective approach, as they replace one PPI with another (e.g. Herceptin, which is FDA approved for breast cancer). However, they are not cell-permeable and cannot be given orally.

Selection of a tractable PPI is important to success.

"Hot spots" appear to have conformational flexibility, and can adapt from a nearflat surface to a cavity capable of binding a small molecule.

Inhibitors based on Structure for Signal Transduction Proteins

Signal transduction: cellular process in which a 'signal' is sent from the outside of the cell to the nucleus. The signal is initiated after a molecule binds to a receptor in the cell surface, which is followed by a cascade of protein-protein interactions.

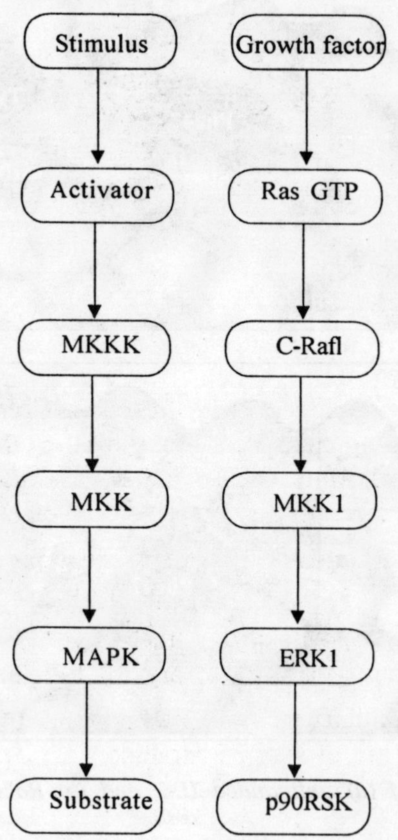

Figure 8. MAP phosphorelay systems.

— *very complex:* a protein can be activated by several proteins, and that active protein can then activate several other proteins (figures 8).

Mitogen Activated Protein Kinase (MAPK) signaling pathway

Extracellular signal-regulated kinase-1 and 2 (ERK1 and ERK2): Serine/Threonine Kinases

A stimulus such as a growth factor binds to the receptor RasGTP. Active Ras activates Raf kinase, which then activates (through phosphorylation) MAP kinase kinase 1 and 2 (MKK), which then activates (through phosphorylation) ERK. When ERK is phosphorylated, it forms a dimer with another ERK protein, which might or might not be phosphorylated. ERK then phosphorylates a variety of substrates: ribosomal S6 kinase proteins (RSK), transcription factors such as the p62 ternary complex factor (p62TCF/ELK-1)...

— why ERK?

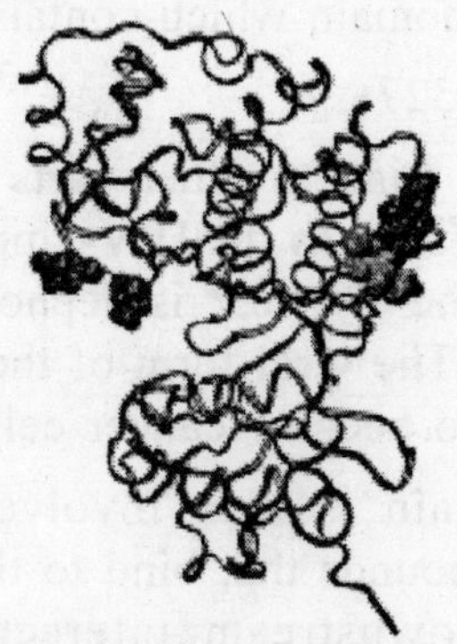

Figure 9. ERK2. Active site: phosphorylation residues Thr183 and Tyr185.

ERK is active in cell proliferation in many types of cancers. Crystal structures of the active and inactive form are available revealing structural info as well as the conformational changes that occur after phosphorylation (fig 9). Mutagenesis studies have discovered residues important for binding to its substrates (blue and green).

— the active site involved in the kinase (phosphorylation) activity is not the target for inhibition.

— the CD and ED sites on the opposite side of the active site are the targets. Point mutation experiments showed that they where necessary for PPI interactions.

— inhibit ERK's ability to bind to its substrate proteins by identifying an effective PPI inhibitor from a large database of lead compounds.

Hck: a protein from the Src family of tyrosine kinases

Hck is a nonreceptor tyrosine kinase that is part of signal transduction pathways and is therefore important in cell proliferation. Src proteins are also involved in the immune response. Src is the name of the gene which codes for these proteins. Peyton Rous (Nobel prize) discovered the virus in 1911 which causes cancer in chickens and contains a 'mutated' version of the Src gene.

This example illustrates the complexity of PPI (both intramolecular and intermolecular PPI are occurring).

— several regions:

— N-terminal (anchors proteins to membranes)

— SH3 (through intramolecular interactions, it binds the linker between the catalytic domain and the SH2 domain in the inactive protein)

— SH2 (through intramolecular interactions, it binds the phosphorylated Tyr527 found in the C-terminal tail inhibiting the protein; when the protein is active, it binds through intermolecular interactions to the phosphorylated tyrosines of downstream proteins)

— SH1 (catalytic or kinase domain which contains two lobes)

C terminal containing Tyr527

In the inactive state, SH2 and SH3 bind to other parts of the protein through intramolecular interactions. When external ligands (such as the HIV-1 protein Nef) bind to the SH3 domain (or SH2) through intermolecular PPI, the Tyr 527 is dephosphorylated, SH3 no longer binds the linker, and the protein is activated. The viral form of the protein is missing Tyr527 (protein is active) which causes normal cells to become cancer cells.

Alternatively, the SH2 domain is also involved on PPI with other proteins (i.e. intermolecular PPI), such that compounds that bind to the SH2 domain may also inhibit these interactions, thereby blocking downstream interactions. Both the intramolecular and intermolecular interactions must be considered when designing compounds to block PPI via the SH2 domain.

Future Perspectives

The successful stories of proteomics application in drug discovery in recent years have demonstrated the potential value of proteomics in drug development. Proteomic approaches can provide valuable information for target identification and validation, lead selection, small-molecular screening and optimisation. In particular, those subdisciplines of proteomics have demonstrated promising application for CADD. However, application of proteomic approaches is rather limited at present due to its inefficiency in detecting low abundant or post-translationally modified proteins. With the development of related techniques, proteomics is sure to play a more important role in rational drug design. The key point to drug development in the future is the integration of proteomics with CADD to use the vast amount of information and techniques available for accelerating drug discovery process.

The field of proteomics faces some daunting challenges, in comparison to genomics, for several reasons. First, protein science lacks an analogue of the polymerase chain reaction (PCR), which can generate many copies of a single, native molecule in vivo (nucleic acids in the case of PCR). However, several recent approaches have been applied in an effort to ameliorate this quandary. Methods of chemical synthesis exist, being limited by yield, particularly when it comes to synthesizing lengthy peptides. In-vivo expression synthesis methods exist as well, however, this approach cannot be applied to producing proteins which may alter normal cellular function. Also, cell-free synthesis ribosome kits can also be employed for accurate and rapid protein synthesis, though the intrinsic presence of ribosome inactivating enzymes contributes to the instability of these systems. Second, in contrast to DNA, protein levels vary significantly depending on cell type and environment. Third, protein abundance is not directly correlated to protein activity. Protein activity is often determined by post-transcriptional modifications such as phosphorylation. Protein activity, not protein abundance, is of interest in the drug discovery process. Finally, proteins form many interactions with other proteins or small molecules. Elucidation of these interactions would greatly speed up the drug discovery process. One way this is currently being done is through ligand bound x-ray crystallographic studies.

The ideal proteomics technique suited for drug discovery would have the following features: it should be able to separate membrane proteins and detect low abundance proteins, two abilities not quite yet realized, yet required in current separations and analytical techniques. Furthermore, it should be able to identify protein activity independent of protein abundance. It also should reveal protein-protein and protein-small-molecule interactions. This method should also be implemented easily, be automatable, and perform at high-throughput speed. Proteomics researchers are addressing these issues, and new methods are being developed.

Virtual drug libraries are being developed, both in the public and private sectors. These databases contain potential drug compounds; these compounds may or may not exist outside of a computer database, and new compounds developed through various methods of synthesis are continually added. Methods of modifying existing database entries to create new isomers and derivatives are also used, to more adequately cover a range of potential drug compounds. Docking and scoring are implemented using known and hypothetical drug targets on a protein, coupled with the databases of virtual chemical compounds. In docking, various computational methods are used to position a chemical properly within a protein binding site. Genetic algorithms and Monte Carlo methods are two popular algorithms for evolving an optimum binding position. This process screens for chemicals that are potential drugs, which initially are termed as hits. After docking, scoring is carried out using mathematical models. These models determine the chemical binding strength and energy state of the drug-protein complex. Those hits with high ranking scores are suqsequently subjected to in-vivo tests; hits with positive scores in both areas are then known to be leads.

Evaluation of docked and scored complexes are then made, selecting an arbitrary number of top hits to be further screened manually. The first two steps are done entirely in silico; however, the best complexes now need to be examined using software visualization, often in three-dimensional setups. This allows scientists to ensure that the determined docking orientation looks acceptable, and that the scoring is correct based on known interaction energies such as hydrogen bonds and ionic interactions.

The compounds that make it through docking, scoring, and evaluation become drug leads, and are then passed on to undergo drug testing techniques by scientists in a wet lab, to ensure that only compounds with effects relatively unique to the target system and safe to the rest of organism are considered. However, the drug company has already saved much time and money up to this point by having computers do chemical screening, rather than human scientists.

Bibliography

Agnihotri S.A., Mallikarjuna N.N., Aminabhavi T.M., *"Recent advances on chitosan-based micro- and nanoparticles in drug delivery"*, *Journal of Controlled Release*, 100, 5-28, 2004.

Alvarez-Lorenzo C., Concheiro A., "Molecular imprinted polymers for drug delivery", *Journal of Chromatography* B, 804, 231-45, 2004.

Bae Y., Fukushima S., Harada A. and Kataoka K., "Design of Environment-Sensitive Supramolecular Assemblies for Intracellular Drug Delivery: Polymeric Micelles that are Responsive to Intracellular pH Change", Angew. Chem. Int. Ed., 42, 4640-43, 2003.

Benita S (ed), *Microencapsulation: Methods and Industrial Applications*, New York, Marcel Dekker, 1996.

Byrne M. E., Park K., Peppas N., "Molecular imprinting within hydrogels", *Advanced Drug Delivery Reviews*, 54, 149-61, 2002.

Charman W.N., Chan H.-K., Finnin B.C. and Charman S.A., "Drug Delivery: A Key Factor in Realising the Full Therapeutic Potential of Drugs", *Drug Development Research*, 46, 316-27, 1999.

Chasin M, and Langer R (eds), *Biodegradable Polymers as Drug Delivery Systems*, New York, Marcel Dekker, 1990.

Chien Y.W, *Novel Drug Delivery Systems*, New York, Marcel Dekker, 1982.

Cleary G.W, "Transdermal Drug Delivery," *Cosmetics and Toiletries*, 106:97–107, 1991.

Domb AJ (ed), *Polymeric Site-Specific Pharmacotherapy*, Chichester, UK, Wiley, 1994.

Donbrow M (ed), *Microcapsules and Nanoparticles in Medicine and Pharmacy*, Boca Raton, FL, CRC Press, 1992.

Haag R., "Supramolecular Drug-Delivery Systems based on Polymeric Core-Shell Architectures", Angew. Chem. Int. Ed., 43, 278-82, 2004.

Heller J., "Controlled Drug Release from Poly(ortho esters)—A Surface Eroding Polymer," J Controlled Release, 2:167–177, 1985.

Kim S.W, "Temperature Sensitive Polymers for Delivery of Macromolecular Drugs," in *Advanced Biomaterials in Biomedical Engineering and Drug Delivery Systems*, Ogata N, Kim SW, Feijen J, et al. (eds), Tokyo, Springer, pp 126–133, 1996.

Kopecek J., "Smart and genetically engineered biomaterials and drug delivery systems", *European Journal of Pharmaceutical Sciences*, 20, 1-16, 2003.

Manabe T., Okino H., Maeyama R., Mizumoto K., Nagai E., Tanaka M., Matsuda T., "Novel strategic therapeutic approaches for prevention of local recurrence of pancreatic cancer after resection: trans-tissue, sustained local drug-delivery systems", *Journal of Controlled Release*, 100, 317-30, 2004.

Mikos AG, Murphy RM, Bernstein H, et al. (eds), *Biomaterials for Drug and Cell Delivery*, Pittsburgh, Materials Research Society, 1994.

Muller-Goymann C.C., "Physicochemical characterization of colloidal drug delivery systems such as reverse micelles, vesicles, liquid crystals and nanoparticles for topical administration", *European Journal of Pharmaceutics and Biopharmaceutics*, 58, 343-56, 2004.

Niculescu-Duvaz I., Springer C.J., "Andibody-directed enzyme prodrug therapy (ADEPT): a review", *Advanced Drug Delivery Reviews*, 26, 151-72, 1997.

Packhaeuser C.B., Schnieders J., Oster C.G., Kissel T., "In situ forming parenteral drug delivery systems: an overview", *European Journal of Pharmaceutics and Biopharmaceutics*, 58, 445-55, 2004.

Park K, Shalaby WSW, and Park H, *Biodegradable Hydrogels for Drug Delivery*, Lancaster, PA, Technomic, 1993.

Peppas NA (ed), *Hydrogels in Medicine and Pharmacy*, Boca Raton, FL, CRC Press, 1986.

Ratner BD, Hoffman AS, Schoen FJ, et al. (eds), *Biomaterials Science: An Introduction to Materials in Medicine*, San Diego, Academic Press, 1997.

Robinson JR, and Lee VHL (eds), *Controlled Drug Delivery: Fundamentals and Applications* (2nd ed), New York, Marcel Dekker, 1987.

Rosler A., Vandermeulen G. W. M., Klok H.-A., "Advanced drug delivery devices via self-assemply of amphiphilic block copolymers", *Advanced Drug Delivery Reviews*, 53, 95-108, 2001.

Santini Jr, J.T., Richards A.C., Scheidt R., Cima M.J. and Langer R., "Microchips as Controlled Drug-Delivery Devices", Angew. Chem. Int. Ed., 39, 2396-407, 2000.

Shalaby SW, Ikada Y, Langer R, et al. (eds), *Polymers of Biological and Biomedical Significance*, Washington DC, ACS Symposium Series, 1994.

Sood A. and Panchagnula R., "Peroral Route: An Opportunity for Protein and Peptide Drug Delivery", *Chemical Reviews*, 101, 3275-303, 2000.

Soppimath K.S., Aminabhavi T.M., Kulkarni A.R., Rudzinski W.E., "Biodegradable polymeric nanoparticles as drug delivery devices", *Journal of Controlled Release*, 70, 1-20, 2001.

Torchilin V.P., "Structure and design of polymeric surfactant-based drug delivery systems", *Journal of Controlled Release*, 73, 137-72, 2001.

Vasir J. K., Tambwekar K., Garg S., "Bioadhesive microspheres as a controlled drug delivery system", *International Journal of Pharmaceutics*, 255, 13-32, 2003.

Winterhalter M., Hilty C., Bezrukov S. M., Nardin C., Meier W., Fournier D., "Controlling membrane permeability with bacterial porins: applications to encapsula' d enzymes", Talanta, 55, 965-71, 2001.

Index